ADULT PSYCHIATRIC NURSING

Current Clinical Nursing Series

JEANETTE LANCASTER, R.N., Ph.D.
Associate Professor
Community Mental Health Nursing
School of Nursing
University of Alabama
Birmingham, Alabama

 Medical Examination Publishing Co., Inc.
an Excerpta Medica company

969 Stewart Avenue • Garden City, New York 11530

Copyright © 1980 by
MEDICAL EXAMINATION
PUBLISHING CO., INC.
an **Excerpta Medica** company

Library of Congress Card Number
78-78020

ISBN 0-87488-577-9

January, 1980

All rights reserved. No part of this
publication may be reproduced in any
form or by any means, electronic or
mechanical, including photocopy,
without permission in writing from
the publisher.

Printed in the United States of America

SIMULTANEOUSLY PUBLISHED IN:

United Kingdom : HENRY KIMPTON PUBLISHERS
London, England

Contents

PART I: BASIC CONCEPTS AS A FOUNDATION FOR ADULT PSYCHIATRIC NURSING

1 : Student Expectations and Reactions to Psychiatric Nursing
Jeanette Lancaster, R.N., Ph.D.

    Introduction / *1*
    Specific Reactions to Psychiatric Nursing / *2*
    Principles / *15*

2 : Theories of Personality Development
Gail Davis, R.N., Ed.D. and Allene Jones, R.N., M.N.

    Introduction / *16*
    Psychoanalytic Theories / *17*
    Cognitive Theory / *36*
    Behaviorist Theory / *38*
    Humanistic Theory / *44*
    Existentialistic Theory / *50*

3 : Personality Development: Stages of Growth
Gail Davis, R.N., Ed.D. and Allene Jones, R.N., M.N.

    Introduction / *54*
    Infant / *58*
    Toddler / *63*
    Preschool Child / *66*
    School-age Child / *70*
    Adolescent / *72*
    Young Adult / *78*
    Middle-aged Adult / *81*
    Older Adult / *89*

PART II: THE NURSING PROCESS IN PSYCHIATRY

4 : Therapeutic Communication
Jeanette Lancaster, R.N., Ph.D.

    Introduction / *97*
    Process of Communication / *99*
    Verbal and Nonverbal Communication / *100*
    Tools of Communication / *103*
    Modes of Communication / *109*
    Aspects of Conversation / *110*
    Techniques that Facilitate Communication / *111*
    Blocks to Communication / *117*
    Criteria for Evaluating Nurse-Patient Communication / *122*
    Principles / *124*

5 : Aspects of the Nurse-Patient Relationship
Jeanette Lancaster, R.N., Ph.D.

    Introduction / *127*
    Confidentiality / *129*
    Involvement / *130*
    Empathy / *131*
    Acceptance / *133*
    Anxiety / *139*
    Trust / *142*
    Responsibility / *146*
    Aggression / *149*
    Shame / *152*
    Humor / *153*
    Orientation Phase / *154*
    Working Phase / *155*
    Termination Phase / *159*
    Principles / *161*

6 : The Nursing Process as a Framework for Psychiatric Nursing
Jeanette Lancaster, R.N., Ph.D.

    Introduction / *163*
    Assessment Interview Tool / *171*
    Principles / *187*

PART III: CLINICAL ENTITIES IN PSYCHIATRIC NURSING

7: Depression and Suicidal Behavior
Linda Colvin, R.N., M.S.

    Depression and Physiological Diseases / *197*
    Symptoms of Depression / *198*
    Suicide / *207*
    Case Study: Depressive Behavior / *212*
    Principles / *218*

8 : Psychophysiological Disorders
Joan Goe, R.N., M.N.

    Introduction / *220*
    Overview of Systems Theory / *220*
    The Nature of Health and Illness / *223*
    Psychophysiological Disorders / *225*
    Nursing Management of Psychophysiological Disorders / *237*
    Case Study / *240*
    Principles / *245*

9 : Neuroses
Ann K. Kirkham, R.N., M.S.

    Introduction / *247*
    Anxiety: The Common Denominator / *249*
    Theories of Etiology / *255*
    Classification of Neurosis / *257*
    Case Study / *266*
    Principles / *272*

10 : Personality Disorders and Sexual Deviations
Ann K. Kirkham, R.N., M.S.

    Personality Disorders / *273*
    Sexual Deviations / *295*
    Case Study / *316*
    Principles / *324*

11 : Alcoholism and Drug Dependence
Anne Lind, R.N., M.S.

    Alcoholism / *328*
    Drug Dependence / *335*
    Case Study / *342*
    Principles / *352*

12 : Psychoses
Frances K. Richardson, R.N., M.S.

    Introduction / *354*
    Paranoia / *358*
    Affective Disorders / *360*
    Involutional Psychotic Reaction / *363*
    Schizophrenia / *364*
    Nursing Management / *371*
    Case Study: Psychosis / *377*

13 : Organic Brain Syndromes
Judith R. Lentz, R.N., M.S.N.

    Introduction / *384*
    Variables Affecting the Expression of Brain Damage / *395*
    Tissue Destruction / *395*
    Location of the Lesion / *396*
    Nature of the Disease Process / *403*
    Delirium / *405*
    Dementiform Syndromes or Dementia / *406*
    Deliriform Syndromes / *425*
    Epileptiform Syndromes / *435*
    Hydantoins / *447*
    Barbiturates / *448*
    Succinimides / *448*
    Oxazolidines / *449*

PART IV: TREATMENT APPROACHES

14 : Somatic Therapy
David P. Colvin, M.S., D.O.

    Introduction / *461*
    Somatic Intervention / *462*

Antipsychotic Drugs / 462
Guidelines for Nursing Intervention / 468
Antidepressant Drugs / 469
Lithium Carbonate Treatment of Acute Mania / 473
Anti-Anxiety Drugs / 474
Sedative-Hypnotic Drugs / 475
Electroconvulsive Therapy / 475
Insulin Shock Therapy / 477
Indoklon Therapy / 477
Psychosurgery / 477
Physiotherapy / 478
The Nurse's Role in Somatic Therapy / 478

15 : Treatment Modalities in Psychiatric Nursing
Linda Colvin, R.N., M.S. and Jeanette Lancaster, R.N., Ph.D.

Introduction / 480
Psychoanalysis / 481
Psychoanalytic Psychotherapy / 482
Behavior Therapy / 483
Hypnosis / 484
Group Psychotherapy / 484
Family Therapy / 486
Other Approaches to Psychotherapy / 487
Activity Group Therapy / 494
Psychodrama / 497
Therapeutic Community / 500
Values Clarification / 503
Principles / 508

16 : Psychiatric Nursing in the Community
Jeanette Lancaster, R.N., Ph.D.

History and Development of Community Mental Health Nursing / 510
Human Ecological Approach to Community Mental Health Nursing / 516

17 : Crisis Intervention
Brenda Riley, R.N., M.S.

Case Study / 528
Nursing Intervention / 535
Principles / 546

18 : Case Presentations for Application of the Nursing Process

Directions for Case Presentations / *549*

APPENDICES

Appendix A: Diagnostic and Statistical Manual of Terms / *557*

Appendix B: Standards of Psychiatric-Mental Health Nursing Practice / *571*

Appendix C / *583*

INDEX / *590*

Preface

According to the American Nurses' Association Standards of Psychiatric and Mental Health Nursing Practice, the field of psychiatric nursing is a specialized area which utilizes theoretical formulations from the sciences as its scientific base and purposeful use of self as its art (ANA, 1973). The intention of this book is to operationalize the Standards of Practice in a concise, yet comprehensive fashion. It is hoped that both students and practitioners of psychiatric nursing can benefit from the theoretical, as well as from the illustrative information provided.

The central purpose of the book is to describe the client who presents with coping difficulties so that practitioners may respond with a high level of humane and informed nursing interventions. This task is accomplished by directing the nurse to become aware of her own needs and responses based on personal experiences which influence her behavior toward clients. Secondly, content is provided which comprises foundational support for understanding human behavior in both its adaptive and maladaptive dimensions. Thirdly, illustrative cases are presented throughout to provide focus for the reader.

The book is divided into four major categories. The first category presents basic concepts which constitute a foundation for nursing interventions. Content related to initial reactions to psychiatric nursing, theories of personality, and growth and development are discussed. An awareness of self often precedes understanding of others; therefore, a description of typically observed reactions to the psychiatric nursing experience seems relevant. An understanding of normal patterns of behavior and stages of human development is essential in recognizing deviations from normal.

The second section describes the nursing process in psychiatric nursing. Prior to an actual application of the nursing process in the psychiatric clinical area, therapeutic communication and aspects of the nurse-patient relationship are detailed. Since psychiatric nursing constitutes a problem-solving approach to nurse-client interaction, the nursing process provides an applicable framework. Assessment, planning, implementation and evaluation constitute the cognitive steps which determine nursing actions. Documentation of the nursing process is accomplished by utilizing the problem-oriented record. The Standards of Practice are an integral part of the utilization of the nursing process in psychiatric nursing.

Part III, "Clinical Entities in Psychiatric Nursing" applies the nursing process to a wide range of presenting clinical pictures. Both theories and examples comprise each clinical section. It is expected that a blending of theoretical information and a description of its application will provide guidelines for the student and nurse practitioner.

The fourth section of the text outlines treatment approaches and trends in psychiatric nursing. It is essential for psychiatric nurses to understand the relevance of somatic, as well as interactional therapy in actual practice. Nurses have considerable impact on the choice of treatment approaches; therefore, informed participation in decision-making is necessary for patient care. Crisis Intervention is described as a specific approach to the acutely disturbed client. In addition, nursing approaches outside the arena of in-patient care are discussed. The community is increasingly becoming a major treatment milieu. Recognition of available treatment approaches applicable to an outpatient setting is essential.

The use of female pronouns to refer to the nurse is not meant to be discriminatory, but rather to facilitate clarity of presentation. In general, the nurse is referred to as "she," while the client or patient is depicted as "he."

                                             Jeanette Lancaster

Contributors

DAVID P. COLVIN, M.S., D.O.
Detroit Osteopathic Hospital, Detroit, Michigan

LINDA COLVIN, R.N., M.S.
Formerly Assistant Professor, Psychiatric Nursing, Texas Christian University, Harris College of Nursing, Fort Worth, Texas

GAIL DAVIS, R.N., Ed.D.
Associate Professor, Pediatric Nursing, Texas Christian University, Harris College of Nursing, Fort Worth, Texas

JOAN GOE, R.N., M.N.
Associate Professor, Psychiatric Nursing, Texas Christian University, Harris College of Nursing, Fort Worth, Texas

ALLENE JONES, R.N., M.N.
Assistant Professor, Psychiatric Nursing, Texas Christian University, Harris College of Nursing, Fort Worth, Texas

ANN K. KIRKHAM, R.N., M.S.
Assistant Professor, Psychiatric-Community Health Nursing, Texas Christian University, Harris College of Nursing, Fort Worth, Texas

ANNE LIND, R.N., M.S.
Assistant Professor, Maternity Nursing, Texas Christian University, Harris College of Nursing, Fort Worth, Texas

JUDITH R. LENTZ, R.N., M.S.N.
Assistant Professor, Psychiatric-Community Health Nursing, School of Nursing, University of Texas at Houston, Houston, Texas

JEANETTE LANCASTER, R.N., Ph.D.
Associate Professor, Community Mental Health Nursing, School of Nursing, University of Alabama, Birmingham, Alabama

FRANCES K. RICHARDSON, R.N., M.S.
Assistant Professor, Psychiatric Nursing, Texas Christian University, Harris College of Nursing, Fort Worth, Texas

BRENDA RILEY, R.N., M.S.
Assistant Professor, Psychiatric Nursing, Texas Christian University, Harris College of Nursing, Fort Worth, Texas

Acknowledgments

Thanks and special recognition are due to many individuals, including the friends and family members of each contributor who tolerated a number of inconveniences so that this text could reach fruition. Special thanks go to the secretarial staff at Harris College of Nursing, Texas Christian University who diligently and patiently typed the manuscript. Without the support and encouragement of Dr. Virginia Jarratt, Dean of Harris College of Nursing, the text would never have become a reality. Her continuing enthusiasm for the project will long be remembered.

notice

The editor(s) and/or author(s) and the publisher of this book have made every effort to ensure that all therapeutic modalities that are recommended are in accordance with accepted standards at the time of publication.

The drugs specified within this book may not have specific approval by the Food and Drug Administration in regard to the indications and dosages that are recommended by the editor(s) and/or author(s). The manufacturer's package insert is the best source of current prescribing information.

PART I: Basic Concepts As A Foundation For Adult Psychiatric Nursing

CHAPTER 1

Student Expectations and Reactions to Psychiatric Nursing

Jeanette Lancaster, R.N., Ph.D.

INTRODUCTION

"Psychiatric nursing is a specialized area of nursing practice employing theories of human behavior as its scientific aspect and purposeful use of self as its art. It is directed toward both preventive and corrective impacts upon mental illness and is concerned with the promotion of optimal health for society " (Congress for Nursing Practice, 1973). This sounds like an awesome task for any student. The first step is to break the task down into small, manageable components. This text will identify and describe the various aspects of psychiatric nursing by focusing first on the expectations a student might hold and on frequent reactions of the student as she approaches the experience of psychiatric nursing. The student must be aware of herself: aware of what she is thinking, feeling and desiring to do before she can use herself as a psychotherapeutic agent. Once an awareness of self is discussed, theories of human behavior are presented, so that the nursing student has access to normal developmental patterns. Normal patterns of behavior are defined in order to recognize deviations from the norm.

Psychiatric nursing is viewed as a problem-solving approach to interactions with patients. The nurse uses problem-solving skills to define her role; she also assists the patient in using problem-solving skills to determine new, more facilitative ways of relating to both his internal and external environments. Each person's health status is the result of a dynamic interaction between his internal environment and the external multi-environments in which he exists. Man is viewed as an open system in continuous interaction with his environment.

The nursing process provides the framework in the text for facilitating more productive patient-environment interfaces. The nursing skills of assessment, planning, implementation and evaluation provide preventive and corrective measures in psychological coping. The problem-oriented record comprises the format for the written component of the nursing process. The components of the problem-oriented record include the data base, problem list (secured in the nursing assessment), plan (formulated in the planning stage and carried out in the implementation phase of the nursing process) and follow-up (completed in evaluation of the nursing process).

Students entering the psychiatric clinical setting are confronted with a wide range of feelings. For many, the psychiatric setting is strikingly different from the familiar clinical areas characterized by machinery, techniques, hustle and bustle, and patients garbed in traditional hospital attire. A student's initial visit to an inpatient psychiatric setting triggers a spectrum of reactions ranging from shock to relief. One student described her first day in psychiatric nursing as follows:

> Well, the first day on psych wasn't as bad as I thought—having feared that rotation throughout school. Strange, but not a threat to life and limb. In fact it was a lot easier than walking onto an intensive care unit. Really, I can't believe what a relaxed, normal atmosphere it is.

SPECIFIC REACTIONS TO PSYCHIATRIC NURSING

Feelings of Anxiety

Each student comes to psychiatric nursing with varied personal experiences and at differing stages of developmental mastery. Each is unique in the ability to cope with problems presented in nursing. The universal reaction to the first day in psychiatric nursing is anxiety. Anxiety is defined as a state of uneasiness, apprehension or tension caused by a non-specific danger or threat. The principle that unknown, untried new situations or roles cause an increase in anxiety certainly applies in this situation. Most students have preconceived notions about what to expect in psychiatric nursing. Many are well acquainted with popular literature, movies or myths describing psychiatric treatment approaches. Fictional literature such as *One Flew Over the Cuckoo's Nest* by Ken Kesey (and the subsequent movie), as well as books based on factual data such as *I Never Promised You a Rose Garden* by Hannah Green, and *Sybil* by Flora Schreiber, have influenced public opinion and sentiment regarding mentally disturbed individuals. Some students have also dealt with emotional problems personally or in immediate family members.

Role Threat

The role of student or learner is threatening and anxiety-producing in and of itself, in that the student is often on the lowest rung of the hospital hierarchy of power (See Figure 1-1).

The student, beset with sensory input from staff and instructors, may feel threatened even in familiar clinical settings. Role threat is compounded in the psychiatric area in that patients behave in ways contrary to many other areas of nursing. First, few psychiatric patients wear hospital garb or remain in bed. Instead the patients are up and about, often looking no different than the staff. In units where staff wear street clothes rather than uniforms, students often feel an immediate threat to role identification. One student described her first reaction: "When I first walked in the door, I saw all those new faces, and what really scared me was that I couldn't tell which ones were the patients and which were the staff." It is a fearful and embarrassing situation to practice newly learned communication techniques on the staff, yet one which happens to students as well as instructors when new staff are hired. Moreover, to give up one's uniform, name tag, stethoscope and bandage scissors can be overwhelming, for then all that is left to effect nursing intervention is one's ability to communicate, convey empathy and apply the problem-solving approach. The principle of behavior which states that a threat to one's role leads to increased anxiety describes the initial role threat encountered when students approach the psychiatric clinical area for the first time.

Lack of Structure

The lack of traditionally structured activities such as giving bed-baths, treatments and medications provides sources of anxiety for

4 / ADULT PSYCHIATRIC NURSING

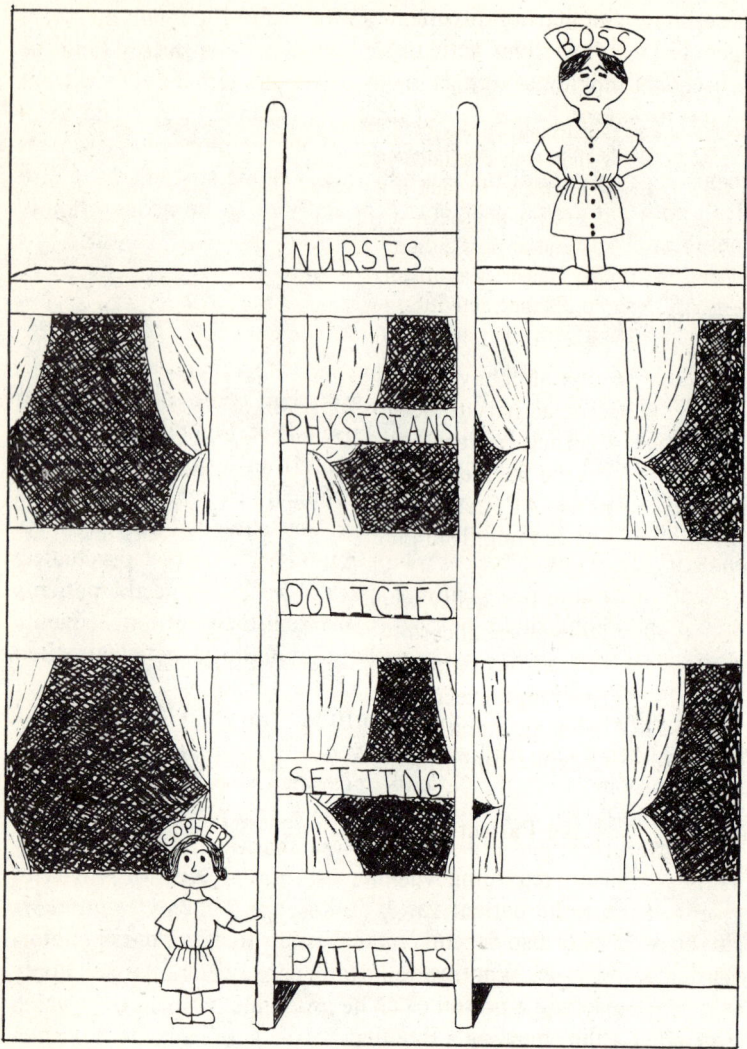

Figure 1-1

students. At first, students fail to recognize the structure of the unit. They do not see the many activities of patient participation on units offering a therapeutic program. Activities such as occupational, recreational and vocational therapy add structure to the patient's day. Initially, students may only see people milling around in what appear to be haphazard directions. Few students immediately know how to "fit in" the unit activities. One student reacted to the first day on the unit by saying,

> I found myself feeling uneasy because of the nature of the patients' illnesses. They didn't have a tangible, physical illness that I could actually view or palpate. In fact, my general feeling that first evening was more of self-conciousness—as if there was absolutely no place for me to sit, stand or pass out on. It was fine when the patients went down to dinner. Then I was able to sit and talk with them, *but* afterwards with no planned activities, I felt an urgent pressure to try and do something with the patients other than merely sitting.

This student would have felt a decrease in anxiety had she been able to find some activity to occupy herself. An additional reaction to the lack of structure was: "At first it was really hard for me to just come up to the people and talk, but after a little while I didn't have any trouble. At first I felt like I was just goofing around, because I wasn't running from pillar to post getting medications and making beds."

A student may feel guilty when not required to exert considerable energy giving physical care. At first glance the energy expended in "just talking" seems minimal, until the student actually becomes involved in a meaningful relationship with a patient and experiences the drain of listening intently and thinking carefully before speaking. Figure 1-2 depicts the principle that activity decreases anxiety.

Need to Know the Patient's History Before Meeting Him

The decision regarding whether students read patient charts before meeting the patient varies from one instructor to another. The decision may also depend on the student's level of anxiety about the new experience. Wanting to know an extensive patient history before approaching a person often indicates that the student is anxious about the meeting. Reading patient records, a familiar procedure in most clinical areas prior to the onset of nursing care, often helps an anxious student structure her time and appear less conspicuous. The increased information from the record may enhance the student's ability to predict how the patient might react to her and thus decrease the student's anxiety.

In psychiatry, it may be beneficial for the student to meet the patient before reading the record, although for many the uncertainty

6 / ADULT PSYCHIATRIC NURSING

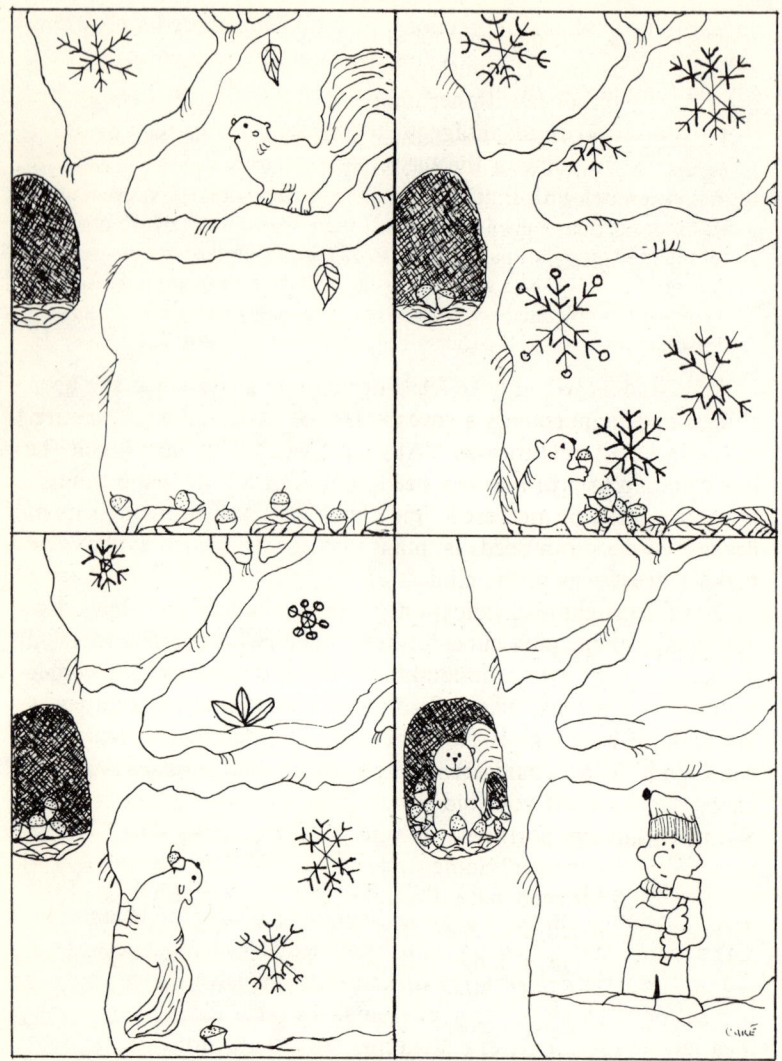

Figure 1-2

is stressful. Since students do not always give direct patient care in the psychiatric setting in the form of treatments, the need to know technical information is lessened. By not reading the record prior to meeting the patient, the student has an opportunity to assess the patient and consider his needs with a minimum of bias from the opinions of others. Preconceived ideas tend to impede the development of the nurse-patient relationship in that the nurse compares what the patient says and does with her impressions of what she expects him to do and say. It is advantageous for students to read the patient's record at some point in the nurse-patient relationship to validate their assessment with that of others on the health care team. If students provide direct care or write on the patient's record, then the record must be read early in the relationship.

Self-awareness

Psychiatric nursing is a voyage into self-exploration and awareness. A first step is to ask, "Why do I want to be a nurse?" The question, "Which of my own needs will be met by being a nurse?" must ultimately be answered. One approach to looking at how nursing meets one's own needs is to ask, "What caused me to feel good the last day I was in the clinical area?" Was it the patient's smile when you brought his medication, his thanks or his comment, "You are going to be a good nurse," when you rubbed his back; or was it the great feeling you experienced upon completing a difficult drug equation? Next, ask who influenced your decision to be a nurse. Was it your aunt who is the ICU supervisor and seems to like her work so well? Did your parents urge you to go to law school and, in an attempt to exert your independence, you chose nursing instead? Was it the image portrayed of nursing in the media which helped you decide on a career? Some students recognize on the first day of the clinical experience that self-awareness can no longer be avoided. The urgency of self-awareness is pointed out in this student's comment: "I went on a long walk after clinical—I felt sad, mad, frustrated, scared and excited all at the same time. Most of all, I saw the need for a lot of introspection on my part."

Self-awareness assists a student in recognizing her limitations as well as her strengths. There is no easy way to attain self-awareness. For students still struggling with the pressures and developmental tasks of adolescence, the predominant feeling may be self-conciousness. The first step in gaining awareness is to identify feelings in oneself. This is facilitated by keeping a diary of the feelings elicited in the clinical setting, writing process recordings, sharing in groups or discussing clinical experiences in individual supervisory conferences. One student's response to the idea of keeping a diary while in the psychiatric clinical area was:

> I've kept a journal before when I've been amidst stressful times, and it has always helped me to sort things out and to put them in a new perspective. Having to write things down forces me to analyze them more fully. It also provides an almost physical release.

The diary format used by this student was that of writing a letter to a friend. Each week she would add a postscript to her letter describing her subjective reaction to the clinical experiences of that week. The diary can serve to alert the instructor, who reads it weekly, to stressful areas, fears and fantasies, as well as to pleasant occurrences. It is often easier to write a note than to verbally initiate a discussion of intense feelings. In reading the diary, the instructor picks up topics needing discussion.

Process recording refers to a format for analyzing nurse-patient interaction. The student writes verbatim notes of her conversation in order to examine her approach and consider alternative ways of interacting. A useful process recording format is:

Data / Thoughts / Feelings / Needs / Principles and Revisions

Data refers to what the patient says and the nurse's replies. If the student does not use a tape recorder or take notes during the conversation or interview, the data may not be verbatim but will be the student's recollection. In general, students recall interactions clearly enough to analyze, although aids are helpful. Some clinical settings discourage the use of tape recorders or note taking; thus the student must rely on her memory.

Thoughts refers to the nurse's thoughts at the time of the interaction, as well as to her perception of what the patient may have been thinking. Likewise, *Feelings* and *Needs* pertain to those of the nurse and those perceived for the patient. The nurse ascertains the thoughts, feelings and needs of the patient by observing his nonverbal behavior, as well as listening carefully to what he says and the way in which he speaks. *Principles* of behavior are essential in the process recording in determining the usefulness of the nursing approach and planning *Revisions* based on the outcome of the interaction. (See Appendix C for a sample process recording.)

Student, faculty and peer group conferences are important in psychiatric nursing to help students assess interactions, evaluate approaches and consider future action alternatives. Conferences also provide valuable information for the instructor. Due to the subjective nature of the clinical experience in psychiatric nursing, the student often has to tell the instructor what she did, rather than show her by demonstrating techniques and treatments.

Next in the pursuit of self-awareness is to examine one's expectations of psychiatric nursing. Some students have heard, read or seen movies about psychiatry. Some wonder if something is wrong with them and feel at times as though they are hanging onto their sanity "by the toenails." One student, when asked to describe her reactions to the first day on the psychiatric unit, said, "My feelings right now are fright and depression. Sometimes I feel under pressure, because I try so hard to do well in school. It scares me to see what can happen to a person under stress."

A student may feel inadequate to interact with patients. Few students realize that they have been interacting in a generally productive manner for a number of years and have many tools at their disposal. A purpose of psychiatric nursing is to refine existing skills and develop additional ones suitable for a wide range of clinical and personal experiences.

Fear of Being Hurt or Hurting

A common reaction to psychiatric nursing is fear. Students are afraid that patients will hurt them physically or psychologically, or that they will harm a patient. A frequently held fear is that the student will say the wrong thing to a patient. One student expressed this fear by saying, "I didn't know what to say that would be therapeutic." Students need to recognize that their comments are unlikely to do irreparable damage to a patient. At the same time, communication skills are important in that thoughtless, hurtful remarks have no place in psychiatric nursing.

This fear of the unknown may come from preconceived ideas not readily accessible to consciousness. Each student learns to cope with his fearful feelings by discovering their source. Whose voice or face is associated with the preconceived notion? Is it something a family member said? Was it heard or seen on television or read in a book? Much anticipatory fear is generated from cultural attitudes and beliefs passed down from one generation to another.

Fear of Loss of Control

Students may fear losing control themselves. Some question what they will say if patients verbally abuse them or use profanity in their presence. Others fear their responses to physical abuse. What if a patient strikes me? Will I hit him back? In reality, patients seldom are abusive to students either physically or verbally; yet the initial fear is real.

Male students may have more fear of losing control than females do, since fighting and using profanity are traditionally considered more acceptable for males than females. One male student said, "I just don't know how I will react if one of those adolescents comes up and punches me." It helps the student to examine past ways of reacting to sudden movements or being hit; to look at the feelings attached to the threat to body integrity and territory; and to consider possible reactions and rank them in order of acceptability to the hospital setting.

Fear of Being Rejected by Patient

A nurse's needs may be met when a patient expresses approval or gratitude. Physically ill patients need the nurse; they need treatments and care. In contrast, psychiatric patients are often shy and afraid that the nursing student will reject them. Some are hostile or withdrawn. A student may feel rejected when, actually, the patient fears approaching her. Students are at times surprised at the receptivity of the patients in contrast to the rejection anticipated. One student remarked, "This week was a new experience—people actually wanted to sit and talk for a while. People for the most part did talk about themselves, especially those who were emotionally hurting, for that seems to be the loneliest time of all."

Although students are generally accepted by patients, consideration of one's possible reactions to rejection is important. For example, some students feel threatened when a patient of the opposite sex is rejecting; they may feel threat to role as well as to self-image as a sexually attractive person. Others experience insecurity and role threat when rejected by any patient.

Students are occasionally rejected by patients, when the anger motivating the rejection is toward the staff. For example, when staff members are experiencing stress, patients—anxious and angry—feel helpless to demonstrate anger toward staff for fear of retaliation.

Thus the anger is displaced onto "those nursing students who are always in the way." When rejection occurs, it is important to distinguish the cause. Is the patient shy and afraid? Have the students inadvertently alienated the patients? Are the patients angry at the staff and handling these feelings by scapegoating the students?

Identification with Patients

At times a student observes patients who are experiencing conflicts and stress similar to her own. The student may become either depressed or afraid, thinking, "Good grief, maybe my problem is worse than I thought," or feel relief that her problem was handled in a growth-producing manner. Students question whether chance or a miracle saved them from psychological disintegration, until they learn to detect the subtle differences between their situation and that of the patient.

One student's reaction to participating as an observer in a family therapy session was:

> It was incredible how much their problems resembled the problems my mother and I had at that time of my life. My mother's personality was so very close to the mother at family therapy, and the daughter was so much like me. The subject was almost identical to something that happened in my youth. I sat there watching them interacting, knowing what each was going to say before she said it—I was right every time. I had to keep pulling myself off the edge of the chair. The mother reacted to things the daughter said just as my mother would have. The daughter was trying to give a message to her mother and the therapist but could not express the words; I think I'm sure I know what she was trying to say. No one picked up on what she wanted to say, and I was hesitant to say anything. I kept wondering if I was over-identifying. She (the daughter) finally became quiet—she gave up (as I had), defeated and misunderstood. She just could not express her needs. Soon the topic died out, and everyone left in tears, but nothing was really resolved. Maybe I should have said something. . . .

As noted in the example, the similarities between patients' problems and those experienced by students are occasionally obvious. Students have often learned ways to handle conflict and stress so as to maintain homeostasis, in contrast to patients whose need for hospitalization represents a disruption to equilibrium.

Anger at Patient for Blocking Student's Goals

Unmet goals or expectations may lead to increased anxiety for either the student or the patient. Often in psychiatric nursing, students write weekly process recordings. Since a considerable portion of the clinical grade is determined by the process recordings, students attempt to obtain "a good conversation to write up" and subsequently arrive on the unit with an agenda for the day's communications. Occasionally, limited patients are available for conversation, as when activities are scheduled allowing minimal verbal interaction. On other days, the student cannot seem to begin and/or sustain an interaction; each time she approaches a patient her overtures are met with silence, social conversation or withdrawal by the patient. One student aptly described such a day: "Frustration capitalized this week of many blocked goals. I wanted to promote conversation with P., but she didn't cooperate. In striving for my goal, I showered her with 'therapeutic questioning' which, in looking back, blocked out conversation even more." When one's goals are not met, reevaluate them to see if they are consistent with the assessment of the patient, the setting or one's ability. Also examine the approach used to make contact with the patient. Perhaps the student appeared anxious, insecure, aggressive or afraid. Patients, being sensitive to the feeling tone of others, frequently respond with like behavior. That is, if the student appears scared and afraid to approach the patient, he may back away and become unapproachable.

Cost of Involvement

Nursing students are taught to utilize a holistic approach in patient care—to care for the entire person, not merely a group of disorganized symptoms. The nurse is likewise a person with needs; often little consideration is given to meeting her needs in ways not interfering with the patient's need attainment. What cost must the nurse pay for "therapeutic use of self"? She is expected to be knowledgeable, caring, supportive and objective. What does she do with her feelings and reactions toward patients and toward nursing in general? When a patient experiences stress, he displays anger, denial, hostility or withdrawal. How can the nurse handle anger? What options are acceptable? The nurse is viewed differently from the patient when she reacts to stress with one of the mechanisms considered acceptable for a patient. She is often described as coping poorly if she expresses anger outwardly, appears sad or talks with colleagues about her negative feelings toward a patient.

What is the price one pays for nursing involvement? Caring, empathy and availability are costly to the nurse with limited supportive systems for meeting her needs. The nurse is likened to a pressure cooker. Each time she becomes involved with a patient and provides empathetic care, the pressure increases. How can this energy be dissipated? Each nurse must find a pressure release valve which allows the energy to be dissipated before the cooker (nurse) explodes.

To be open and involved with a patient means to share both sorrow and happiness. Nurses become tired and anxious when continuously interacting with patients. At least three sets of reactions to intense involvement with patients are observed: (1) battle the problems alone, (2) seek help from other health team members, (3) avoid the problem by ignoring the increasing feelings of stress.

Several specific reactions are seen in nurses feeling the stress of involvement, as well as in students struggling to cope with an adjustment to psychiatry. First, the nurse experiences the same physiological and psychological reactions as the patient: she reacts by crying, having outbursts of anger or experiencing difficulty eating or sleeping. Nursing students, as well as graduate nurses, use defense mechanisms unconsciously to cope with feelings of insecurity, anxiety and lack of self-confidence. Displacement is often seen when the student takes out feelings on someone or something in the environment, rather than on the actual source of the feeling. Examples include being noisy on the unit or berating others.

Projection is seen when the student attributes her feelings to someone else: when she says the instructor did not adequately orient the students; that the doctor doesn't care for his patients; that all the staff nurses are incompetent. Other students use overcompensation to deal with the intrapsychic reaction to psychiatric nursing; that is, they arrive early, ask to stay late or come to the hospital at unscheduled times. Denial is another frequently used defense mechanism. Denial is seen when students repress the stress they experience in the clinical setting. The student says, "Psychiatric nursing is really a breeze—all you do is sit around and talk or play games."

Whenever a student utilizes a defense mechanism to cope with the stress of psychiatric nursing, the instructor and classmates assist her toward greater self-awareness. The student is encouraged to assess her own situation, determine the cause of the stress and define a plan for coping more effectively with her internal environment or the external environment of the clinical area.

Normal coping mechanisms are available to nurses as well as to patients. There are both appropriate and inappropriate times and settings to express feelings openly. The patient's room is no place to engage in a tirade about hospital policy, whereas the conference room provides a suitable setting for expression of negative thoughts and feelings. Nurses, like patients, are encouraged to handle feelings and reactions directly rather than bottling them up or displacing them.

The following example expresses one student's subjective progression through the psychiatric nursing experience:

Walking through the psychiatric unit that first day left me with mixed feelings. I was very unsure, more like scared, about myself, about how I would react and about my ability to use communication skills in an atmosphere totally foreign to me. At the same time, I was excited and halfway looking forward to the psychiatric experience. Could I handle this or not? How would I handle it when I actually was on the unit with the patients?

My first impression of the unit was of the casual atmosphere—no men in white coats, no zombies. Nurses were actually wearing blue jeans! The place couldn't be all that threatening with nurses in blue jeans! After the first two days on the adolescent side, I was feeling very inadequate—I just couldn't get a "therapeutic" interaction going. I felt so awkward knocking on a stranger's door and saying, "Could we talk a minute?" I tried to find residents in places where I wouldn't have to talk much—like in the dayroom, the hall, etc. I didn't realize that I was avoiding really getting to know the residents, until I finally made myself walk down the hall and go in a resident's room. Once I got inside the room alone with the patient, we actually talked—boy, was I elated! I had succeeded! It hadn't been perfect, but I hadn't blown it either.

I learned a lot about myself in psych. I'd always thought I was outgoing, so sure of myself, but I came to realize I wasn't as outgoing and confident as I had thought! Once I realized that most of the patients would talk with me and wouldn't run away when I walked up, I had more confidence and felt more comfortable on the unit.

From this clinical experience, I was able to improve my communication skills and become more aware of myself—maybe that's why I have developed the really positive feelings about being a part, even if only a temporary part, of a psychiatric unit. Once I got over the fear of being in a one-to-one with a patient, I was much more comfortable and actually enjoyed being on the unit. I can understand my initial hesitancy: it's not everyday that you approach a total stranger with the intent of getting him to talk about "deep" subjects. I still believe talking is difficult, but I'm not afraid of it anymore.

SUMMARY

For many, psychiatric nursing proves a strange and unknown situation. Familiar vestiges of power are removed to varying degrees depending on the setting. In some psychiatric units, staff wear street clothes and are barren of typical hospital accessories such as stethoscopes, scissors or even name tags. Students react to the clinical experience with fear and anxiety, largely due to the unfamiliar setting and preconceived notions. Once the student is comfortable in the setting, she recognizes it as less threatening than she feared.

PRINCIPLES

1. Fear of the unknown leads to increased anxiety.
2. All behavior is a response to changed conditions in the individual's total environment.
3. Acceptance by others precedes self-acceptance.
4. Threat to one's role leads to increased anxiety and decreased security and self-confidence.
5. Fear of losing control of the situation leads to increased anxiety, which leads to decreased self-esteem, leading to increased helplessness and decreased ability to assess and problem-solve.
6. High levels of anxiety lead to decreased ability to assess.
7. To reject before being rejected by someone, temporarily increases one's feeling of power.
8. Anxiety is contagious.
9. Unknown, untried or new situations or roles lead to increased anxiety.
10. Activity decreases anxiety.

BIBLIOGRAPHY

Congress for Nursing Practice. *Standards of Psychiatric-Mental Health Nursing Practice.* Kansas City, Mo.: American Nurses' Association, 1973.

CHAPTER 2

Theories of Personality Development

Gail Davis, R.N., Ed.D. and Allene Jones, R.N., M.N.

INTRODUCTION

How does personality development relate to the practice of psychiatric nursing with the adult client? This question has probably been answered best by H. E. Peplau (1952, p. 73) as follows:

> The function of personality is to grow and develop. Nursing is a process that seeks to facilitate development of personality by aiding individuals to use those compelling forces and experiences that influence personality in ways that insure maximum productivity.

Personality, a concept with many interpretations, has been studied and grouped under such diverse headings as theological, sociological, psychological, biological and philosophical. For the purpose of relating personality theory to the practice of psychiatric nursing, selected theories generally categorized as psychological are presented: (1) psychoanalytic, (2) cognitive, (3) behavioristic and (4) humanistic. In addition, the existential theory, usually considered to be in the philosophical grouping, is discussed because of its implications for nursing practice.

Due to the varied approaches to the development of personality theory, a number of definitions of the term "personality" exist. The comprehensive study of personality by G. W. Allport lists 50 different definitions. The final definition originated by Allport (1947, p. 48) states: "Personality is the dynamic organization within the individual of those psychological systems that determine his unique adjustments to his environment."

The early ego or self-oriented psychoanalytic formulations by Freud focus on mental mechanisms, the unconscious, and life and death instincts, thereby implying an internalized approach to the study of personality. Following Allport's theoretical formulations in the 1930s, the scope of personality development expanded to include diverse and more comprehensive definitions and concepts. Later psychoanalytical theorists—Jung, Adler, Fromm, Sullivan and Erikson—gave added consideration to interpersonal and social influences.

Humanistic psychology incorporates selected ideas of earlier theories, basing its beliefs on a holistic view of man. According to the humanists, one's self-concept is the nucleus of the total system. This leads to the belief that in order for an individual to change his behavior, he must change his self-concept. Due to the belief that one can change his self-concept and his behavior, this is a growth-oriented psychology.

The behavior theorists, on the other hand, basically differ from the humanists in their belief that the way to change the self-concept is *first* to change behavior. Basic to their belief is the idea that behavior can be measured, while inner processes cannot. It is desirable, therefore, to be concerned only with that which can be observed and measured.

With this brief introduction to the classification of theories, one can see some of the major approaches and trends in the psychological study of personality development. Certain aspects of these classifications are presented in more depth.

PSYCHOANALYTIC THEORIES

Freud's Psychoanalytic Theory

Three major categories of personality development will be looked at from the Freudian point of view. In describing a theory of personality development, Freud used three major categories: (1) the organization or structure of personality, (2) the dynamics of personality and (3) the development of personality.

The Organization or Structure of Personality

The organization or structure of personality is made up of three major systems: the id, the ego and the superego. Although each of these systems has unique functions and characteristics, they work cooperatively for man to live in harmony with his environment. The overall purpose of these three major systems and their transactions is to fulfill man's basic needs and desires of daily living. Behavior is a result of the interaction of id, ego and superego. When these three systems are not working in harmony, the personality is considered to be maladjusted; thus, the individual's productivity is decreased, and he is unhappy with himself and his environment (Hall, 1954, p. 22; Hall and Lindzey, 1957, p. 32).

The *id* is present at birth, whereas both ego and superego develop from the id (Bischof, 1970, p. 22). The primary function of the id is relief of tension. The id, concerned with the pleasure principle, is intent on keeping the individual in a quiescent state (Hall, 1954, p. 23).

Much of id behavior is seen in the young infant. For example, the young infant expresses his discomfort without regard to time, place or person. When bodily discomforts are relieved by the caretaker, the infant returns to a quiescent state. An individual, however, cannot go through life reducing tension by primitive reflex (id) behavior. The primitive reflex behaviors allow no real psychological development to take place, providing only maintenance functions.

A new development may take place in the id as a result of frustration. This development is known as primary process. This process produces an image of the object that will reduce tension. For example, the infant through repetitious exposure to the bottle, learns to associate food with relieving tension (hunger pangs). The infant then forms a mental image of the bottle; however, he is unable to differentiate between a subjective memory and an objective memory. Obviously, another kind of memory or process is needed, namely, the secondary process, which is characteristic of ego functioning. More will be said about the secondary process in relation to the ego.

Primary process thinking is illustrated in the adult through the example of the thirsty traveler in the middle of the desert who sees a pool of water and forms a mental image which would reduce tension. Wish-fulfillment is the process of accepting the image as real (Hall, 1954, p. 25).

The id has certain characteristics differentiating it from the ego and superego. The id is the primary source of psychic energy and instincts. Unchanging with the passage of time, the id is not governed by logic, laws or reason; yet it is in close touch with bodily processes. Since the id is not in touch with the external world, the individual motivated by id impulses appears selfish, demanding and even odd. Obviously, an individual cannot function effectively in daily living when guided by his id. This inability to function effectively necessitates the development of the ego (Hall, 1954, pp. 24-27; Bischof, 1970, p. 39; Hall and Lindzey, 1957, p. 33).

The *ego*, obtaining psychic energy from the id, comes into existence to assist the individual to cope with reality. Concerned with the reality principle, the ego is described as secondary process functioning. The reality principle, dealing with existing circumstances, holds as its aim the delay of gratification until the need can be appropriately met. The reality principle does not forbid the operation of the pleasure principle, but it postpones its activity in the interest of reality. Meeting needs at the appropriate time and place decreases painful experiences that the individual is likely to experience should he attempt to meet needs at the inappropriate time and place.

The reality principle, operating by the secondary process, is governed by problem-solving and rational thinking; it enables the individual to develop a plan before moving toward action. The secondary process differentiates between the objective world and the subjective world, whereas the primary process is unable to differentiate, thereby functioning only on a subjective level.

The ego or the "I" of the personality allows the individual to distinguish between himself and his world. The ego, serving as the executive of the personality, makes acceptable compromises between the impulsive activities of the id and the demands and requirements of the external world (Hall, 1954, pp. 27-29; Hall and Lindzey, 1957, p. 34; Bischof, 1970, p. 40).

The third personality component, the *superego*, serves as the moral or judicial branch of the personality. The superego is developed from the ego in response to rewards and punishments meted out by parenting figures. The child assimilates parental standards of right and wrong, thereby making them his own.

The superego is composed of two subsystems: the ego ideal and the conscience. The ego ideal is what the child conceives of his parents' behavior as being good. For example, if the child is always rewarded for being kind, kindness will be one of his ideals. Conscience, on the other hand, corresponds to the child's conception of what is morally bad, and this is established through experiences with punishment (Hall, 1954, p. 31). For example, if the child is frequently punished for expressing anger, the expression of anger is considered bad.

Obviously, there are no clearly delineated boundaries between the id, the ego and the superego. The three systems must work in harmony as an integrated whole in order to achieve a stable personality (Hall, 1954, pp. 31-35; Hall and Lindzey, 1957, pp. 35-36).

The Dynamics of Personality

In order for the systems—id, ego, superego—to interact, *psychic energy*, defined as the energy required for psychological work, is required. The conservation of energy principle holds that energy is never lost but is transformed from one state into another. According to Freud, each individual has a specifiable amount of psychic energy which is used efficiently within the three subsystems of the personality in order to cope with the problems of everyday living.

What is the source of psychic energy? According to Freud, psychic energy is derived from the instincts. An instinct is defined as "an inborn condition which imparts direction to psychological processes" (Hall, 1954, p. 37). An instinct has four distinct features: a source, an aim, an object and an impetus. The aim of the instinct is to remove a bodily discomfort. An example of a hungry person is used to describe how an instinct operates:

Source = bodily need → hunger instinct
Aim → reduce hunger
Object = food
Impetus (force) = amount of psychic energy used in seeking food

Obviously, the greater the nutritional need, the greater the psychic energy which will be used in obtaining food in order to decrease the hunger pangs. Once the hunger pangs are relieved, the individual can use this psychic energy for performing other meaningful tasks.

It is not surprising that a starving person has little available psychic energy for performing complicated psychological tasks, since most of his psychic energy is tied up in searching for food to relieve the bodily need of hunger. The instinct is conservative, in that its aim is to return the person to the quiescent state. Keeping the individual in a quiescent state conserves psychic energy.

The id is the original reservoir of instincts and, therefore, of psychic energy. In order for the ego and superego to develop, psychic energy is withdrawn from the id. As previously stated, the energy of the id is used for tension reduction. Examples of tension reduction include urination, defecation, eating and daydreaming.

Energy in the id is fluid and can be displaced easily from one object to another. The investment of psychic energy in the image of an object is known as object cathexis. For example, the hungry infant puts any object resembling a bottle in his mouth until he learns to discriminate between food and objects. The infant and young child's attention span is short, since most of their psychic energy resides in the id. Obviously, an adult cannot cope with the problems of daily living if his energy is still in the id. Thus the ego comes into being.

The young child soon learns that tensions cannot be relieved by impulsive behavior. The energy in the id will remain the same unless help arrives. As a result of repeated frustrations, the ego begins to form. Some of the energy from the id is shunted to the ego. As a result of this shunting of psychic energy, a new kind of cathexis is formed, ego cathexis. Once the ego cathexes are formed, psychic energy is less fluid, attention span is increased and the secondary process is in operation. Thus a more reality-oriented personality can be observed.

Energy in the ego is bound rather than fluid. With its bound energy, the ego is able to control the impulsive actions of the id and the idealistic actions of the superego.

As the child increasingly identifies with parental attitudes of what is morally right or wrong, psychic energy is shunted from the ego to another form—the superego. As with the ego, the processes of identification and anticathexis are responsible for the superego development.

The distribution of psychic energy within the three subsystems of the personality results in a change in personality. An individual with energy primarily controlled by the superego behaves in an overly moralistic manner. Under normal circumstances, the ego monopolizes the store of psychic energy; however, when the ego receives more than its share of psychic energy from the other two systems, the person is overly concerned with himself. An individual's behavior is impulsive if the psychic energy is retained in the id. Obviously, the system monopolizing psychic energy governs the person's behavior (Hall, 1954, pp. 39-47).

Cathexis is known as the urging force, while *anticathexis* is known as the checking force. Cathexis is the process by which the id invests energy into an object in order to satisfy a bodily need, and it is associated with external frustration. For example, an individual hunting food will experience external frustration if no food is within his reach. In looking at external frustration, one must keep in mind that the id cannot curtail its activity. This is where the role of anticathexis comes into play. Anticathexis is the property of the ego and the superego. Since the ego and superego deal with reality and morality, an internal conflict can result when a desired goal is blocked. For example, the hungry person unable to obtain food in a normal fashion might resort to stealing or taking food without permission, if his ego and superego fail to urge him to wait and find another way—even though, for him, stealing is wrong. Obviously, too much cathexis by the id and too little anticathexis can produce a maladjusted person. The same is true if too much anticathexis is employed by the ego and the superego. More will be said about cathexis and anticathexis in relation to the development of personality (Hall, 1954, pp. 49-54).

The Development of Personality

Discussing the development of personality according to Freud's psychoanalytic theory is incomplete without briefly discussing the *levels of consciousness*. Freud described three levels of consciousness: unconscious, pre-conscious and conscious. These levels of consciousness are known as Freud's topographical theory. The topographical theory of the mind is compared to an iceberg. The conscious part of the mind is that part which is aware of the here and now. It is analogous to the tip of the iceberg above the water. The next part is the pre- or subconscious containing thoughts, feelings and ideas that are partially forgotten. With recall, material stored in the pre-conscious can be remembered. The pre- or subconscious portion, just below the conscious level, has a small part submerged and a small part above the water. The unconscious portion, the largest part of the iceberg, is usually submerged under the water. All forgotten and repressed memories, thoughts, feelings and responses are stored in the unconscious. The unconscious portion is the most significant level of consciousness, because of the effect it has upon behavior. Considerable psychic energy is needed to keep unpleasant memories stored in the unconscious part of the mind. In general, psychic energy is utilized in shifting material from one level of consciousness to another (Hall, 1954, pp. 54-57).

Anxiety and the defense mechanisms assume a major portion of Freud's theory of personality development. The relationship of this development to the dynamics of personality is a basic part of Freudian theory. High levels of anxiety, in general, are threatening to the ego. High levels of anxiety cause the ego to use defense mechanisms excessively to preserve the integrity of the individual. Excessive use of ego defense mechanisms requires psychic energy. If too much psychic energy is used by defense mechanisms, not enough psychic energy is left for solving problems of everyday living.

There is no consensus as to the way in which defense mechanisms should be categorized. For example, Corsini (1977) arranges some of the more commonly used defense mechanisms along a hierarchical continuum. The more sophisticated defenses characteristic of an integrated ego would be at the top of the list, while the more primitive ones would be down the list. Corsini gives the following example of categorizing defense mechanisms along a hierarchical continuum (p. 28):

> (1) rationalization, (2) repression, (3) displacement, (4) identification, (5) conversion, (6) isolation or intellectualization, (7) reaction formation or overcompensation, (8) undoing, (9) introjection, (10) projection and (11) denial.

The criterion Corsini uses to determine whether a defense mechanism is more sophisticated than primitive is the amount of the reality testing the defense mechanism retains. For example, rationalization is at the top of the list because it distorts reality minimally, whereas denial at the bottom of the list repudiates reality.

Mereness in her book, *Essentials of Psychiatric Nursing* (1970), categorizes defense mechanisms with the phase of growth and development in which they are initiated. For example, defense mechanisms likely to originate in the oral phase are compensation, displacement, substitution and fixation. Defense mechanisms likely to originate in the anal stage include suppression, sublimation, reaction formation, identification and introjection. Rationalization, repression and regression may originate in the phallic period, whereas projection is thought to originate in the latency period. Symbolization, condensation and conversion are not assigned to any particular stage of growth and development. Mereness does state that any of these defense mechanisms may originate in more than one phase of development.

Although no attempt will be made to arrange defense mechanisms categorically, a general explanation of ego defenses is summarized as follows:

1. Ego defense mechanisms are necessary for assisting one in adjusting to life situations
2. The ego needs defense mechanisms to protect it from becoming overwhelmed by anxiety
3. All human beings use defense mechanisms
4. Defense mechanisms become pathological only when they are overused to the degree that they distort reality
5. True ego defense mechanisms occur unconsciously; they are never planned

Psychogenetically, repression is one of the earliest defense mechanisms available to a human being. Repression occurs when one involuntarily puts unacceptable ideas or impulses into the unconscious. Repression is a kind of unconscious forgetting and is the best known of the ego defense mechanisms. It is exemplified when one suddenly forgets this friend's or relative's name, because the name would remind him of an unpleasant experience which would give rise to anxiety.

Suppression is not considered a true defense mechanism, because it is the voluntary banishment of unacceptable thoughts, feelings, needs and impulses into the pre-conscious. Suppression is conscious forgetting, whereas repression is unconscious forgetting. Although suppression is not a true defense mechanism, it does relieve anxiety. Suppression is commonly used by people with adequately functioning personalities. An example of suppression is seen when one behaves inappropriately and then forgets about his behavior.

Regression is the unconscious return to an earlier developmental level associated with comfort and security. Regression occurs when one is confronted with a conflict that gives rise to anxiety and other associated feelings of discomfort. Retreating to an earlier level of comfort is an unconscious way of handling the conflict. Although individuals in all age groups regress to a certain extent when physically ill or emotionally upset, regression as a way of adaptation is not desirable. When one repeatedly resorts to regression as a method of adaptation, the mastery of developmental tasks decreases or ceases.

A common and normal use of regression is seen when the 3-year-old who is toilet trained loses bladder and bowel control in response to the arrival of a new brother or sister. Why does this 3-year-old return to wetting and soiling? First of all, he is faced with the conflict of hate or resentment over the newcomer and the wish to retain the love of his parents. One must also keep in mind that this 3-year-old has an underdeveloped ego and is unable to use some of the more sophisticated mechanisms of defense; he also has fond memories of being held and cuddled by his parents. The return, therefore, to wetting and soiling of clothing is bound to get his parents' attention. If the parents realize the reason for the change in the child's behavior and act accordingly, the child soon returns to his normal state of being.

Regression is often seen in hospitalized patients. These patients often have unmet dependency needs which become reactivated when they are placed in a dependent state. Obviously, repression of these unmet dependency needs has failed. These patients are usually demanding, attention-seeking and/or helpless.

Identification is a defense mechanism denoted by the unconscious internalization of desirable attributes of an external object—usually those of another person, generally a parent—into one's own personality. Obviously, identification is an important mechanism in the development of a child's personality, especially the development of the superego or conscience (Rowe, 1965, p. 20; Mereness, 1970, p. 23; Hall, 1954, p. 74). The following are four types of identification and their relationships to personality development:

1. Narcissistic, which is defined as the spread of self-cathexis to other people and things that resemble the self

2. Goal-oriented, which is defined as the modeling of one's personality upon that of a person who is achieving goals which the identifier would like to achieve
3. Object-loss, defined as the incorporation of cathected objects that one has lost or has not been able to possess
4. An aggressor, which is defined as the incorporation of prohibitions imposed by an authority figure

Incorporation, a primitive defense mechanism, is sometimes considered a type of identification. It is the psychic representation of a person or parts of a person which are figuratively incorporated into one's own self-perception. Its origin is in the oral phase, and it is related to the infant nursing experience. For example, the infant believes that the mother's breast is a part of his own body (Rowe, 1965, p. 20).

Introjection is the unconscious taking into oneself of a loved or hated person or external object. Like incorporation, introjection is sometimes regarded as a type of identification. Introjection is the opposite of projection. Introjection operates when the child begins to take on attributes of his parents or other significant authority figures and makes them his own. This is important to superego development. In adults, introjection operates when the individual is unable to express anger or aggression against another person but instead turns these feelings against himself. The individual then tends to ridicule, deprecate and accuse himself of acts that belong to another person. In reality, the individual is directing these angry and aggressive feelings towards the characteristics of the other person or object in himself. As might be expected, introjection is often observed in depressive reactions and in suicidal thoughts and tendencies (Rowe, 1965, p. 20; Mereness, 1970, p. 23).

Projection is the unconscious attributing to another person or object of one's own unacceptable thoughts, feelings, desires and motives. All individuals use projection to a mild degree in everyday living. Sometimes people cannot accept their failures and shortcomings, so they tend to blame someone else. For example, the student who blames the teacher for his poor grade is utilizing projection. Obviously, if projection is carried to the extreme, it can be pathological. This pathological use of projection is seen in all types of paranoid reactions. The individual often exhibits delusions of persecution, hallucinations and ideas of reference (Rowe, 1965, p. 21).

Rationalization is the unconscious invention of an acceptable reason for one's behavior, thoughts, feelings and motives. Rationalization differs from lying or pretending, because it is an unconscious process, whereas lying and pretending are conscious processes.

Like projection, rationalization is a commonly used defense mechanism, but it can be dangerous when overused. Overuse of rationalization is dangerous, because it prevents the individual from facing the problem at hand. There are many common examples of rationalization. One example is that of the student who has done poorly on an examination, even though he wanted to do well and had studied hard. He may explain his poor performance by saying that he just did not study enough, because he fails to face the fact that he did the best he could (Rowe, 1965, pp. 21-22).

Compensation is the conscious or unconscious attempt to overcome real or imagined weaknesses. It is used more extensively when one's status is threatened. Since the maintenance of one's status is important, compensatory behavior is a common occurrence in all people. Compensatory behavior can be seen in individuals who are physically handicapped, but who become quite proficient at using their minds. Compensatory behavior is not always socially acceptable; for example, a person who is small in stature may become aggressive, hostile and domineering ("the small man syndrome"). The person suffering from the "small man syndrome" is heard and seen by the individuals in his environment, but seldom gets the respect he is seeking; thus, his status is constantly threatened (Rowe, 1965, p. 22).

Reaction formation occurs when an individual behaves in direct opposition to his actual thoughts and feelings. People who are overly polite, friendly, courteous and overprotective usually have feelings of hostility, anger and aggression toward others. The meticulous individual may also be covering up the impulse to be messy. Some adult individuals become untidy in their home and personal hygiene as a reaction formation to earlier rigid and meticulous toilet training experiences (Rowe, 1965, p. 22; Mereness, 1970, p. 32).

Obviously, reaction formations are irrational adjustments to fear and anxiety. The more an object or person predisposes one to experience fear and anxiety, the more likely reaction formation is to occur. The frequent use of reaction formation distorts reality and causes the individual to be increasingly rigid and inflexible (Hall, 1954, p. 93).

Sublimation is "the diversion of unacceptable, instinctual drives into socially sanctioned channels" (Rowe, 1965, p. 23). Sublimation, the most positive and normal of the defense mechanisms, is commonly used against angry, hostile and aggressive feelings. Strong emotions may be sublimated by physically active sports and games. Certain careers and vocational choices may represent a sublimation of unacceptable impulses (Rowe, 1965, p. 23). The important aspect to remember regarding sublimation is that the person is usually rewarded for his behavior, which occurs as a result of his ability to divert socially unacceptable drives into socially accepted ones.

Denial is the unconscious disclaim of unacceptable thoughts, feelings, needs or certain external factors. Stated simply, denial is the refusal to admit that certain feelings or situations exist. Through the use of denial, the individual is temporarily freed from the anxiety which the denied feelings or situations entailed (Rowe, 1965, p. 23). For example, the alcoholic who refuses to admit that he cannot drink does not have to deal with the anxiety that evolves when he admits he is a "weak individual." Denial also prevents the alcoholic from thinking about treatment for his problem, which would entail anxiety and also the fear of failure. Denial seems to provide the easy way out by allowing the avoidance of anxiety.

Substitution is the replacement of an unattainable or unacceptable activity by one which is attainable or acceptable. For example, an individual with the desire to hurt or destroy someone may be given a punching bag to substitute for the person. In order to be satisfactory, the substitute activity must have a certain resemblance to the original one (Rowe, 1965, p. 23).

Displacement is the redirection of emotions, thoughts, feelings and motives from the primary or original subject to a more acceptable and less threatening substitute subject. A classic example of displacement occurs when a husband who is angry with his boss but is afraid to express his anger comes home and screams at his wife; the wife, in turn, threatened by her husband's unwarranted attack, screams at the child; and the child, who is even more threatened, kicks the dog. Displacement is further seen on obsessive-compulsive reactions.

Isolation is a form of emotional insulation in which the emotional charge or hurt is separated from the traumatic incident. The individual retains the memory of the incident, but the psychic pain associated with the incident is repressed. For example, a mother's hurt over her young child's traumatic death may be reduced by saying, "She was a beautiful child" or "The Lord loved her best." The normal display of grief would not be seen in this situation. Some psychiatric patients appear quite odd, because they overuse isolation, e.g., their affect is inappropriate to the situation encountered (Coleman, 1964, p. 106; Rowe, 1965, p. 24).

Undoing is a form of symbolic atonement designed to undo or erase some socially disapproved act, thought, feeling or desire. Forms of undoing include apologizing, repentance, penance, bringing presents and even undergoing punishment. Pathological symptoms of undoing are seen in obsessive-compulsive disorders and may include such behavior as repetitious and needless handwashing.

Undoing is designed to help one escape rejection and punishment; thus, it is a valuable ego defense mechanism. Like all other defense mechanisms, though, overusage is detrimental to personality growth and development, because the person becomes overladen with guilt combined with an excessive need to apologize and/or to be punished (Coleman, 1964, p. 101; Rowe, 1965, p. 24).

Dissociation is a form of isolation in which there is a detachment of strong emotionally-charged conflicts from the consciousness. Dissociation is seen in sleepwalking, dual personality, automatic writing and dissociative reactions (Coleman, 1964, p. 107; Rowe, 1965, p. 24).

Symbolization is a defense mechanism in which a less threatening object or idea is used to represent another. Symbols in dreams and fantasies are common examples of symbolism. Certain types of speech, dress and gait may be symbolic.

A discussion of the *erogenous zones* is important to an understanding of Freud's theory, and discussion of the Freudian view of personality development is incomplete without a brief summary of the erogenous zones, e.g., the oral, anal and sexual zones. Freud noted that these zones have a great impact upon personality development.

According to Freud, the mouth has five major modes of functioning: "(1) taking in, (2) holding on, (3) biting, (4) spitting out, and (5) closing" (Hall, 1954, p. 104). These modes are important, because each serves as a prototype for certain personality traits. While no attempt is made here to discuss all the personality traits that could occur, selected examples are given.

Taking in through the mouth is the prototype for acquisitiveness; holding on, for tenacity and determination; biting, for destructiveness; spitting out, for rejection and contemptuousness; and closing, for refusal and negativism. Whether these traits develop and become a part of one's character depends upon the amount of anxiety experienced in connection with the prototype's expression. For example, the baby who is weaned too early may develop a strong tendency to hold on to things in order to prevent the repetition of a traumatic experience (Hall, 1954, p. 104).

Other examples of personality traits that can be observed in adult life include (a) individuals who are dependent, gullible and will "swallow" anything and (b) individuals who are sarcastic, e.g., the oral biter (Payne and Clunn, 1977, p. 27).

The anal phase comprises the second eighteen months of life. It is during this period of life that toilet training takes place. Although the mouth is still an erogenous zone, the child becomes more aware of the anal area as an erogenous zone. He receives pleasurable sensations in the anal and bladder area when he freely holds on or lets go of feces and urine, or when he is requested to do so by his parents.

If the parent attempts bowel and bladder training before the child is physically and psychologically ready, the child may react by expelling feces and urine at any time or place; on the other hand, he may hold on and become constipated. Behavior recognizable in adult life from this type of toilet training includes miserliness, compulsive orderliness, disgust, fastidiousness, frugality and strict budgeting of time and money.

The opposite personality traits could occur, however, if the mother pleads with the child to have an elimination, or if she gives him excessive praise for defecating. In such cases, the individual may grow up to be overly generous, a giver of presents, philanthropic and charitable.

Obviously, neither of these methods of toilet training is desirable, the first method being less desirable. The best method of toilet training is the permissive method, which is less rigid and thus leads to a personality that is outgoing, friendly, tries to please others within the bounds of reason and is generally productive (Payne and Clunn, 1977, p. 26; Hall, 1954, pp. 107-108).

The phallic stage includes the second three years of life (3-6 years) in which the genital area is the dominant erogenous zone. It is during this stage that children explore and examine their own bodies. They derive pleasure from manipulation of the penis or clitoris. Such behavior is usually upsetting to parents, and the children are punished for their behavior. They then tend to feel anxious and/or bad, perceiving their sexual organs as dirty.

The phallic stage is a stage of growth and development in which the child also learns to identify with the parent of the same sex. He achieves this sexual identity by the resolution of the Oedipal conflict. If the Oedipal conflict is not resolved, certain undesirable personality traits can result, i.e., sexual deviancy, inability to accept one's sexual role and trouble with authority figures (Payne and Clunn, 1977, p. 28).

Erikson's Psychosocial Theory

Erikson's psychosocial theory of personality development has much in common with Freud's psychosexual theory of personality development; however, some differences do exist. Some of the outstanding *similarities* include the following:

1. Both are psychoanalytic in nature.
2. The first five stages of Erikson's eight stages of growth and development correspond to Freud's five stages of growth and development.
3. Both see growth and development occurring in successive stages.
4. Both stress the importance of the endopsychic conflict and its effect on personality development.
5. Both are detailed in their discussions of each stage of growth and development.

Some of the outstanding *differences* include the following:

1. Erikson's theory is more optimistic than Freud's and thus is easier for many to accept.
2. Erikson places greater emphasis upon the resolution of crises that occur with each stage of growth and development than does Freud.
3. Erikson places less emphasis upon sex as a cause for aberrant behavior than does Freud.
4. Erikson describes eight stages of growth, whereas Freud only

describes five. Freud does not describe the middle-age and older-adult stages in his theory of development.
5. Erikson includes more of the social and environmental factors in describing personality development than does Freud.
6. Erikson emphasizes the healthy aspects of personality, whereas Freud emphasizes the pathological aspects of personality.
7. Erikson's theory is less body-oriented than is Freud's (Craig, 1976, pp. 38-39).

Erikson's eight stages of development are described in polarities. For example, in the first stage—trust versus mistrust—the individual tends to be either trustful or mistrustful, depending upon factors in his environment. Erikson further describes basic virtues that are achieved with each of the eight stages of growth and development. A virtue is a particular moral excellence or commendable quality.

The first stage is *trust versus mistrust*, and the basic virtue is *hope*. This stage corresponds to Freud's oral stage and Piaget's sensorimotor stage. It lasts from birth to eighteen months. Erikson postulates that if the infant's physical and psychological needs are met in a loving and caring manner, he will be a trustful person. If he is shown love during this period, he is better able to give and receive love later in life. The quality of care rather than quantity of care given during this period is important. During this period the parents obviously play an important role in shaping the infant's outlook on life.

The second stage is *autonomy versus shame and doubt*, and the virtue is *willpower*. This stage corresponds to Freud's anal stage and partially to Piaget's preoperational stage. The age span is from one or one-and-one-half to three years, with the stage beginning when the child learns that he can exert some control over his environment. He is able to exert more control over his environment, because he can walk, carry on a limited conversation and control his eliminations to a certain extent. With these newly acquired skills, he is more able to do things for himself. Parents may make the child doubt his abilities and himself, if they try to do everything for him or belittle him when he does his best. Shaming a child does not cause him to act properly. Rather, Erikson observes that excessive shaming causes the child to behave in a shameless manner. If the child develops a sense of shame and doubt, he may disguise his true feelings behind a "reckless bravado"; he attempts to conceal his inner feelings of inadequacy and lack of control over his environment. Summarizing, feelings of shame and doubt undermine the developing ego of the young child.

Erikson's third stage of growth and development is *initiative versus guilt*, and the virtue is *purpose*. The age span is three to six years; thus, this stage corresponds to Freud's phallic stage and Piaget's preoperational and concrete stages. During this stage, the child is increasingly able to exert positive controls over himself and his environment. Since the superego is developing, the child is able to experience guilt. Guilt results when the child's behavior is contrary to what he has learned regarding what is morally good and morally bad.

If the child views his behavior as bad more often than good, he will have an overwhelming sense of guilt instead of initiative. Too much guilt prevents the child from exploring his environment and making decisions. He feels that his explorations and decision-making might be wrong (morally bad). If the emphasis is on initiative rather than guilt, however, the child is able to see his shortcomings in a more realistic manner.

Erikson's fourth stage of growth and development is *industry versus inferiority*, and the virtue is *competence*. This stage corresponds to Freud's latency stage and Piaget's concrete operations. The age span is six to twelve years. The child usually enters school during this stage of life; thus, he is faced with many new tasks which require problem solving. More is expected of him by his parents and other significant adult figures. He also has to interact with his peer group in a less infantile manner.

If the child has met the developmental tasks during the first three stages of life, he is less likely to develop overwhelming feelings of inferiority. School activities and play during this stage are considered to be the child's work. If he cannot perform his work in a culturally accepted manner, he tends to withdraw or act out, in order to decrease feelings of inferiority and increase his sense of industry.

Erikson's fifth stage of man is *identity versus role confusion*, and the virtue is *fidelity*. This stage corresponds to Freud's genital stage and Piaget's formal operations. The age span is twelve or thirteen to eighteen or 21 years. With the emergence of bodily changes such as rapid growth and the appearance of secondary sex characteristics, the adolescent is faced with defining or sorting out his ego identity. If a person does not learn who he is, what he can and cannot do, and what others think of him, he does not have a clear sense of identity. A failure to develop ego identity results in role confusion. An individual suffering from role confusion frequently has problems with sexual roles, social roles, choosing a career or vocation and interpersonal relationships.

Erikson's sixth stage of man is *intimacy versus isolation*, and the virtue is *love*. This stage and the last two ages of man discussed by Erikson correspond to Freud's genital stage and Piaget's formal operations. The age span is eighteen or 21 to 35 or 40 years of age. If the individual enters this stage of growth and development with a clear sense of identity, he is able to establish a mature relationship with a member of the opposite sex, choose a suitable marital partner and perform work and social roles in a socially acceptable manner. If an individual is unable to achieve a basis for intimacy, he tends to isolate himself from others and is frequently unable to share thoughts, feelings and needs on an emotionally mature level.

Erikson's seventh stage of man is *generativity versus stagnation*, and the virtue is *care*. The age span is 35 or 40 to 65 years. This stage is commonly called middle age. Erikson states that an individual during this stage has a need to be needed by others. It is during this stage that children begin to leave home. Parents may find themselves feeling lonely and somewhat useless, if this extra time is not spent wisely. This time can be spent wisely by becoming engaged in helping activities, such as teaching, counseling, community activities and volunteer work. If the individual does not become overly concerned with himself and the bodily changes that occur during this stage, Erikson feels that he can be a creative, caring and productive person.

Erikson's eighth stage of man is *ego integrity versus despair*, and the virtue is *wisdom*. The age span is 65 until death. This stage is known as old age. During this stage the individual should be able to review his life realistically. He should be able to accept his past failures and his future limitations. If he sees his past life as a total failure, he is likely to sink into despair. An individual who has a sense of integrity experiences wisdom. With wisdom, he is able to help members of the younger generations view life more realistically. Also, the individual with integrity is able to accept death with dignity (Lidz, 1968, pp. 80-83; Craig, 1976, pp. 39-42).

Implications for Psychiatric Nursing Practice

Psychoanalytic theory is closely related to chronological growth and development. While Freud's theory covers the period of life extending through adolescence, Erikson's theory extends throughout the life span.

The primary implications of psychoanalytic theory for nursing practice, then, are based on the major problem areas which may occur and the related tasks to be accomplished at each stage of growth and development. An understanding of Freudian theory is helpful to parents and/or other adults responsible for the rearing of children, and the nurse can assist those responsible adults in the understanding and application of this theory. In addition, an understanding of the major tasks designated by Erikson for each of the eight stages throughout the life span can provide the nurse with a focus for assessment and intervention with the client's development at each stage.

The application of psychoanalytic theory through psychotherapy (psychoanalysis) is not a nursing responsibility per se. The nurse participates in the client's treatment primarily in three ways:

1. through close observation and assessment of the client's status and the developmental tasks which have or have not been resolved
2. through interventions which will assist the client in understanding his problem area(s) and which will interrupt the continuance of maladaptive behavior
3. through evaluation of the client's progress during the course of treatment.

In order to implement the nursing role successfully, the knowledge and understanding of defense mechanisms is most important. An understanding of how, why and to what extent different defense mechanisms are used is an essential part of assessment. When the use of these mechanisms is supporting a client's maladaptive behavior, nursing intervention is aimed at *not* providing support for the continued use of those mechanisms. Evaluation can be based upon the client's ability to adapt without the continued overuse of those defense mechanisms upon which he had become dependent.

COGNITIVE THEORY

Cognitive theory is not as well known or accepted in the United States as it is in Europe. The psychologist most immediately associated with cognitive theory, and whose work will be considered here, is Jean Piaget. The work of Piaget (1969), a Swiss psychologist who began his career as a biologist, has become increasingly accepted in recent years.

Piaget's cognitive theory is mainly concerned with the study of the development of intelligence. In order to present a theory of cognitive development, Piaget studied normal children. Much of his research was with his own children. By carefully observing and recording their growth, Piaget was able to present a coherent picture of the mental growth of children. This research with his own children provided a background for his later studies of intellectual development.

How the child learns and how he adapts what he learns to the adult world is the major concern of most of Piaget's research. Listed below are the four stages of intellectual growth that the child passes through according to Piaget.

1. *The Sensorimotor Stage.* This stage occupies the first two years of the child's life. During this time, the infant explores his environment with his body and senses. He explores persons and objects in his environment by smelling, touching, tasting and listening. His mouth and lips are the main organs of exploration.

During this stage the infant develops schemata, which are methods for assimilating and accommodating incoming information. The schemata are named for the senses they represent; examples include the sucking schema, looking schema and hearing schema. Piaget states that these schemata must be practiced by the infant if he is to learn about his world.

2. *The Preoperational Stage.* This period begins at about age two and lasts until about age seven. During this time, the child acquires language. He learns that words are symbols for objects; thus, he begins to develop symbolic images. He is able to make some simple abstractions from concrete reality, but his intellectual development is hampered by his egocentrism. Egocentrism may cause the child to appear selfish. He is really not selfish; he is just seeing things from his own point of view. He feels that others see his world

as he does. As the child matures and interacts with others, he begins to understand that other people see things differently.

3. *Concrete Operational Stage.* The period of concrete operations begins at about age seven and extends until age twelve. During this period, the child is more logical in his thinking. His ability to think in a more abstract manner is increased.

His egocentrism is declining, and his ability to play with other children in a more cooperative manner is increasing. He usually understands and abides by rules.

4. *Formal Operational Stage.* This last period begins between the ages of twelve to fifteen. It is during this time that an individual develops adult logic which continues through the rest of his life. The individual is now able to reason, plan for the future, think in an abstract manner and build ideals. The egocentrism that occurs with adolescence may, however, continue to color his logical and abstract thoughts (Stagner, 1961, pp. 149-152).

Implications for Psychiatric Nursing Practice

While much of the application of Piaget's cognitive theory has been to learning and education, it does hold some implications for nursing practice. The logical sequence through which cognitive development occurs provides a basis for assessing *where* an individual is in relation to "normal."

In working with the adult client, the nurse knows that the individual should be functioning at the level of "formal operations" characterized by logical and abstract thinking. If the client's consistent mode of thinking is not marked by both logical and abstract thinking, then the nurse may assess that a problem does exist. Whether the problem is related to some failure of cognitive development or to a distorted perception of reality will need further assessment and study.

The nursing role also includes working with parents and others involved with the cognitive development of children, since Piaget's theory is primarily concerned with development from infancy through adolescence. This role might include:

1. assessing and evaluating opportunities which parents and other concerned adults are providing for positive cognitive development

2. assessing and evaluating outcomes of the child's cognitive growth related to his experiences
3. making recommendations (and providing teaching, as appropriate) concerning ways in which cognitive development can be fostered and enhanced.

BEHAVIORIST THEORY

The person most commonly associated with behaviorism in the United States is B.F. Skinner, whose theory is based on operant conditioning. Skinner's work has followed the work of earlier behaviorists—E.L. Thorndike, I.P. Pavlov, E.R. Guthrie and J.B. Watson. Almost everyone is familiar with Pavlov's classical conditioning experiments, such as the one described here:

> When meat powder is placed in a dog's mouth, salivation takes place; the food is the *unconditioned stimulus* and the salivation the *unconditioned reflex*. Then some arbitrary stimulus, such as light, is combined with the presentation of food. Eventually, after repetition and if time relationships are right, the light will evoke salivation independent of the food; the light is the *conditioned stimulus* and the response to it is the *conditioned reflex* (Hilgard and Bower, 1966, p. 48).

Pavlov's work followed that of E.L. Thorndike, who introduced the so-called theory of connectionism. This was the original stimulus-response theory, demonstrating a bond or connection between a stimulus and response. Thorndike formulated three laws important to connectionism: (1) readiness, (2) exercise and (3) effect. The law of readiness takes into account the need for preparation prior to action. Broadly, preparation can include anticipation, physiological readiness and motivation. The law of exercise refers to the importance of practice. A connection is strengthened with practice and weakened without it. A connection is strengthened or weakened as a result of the consequences of a response; this is the law of effect. Thorndike's work includes five subordinate laws, the most important of which is "associative shifting." This refers to the ability of an organism to hold the response through a number of gradual changes in the stimulus. Thus, in the end the same response may occur in the presence of a totally new stimulus. The concept of associative shifting is useful in the implications which it holds for behavior therapy.

Many consider J.B. Watson actually to be the first behaviorist. In 1913 he published *Psychology as the Behaviorist Views It*, arguing that "psychology should be redefined as the study of behavior." This represented a break with most psychologists, who were involved in studying "mental processes in a mental world of consciousness" (Skinner, 1974, p. 5). Watson (1930, p. 5) states:

> This thing we call consciousness can be analyzed only by introspection—a looking in at what takes place inside of us.
>
> As a result of this major assumption that there is such a thing as consciousness and that we can analyze it by introspection, we find as many analyses as there are individual psychologists. There is no way of experimentally attacking and solving psychological problems and standardizing methods.

Watson thus set the stage for behaviorism with the belief that "the subject matter of human psychology *is the behavior of the human being*" (Watson, 1930, p. 2). One's behavior, not his inner processes, is all that can be experimentally and objectively measured.

Skinner's Theory of Operant Conditioning

Skinner's theory of operant conditioning was directly influenced by the earlier behaviorists' work. Especially influential in his work is Thorndike's law of effect, e.g., the connection between the stimulus and response is strengthened or weakened by the consequences of the response. Skinner felt it necessary also to deal with the concept of "probability of response." The probability of a response, of course, is not observable; rather, it is a variable which might result from prior experiences, interest and ability. Though not observable, it might become predictable over a period of time. For example, a person who is interested in music and is able to play the piano is likely to play the piano when provided with the instrument and the right situation. In order to predict when this would happen, an experiment controlling all known variables would be necessary. The frequency of a selected response could be determined through repeated observations.

This concept leads to the defining of "operant" as follows:

> A response which has already occurred cannot, of course, be pre-

dicted or controlled. We can only predict that *similar* responses will occur in the future. The unit of a predictive science is, therefore, not a response but a class of responses. The word "operant" will be used to describe this class. The term emphasizes the fact that the behavior *operates* upon the environment to generate consequences (Skinner, 1953, p. 65).

Whereas in classical conditioning a stimulus and a reinforcer (light and food) were paired to gain a response (salivation), in operant conditioning, the operant behavior is contingent upon a reinforcer. The greatest difference, then, in Skinner's theory when compared to previous behavior theories is his emphasis upon operant, rather than respondent, behavior. Rather than S-R (stimulus-response) theory, it can be diagrammed as S-O-R (stimulus-operant-reinforcement).

There are two types of responses: elicited and emitted. Those responses which are *elicited* by known stimuli are classified as *respondents*. Reflex behavior to stimuli, as pupillary constriction to light, represents respondent behavior. Respondent behavior thus requires eliciting stimuli.

Emitted responses are called *operants*. An operant is related to a stimulus, but the nature of the stimulus is usually environmental, so that one specific incident or action is not identifiable as the stimulus. Reinforcement of operant behavior is essential in determining whether or not it becomes a lasting kind of behavior for the individual. The consequence of the behavior is the reinforcement. Most human behavior, according to Skinner, is operant; and his theory gives more consideration to the variables of human behavior than do the prior behavioristic theories.

The following operant conditioning experiment conducted by Skinner describes operant behavior and some of the associated terminology. For the experiment, a hungry pigeon is placed in an enclosed rectangular box which has a "key" on one side at the height of the pigeon's beak. A "food magazine" is positioned slightly below the "key." The pigeon is hungry when placed in the box, but no stimuli are used.

> The pigeon eventually pecks the small disk-shaped key. The food magazine operates automatically, making food available immediately after a peck (response) on the key. We observe that when the pigeon has pecked the key and received food, it soon pecks again (and receives food and pecks again, etc.); i.e., the *rate* or *frequency* of pecking is increased. Because the rate increases when the response is

followed by food, food is said to reinforce the response. Food is called a *reinforcer,* and the event *reinforcement.* Because the response does not appear to be produced by eliciting stimulus, it is said to be *emitted.* This type of behavior, which operates or acts upon the environment, is called operant behavior (Holland and Skinner, 1961, p. 46).

The emitted response, then, is the operant behavior. It may occur in the presence of a known stimulus, but most often is related to environmental stimuli which are unidentified. The consequence of the behavior is the reinforcer; thus, the consequence determines whether this behavior will be retained as an appropriate one for the individual.

Wolpe's Behavior Therapy

Behavior therapy involves the application of knowledge gained from the behavioristic theories to the treatment of neuroses. This application is based on the premise that "neurosis is accounted for by the learning of unadaptive behavior through normal learning processes" (Goldstein, 1977, p. 207). Behavior therapy is aimed at changing the unadaptive behavior, or responses, to adaptive behavior. Another term used synonymously with behavior therapy is behavior modification.

J. Wolpe (1973, pp. 16-20), primarily responsible for the origination of behavior therapy, states that there are three major principles involved: *counterconditioning, reinforcement* and *extinction.* Counterconditioning is used most often in the treatment of neuroses. A neurosis is produced when a high-anxiety response to environmental stimuli is strongly reinforced (conditioned). The goal of the counterconditioning is to replace the high-anxiety response with a response which will inhibit anxiety. Laboratory experimentation with counterconditioning led to the principle of "reciprocal inhibition": "If a response-inhibiting anxiety can be made to occur in the presence of anxiety-evoking stimuli, it will weaken the bond between these stimuli and the anxiety" (Wolpe, 1973, p. 17). One application of this principle is the use of relaxation techniques along with anxiety-producing stimuli. For example, if relaxation procedures can be paired with a testing situation, the person with high test anxiety may be able to overcome this problem.

Reinforcement is useful in the conditioning of effective behavior. As effective behavior is conditioned through reinforcement, the ineffective behavior may be eliminated. Successful conditioning usually involves the use of rewards or positive consequences for the individual. An example of this approach is its use in the treatment of enuresis nocturna.

> By arranging for the patient to be awakened by an alarm as soon as the first drop of urine is excreted during sleep, the waking reaction is conditioned to the imminence of urination, and this subsequently leads to the development of an inhibition of the tendency to urinate in response to bladder stimulation during sleep (Wolpe, 1973, p. 19).

This approach has been successfully used in psychiatric hospitals where desirable behavior has been reinforced through such rewards as increased freedom of mobility, desired responsibilities and coupons for desired commodities.

The principle of extinction refers to the weakening of a response through withholding reinforcement. If the response occurs again and again without reinforcement, it is likely gradually to cease or become extinct. Skinner's experiment of feeding the pigeon after it had pecked on the key provides an example. If the food was repeatedly withheld after the pecking behavior occurred, the pecking would eventually stop.

The role of the therapist using behavior therapy becomes evident through these behavioral principles. The therapist, not the client, is in control of the situation. Wolpe (1973, p. 9) describes this control:

> The most enviable feature of behavior therapy is in the command it gives to the therapist, both in general planning of his therapeutic campaign and in modifying its details as he goes along. When a particular maneuver fails to accomplish change, another will be tried that, like its predecessor, is logically deductible from an experimentally established principle—sometimes the same principle, sometimes another....
>
> The power to intervene rationally and predictably makes a striking contrast to the uncertainty of the conventional therapist's position. Since the latter directs his procedures at an "inner process" which he regards as responsible for the unadaptive behavior, instead of working on the behavior itself, he can only stand aside passively and hope for favorable effects to follow his efforts.

Behaviorism implies that behavior is predictable. The behavior therapist, therefore, sees the change of behavior as a controlled, objective process. The client need only realize that his behavior is ineffective and seek assistance in making it effective or adaptive.

Evaluation of the effectiveness of behavior therapy is, likewise, straightforward and objective. Success of therapy can be evaluated by simply listing the individual's maladaptive behaviors (habits) prior to therapy and assessing the status of each of these behaviors when therapy ends. Assessment might include observation, client interpretation and/or psychophysiological studies.

Implications for Psychiatric Nursing Practice

The behaviorists make limited assumptions about man's behavior. Simply, their beliefs are described by such major theoretical terms as stimulus, response, reinforcement and conditioning. Behavior represents a response to stimuli in one of these two ways: (1) a reflex response is elicited by a specific stimulus or (2) operant behavior (response) is emitted as a result of more generalized environmental stimuli. Whether or not this behavior becomes a pattern (habit) for the individual depends upon the reinforcement (consequences) he experiences.

Conditioning provides the explanation of personality development. The unconsciousness and the thoughts of an individual are not of concern, because these are not observable. If they are important, their influence will be evidenced through one's behavior. To assess why one behaves as he does, his reinforcement history must be evaluated.

The ability of one individual (the therapist) to control the behavior of another (the client) through conditioning techniques has been the subject of much debate. The question frequently occurs as to whether this approach allows for individual freedom of choice. This question received added debate following the publication of Skinner's (1971) *Beyond Freedom and Dignity* in which he proposes a "behavioral technology" which could alleviate many of the humanly created world problems.

The behavioristic theories do hold implications for psychiatric nursing practice. The technique of conditioning easily lends itself to use in certain therapeutic situations. The behavioral approach to nursing practice is evidenced in the following ways:

1. Assessment and planning is based on the client's presenting maladaptive behavior(s) and the reinforcement history of this behavior.

2. A written documentation of the maladaptive behavior to be treated is made.
3. A decision is made by the nurse therapist* concerning the type of treatment to be used: counterconditioning, reinforcement or extinction.
4. A specific technique for treatment, based on one of the three approaches above, is formulated.
5. Techniques are used, reused and changed as the nurse therapist deems appropriate.
6. Therapy is discontinued when the nurse therapist determines that adaptive behavior has replaced the maladaptive behavior.
7. Evaluation is performed by the nurse therapist and/or requested colleagues through observation, client self-reporting and/or psychophysiological techniques, using the initial written documentation of maladaptive behavior as a guide.

HUMANISTIC THEORY

Although a number of theorists are classified as "humanists," the representative work of Carl Rogers and Abraham Maslow is presented. The following statement describes the humanistic intent:

> The term humanism identifies a wide variety of persons and groups ... persons in the humanist endeavor so describe themselves only to indicate that the focus of their work is the whole person as an integrative and interactive human organism, the qualities that make people distinctly human, and the process by which they develop those qualities (Combs, Richards, and Richards, 1976, p. 6).

Rogers' Self-Theory

A person immediately associated with humanistic psychology is Carl Rogers. In his work as a psychotherapist, Rogers developed a person-centered approach called client-centered therapy. In discussing the character of this therapy, Rogers (1942, p. 28) states:

> The individual and not the problem is the focus. The aim is not to solve one particular problem, but to assist the individual to *grow*, so that he can cope with the present problem and with later problems in a better integrated fashion.

Nurse therapist refers to the nurse primarily responsible for direction of the client's treatment. Other nurses providing treatment consistently follow the set approach.

Client-centered therapy "is based on the premise that the human being is basically a trustworthy organism" (Rogers, 1977, p. 15). This premise is in opposition to Freud's less optimistic view of man as predatory and destructive. Since the person is trustworthy, the person-centered approach places the responsibility for decision-making and the consequences and evaluation of these decisions upon the client. Power, then, is in the hands of the client, not the therapist. This represents a break in the traditional therapist role.

Feelings and honest interactions are essentials of the humanistic approach. Rogers stresses the interrelatedness of three therapist attitudes necessary to establish sincere and caring relationships: (1) empathy, (2) positive regard and (3) genuineness (Meador and Rogers, 1973, pp. 137-139).

Rogers' emphasis is upon growth of the individual; thus he sees growth as entirely possible. The growth theme permeates his theory of personality known as self-theory and developed primarily as a result of his work as a client-centered therapist. Rogers' formulations have continued to develop and change as he has gained more data about personality, through therapeutic observations.

Rogers' development of a theory of personality is based on a broad foundation with a focus on the growth-oriented individual rather than on the maladjusted individual. The desired goal of therapy is that of becoming a fully functioning person. Rogers describes three additional characteristics of trends of the person growing toward optimum function:

1. An increasing openness to experience...
2. A process toward becoming...
3. An increasing trust in his organism (Rogers, 1962, pp. 23-29).

The person in the process of becoming more open to experiences is, then, becoming less defensive in his responses. Realistic awareness is increased. In other words, "self and personality emerge *from* experience, rather than experience being translated or twisted to fit a preconceived self-structure" (Rogers, 1962, p. 26). The growth-oriented person becomes increasingly able to trust his reaction to a situation and to utilize this reaction as a basis for his related behavior. This degree of trust seems closely bound to one's ability to be open to his experience as well as to the awareness of his own individuality at any point in time.

Maslow's Theory of Self-Actualization

Whereas Rogers refers to the fully functioning person as the end product in the process of becoming, A. H. Maslow cites the self-actualized individual (Being) as the desired outcome. There are many similarities in the growth-oriented process and in becoming and its goals as described by both Rogers and Maslow. Basically, Maslow's theory is a motivational one, based on the concepts of "growth-needs" and "basic needs." A need is "basic" if:

1. its absence breeds illness
2. its presence prevents illness
3. its restoration cures illness
4. under certain (very complex) free choice situations, it is preferred by the deprived person over other satisfactions
5. it is found to be active, at a low ebb, or functionally absent in the healthy person (Maslow, 1968, p. 22).

An individual's basic needs must be met if he is to be involved with "growth needs."

In formulating his theory, Maslow studied persons whom he felt to be self-actualized individuals. These persons were primarily older adults. The fact that so-called self-actualized or "healthy" individuals rather than "sick" individuals were studied makes this theory one of a positive nature. He studied individuals whose achievements provide guidelines for facilitating the growth-oriented process.

Maslow (1968, p. 26) describes the clinically observed characteristics of healthy people as follows:

1. Superior perception of reality
2. Increased acceptance of self, of others, and of nature
3. Increased spontaneity
4. Increase in problem-centering
5. Increased detachment and desire for privacy
6. Increased autonomy and resistance to enculturation
7. Greater freshness of application and richness of emotional reaction
8. Higher frequency of peak experiences
9. Increased identification with the human species
10. Changed (the clinician would say, improved) interpersonal relations

11. More democratic character structures
12. Greatly increased creativeness
13. Certain changes in the value system

Maslow has identified a hierarchy of needs through which the person advances in the growth process: (1) physiological, (2) safety, (3) love and belongingness, (4) self-esteem and (5) self-actualization. Generally, an individual in the process of growth is advancing up the needs hierarchy. Certainly, though, depending upon the person's life situation at any point in time, his position in relation to the hierarchy may fluctuate.

Growth toward self-actualization is not a short-term process, it may involve most of a lifetime. The growth-motivated individual finds satisfaction in working toward a higher-level goal. The attainment of a goal usually is motivation for setting additional goals, because, as Maslow (1968, p. 30) states, "Growth is, *in itself*, a rewarding and exciting process...."

The physiological needs represent the beginning of motivation theory. The list of physiological needs is potentially vast; the classic ones are hunger, sex and thirst. These needs are generally easy to pinpoint and occur independently rather than in combination. Other needs are nonexistent until the physiological needs are met. Satisfying the present need is all-consuming; for example, the man who is hungry defines almost every life occurrence in the context of food.

When the physiological needs have been met, safety needs emerge. Generally, adults do not experience too many problems in this area. The adult's prior experiences determine what he perceives as safety; this could include religion, a savings account, insurance and/or a good job. Occurrences such as war, natural disasters or a persistent high-stress situation may cause one to focus on safety.

The love and belongingness needs emerge when the physiological and safety needs are pretty well met. Love is not synonymous with sex; rather, sexual behavior is one aspect of love. The person becomes extremely concerned with loving relationships—wife, children, sweethearts, friends. In addition, he may strive in his work for the feeling that he is indispensable. The thwarting of this need, more than any other, may be related to severe cases of maladjustment and psychopathology. Maslow stresses its importance to one's behavior:

> The fact is that people are good, if only their fundamental wishes are

satisfied, their wish for affection and security. Give people affection and security, and they will give affection and be secure in their feelings and behavior (International Study Project, Inc., 1972, p. 95).

The esteem needs include the need for self-esteem from others. A good self-concept based on realistic perceptions is important to adequate functioning. Also important is the recognition and appreciation of others.

The need for self-actualization is interpreted as the need to be what one is. What one can be, he must be. Maslow describes self-actualizers as "psychologically healthy, fully human, highly evolved, fully mature persons" (International Study Project, Inc., 1972, p. 52). The emergence of this need is dependent upon the satisfaction of the prior needs. The self-actualized person is the exception, not the rule.

Maslow refers to the occurrence of peak experience in describing the healthy person. A frequently occurring question is, "What is meant by peak experiences?" As the person grows closer to becoming self-actualized, he is aware of more frequent peak experiences. In order to be aware of these, one must be open to his experiences. Probably most persons have peak experiences, but some deny or repress them. There may also be a difference in the degree to which these experiences are felt. "High peakers" are described by Maslow (International Study Project, Inc., 1972, pp. 96-98) as follows:

> ...witnesses of the highest that there is in life, both inner life and witnessing of external reality.... for these people there is simply no question about the validation of living and its worthwhileness and its richness and its beauty.... Such people can be unshakable in their will to life and in their trust that life is beautiful and worthwhile.... are sure, decisive, certain, unshakable.... know their path... resist all efforts to take them away from it....

The peak experience, thus, may involve any variety of situations. A very generalized and simplified explanation is that peak experiences occur when one is functioning at the very optimum of his senses (total awareness—unconscious and conscious) and abilities. There is heightened perception, and this may lead to such results as (1) a creative or aesthetic effort or production by the individual, i.e., a poem, musical composition, work of visual art, solution of a problem and (2) increased self-identity. These peak experiences cannot be planned; rather, they just happen.

Implications for Psychiatric Nursing Practice

The humanistic theories are optimistic in nature, holding that individuals are not bound by their past. While each is influenced by his past, he can change and grow. Maslow states this belief eloquently:

> Everybody born is capable, in principle, of self-actualization. You should never give up on anyone, ever. Man has an instinctoid higher nature. It's possible to grow this or to stunt it. Society can do neither (International Study Project, Inc., 1972, p. 113).

The nurse whose practice is influenced by the humanistic theories holds to this optimistic view of man's nature and capabilities. The nurse, in order to make the best therapeutic use of herself, needs to be growth-motivated, open to her own experiences and trusting of herself. The humanistic approach to nursing practice is evidenced in the following ways:

1. Client planning is based on "where" the client is in the process of his developmental growth. A guide for client assessment is Maslow's hierarchy of needs:

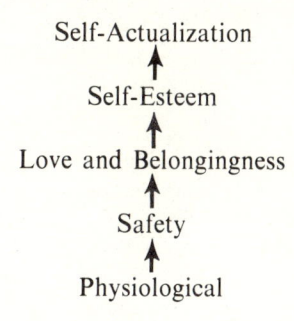

$$\text{Self-Actualization} \uparrow \text{Self-Esteem} \uparrow \text{Love and Belongingness} \uparrow \text{Safety} \uparrow \text{Physiological}$$

2. Nurses must be aware of clients' behavior which indicates an inadequate perception of self, e.g., presence of "basic needs" rather than "growth needs."
3. Setting health-related goals is shared by the client and the nurse.
4. Desired and appropriate activities for reaching defined goals are jointly identified by client and nurse.
5. Ideas for a plan of implementation of care are openly and creatively explored, with an emphasis on problem-solving by the client.

6. Motivation of both the client and nurse is as inner-directed as possible; though, in some instances, the nurse may need to provide motivational forces for the client.
7. The nurse's criticism of a client's behaviors or achievements is constructive, focused on increasing client understanding.
8. The nurse communicates a feeling of honest trust in the integrity and the abilities of the client.
9. Evaluation of the therapeutic plan is carried out jointly by the client and nurse.
10. The nurse is a facilitator of treatment, providing the assistance the client needs to help himself.

EXISTENTIALISTIC THEORY

Although existentialism falls primarily in the philosophical grouping of personality theories, a brief description is included here, because of its therapeutic implications and the applications which have been made to psychotherapy by Rollo May. The existential theories show some similarity to the humanistic, though the focus on the individual is less optimistic. Their similarity is seen in the emphasis upon the individuality of the person. In comparing the self-actualized person to the existential theory, Maslow (1968, p. 174) states:

> Even our most fully human beings are not exempted from the basic human predicament, of being simultaneously merely-creaturely and godlike, strong and weak, limited and unlimited, merely-animal and animal-transcending, adult and child, fearful and courageous, progressing and regressing, yearning for perfection and yet afraid of it, being a worm and also a hero. This is what the existentialists keep trying to tell us.

Maslow does not disagree with this idea; instead, he agrees that opportunities are hierarchically integrated. To move towards the integration of opposites is the goal of therapy.

The philosophy of existentialism needs some interpretation. Since its proponents have been primarily Europeans, its application has not been as great within American society. Existentialistic thought involves a search for Being; thus, there exists a basic difference with the humanists. The humanists are concerned with the process of Becoming, or growth toward the definable and attainable end of Being, while the existentialists are searching for the existence of Being. There is general agreement among existentialists in their belief that "the search for Being is . . . a search for the direction of Being in thought and in action" (Kimmel, 1962, p. 12). Existence is a given, but Being determines one's movement toward self-fulfillment. Morris (1966, p. 135) describes this with three propositions:

1. I am a *choosing* agent, unable to avoid choosing my way through life.
2. I am a *free* agent, absolutely free to set the goals of my own life.
3. I am a *responsible* agent, personally accountable for my free choices as they are revealed in how I live my life.

Rollo May, like Rogers and Maslow, largely developed his theory of personality through data collected from persons in therapy. Unlike the humanists, May focused not only on the person's individual problems or characteristics but also on "the universal characteristics of man." His therapy includes treatment aimed toward the givens within the situation. A descriptive example is that of a neurotic individual:

> First, certain traumatic or unfortunate experiences have occurred in his life which make him more sensitive than the average person and less able to live with and manage his anxiety. Second, he may possess a greater than ordinary amount of originality and potential which pushes for expression and, when blocked off, make him ill (May, 1969, pp. 20-21).

May (1969, p. 289) describes his concept of care, also based on an existentialistic view of man:

> It is a state composed of the recognition of another, a fellow human being like one's self; of identification of one's self with the pain or joy of the other; of guilt, pity, and the awareness that we all stand on the base of common humanity from which we all stem.

This concept of care certainly implies an empathetic approach to the therapeutic relationship. In fact, May (1969, p. 120) states that "personal counseling is any deep understanding between persons which results in the changing of personality."

Implications for Psychiatric Nursing Practice

1. Establishment of rapport is basic to any communication

between client and nurse. It is essential that there be a feeling of "working together."
2. The client sets his own goals. The nurse identifies with the client as much as possible, in order to assist him in perceiving realistic alternatives.
3. The client selects what he sees as the appropriate plan of care. The nurse provides guidance but does not make the decision for him.
4. The nurse allows the client, at some point during treatment, to accept responsibility for himself.
5. There is periodic evaluation, allowing the client and nurse to determine objectively the progress being made toward identified goals. In this case, the nurse may serve as a consultant to the client.
6. Any revision of goals or change in plan of care is the client's decision. Again, the nurse may be a consultant.

BIBLIOGRAPHY

Allport, G.W. *Personality: A Psychological Interpretation.* New York: Henry Holt & Co., 1947.
Bischof, Ledford. *Interpreting Personality Theories.* 2d ed. New York: Harper & Row Publishers, 1970.
Coleman, James C. *Abnormal Psychology and Modern Life.* Glenview, Ill.: Scott Foresman & Co., 1964.
Combs, A.W., Richards, A.C., and Richards, F. *Perceptual Psychology: A Humanistic Approach to the Study of Persons.* New York: Harper & Row Publishers, 1976.
Corsini, Raymond J. *Readings in Current Personality Theories.* Itasca, Ill.: F.E. Peacock Publishers, Inc., 1977.
Craig, Grace J. *Human Development.* Englewood Cliffs, N.J.: Prentice-Hall, Inc., 1976.
Goldstein, Alan. "Behavior Therapy," in *Current Psychotherapies.* Edited by R. Corsini. Itasca, Ill.: F.E. Peacock Publishers, Inc., 1977, p. 207-249.
Hall, Calvin S. *A Primer of Freudian Psychology.* New York: The New American Library, 1954.
Hall, Calvin S., and Lindzey, Gardner. *Theories of Personality.* New York: John Wiley & Sons, Inc., 1957.
Hilgard, E.R., and Bower, G.H. *Theories of Learning.* New York: Appleton-Century-Crofts, 1966.

Holland, J. G., and Skinner, B. F. *The Analysis of Behavior.* New York: McGraw-Hill Book Co., Inc., 1961.

International Study Project, Inc. *Abraham H. Maslow: A Memorial Volume.* Monterey, Cal.: Brooks/Cole Publishing Co., 1972.

Kimmel, William. "Introductions," in *The Search for Being: Essays from Kierkegaard to Sartre On the Problem of Existence.* Edited by J. T. Wilde and W. Kimmel. New York: Twayne Publishers, Inc., 1962, pp. 9-26.

Lidz, Theodore. *The Person: His Development Throughout The Life Cycle.* New York: Basic Books, Inc., 1968.

Maslow, A.H. *Toward A Psychology Of Being.* 2d ed. New York: Van Nostrand Reinhold Co., 1968.

May, Rollo. *Love and Will.* New York: W. W. Norton & Co., Inc., 1969.

Meador, Betty O., and Rogers, C. R. "Client-Centered Therapy," in *Current Psychotherapies.* Edited by R. Corsini. Itasca, Ill.: F. E. Peacock, Publishers, Inc., 1973, pp. 119-165.

Mereness, Dorothy. *Essentials of Psychiatric Nursing.* St. Louis: The C. V. Mosby Co., 1970.

Morris, V. C. *Existentialism in Education.* New York: Harper & Row Publishers, 1966.

Payne, Dorris, and Clunn, Patricia (eds). *Psychiatric-Mental Health Nursing.* Garden City, N.Y.: Medical Examination Publishing Co., Inc., 1977.

Peplau, Hildegarde E. *Interpersonal Relations in Nursing.* New York: G.P. Putnam's Sons, 1952.

Piaget, J. *The Theory of Stages in Cognitive Development.* New York: McGraw-Hill Book Co., 1969.

Rogers, Carl R. *Counseling and Psychotherapy: Newer Concepts in Practice.* Boston: Houghton Mifflin Co., 1942.

———. *On Personal Power.* New York: Delacorte Press, 1977.

———. "Toward Becoming a Fully Functioning Person," in *Perceiving, Behaving, Becoming.* By the Association for Supervision and Curriculum Development. Washington D.C.: National Education Association, 1962, pp. 21-33.

Rowe, Clarence J. *An Outline of Psychiatry.* Dubuque, Iowa: William C. Brown & Co., 1965.

Skinner, B. F. *About Behaviorism.* New York: Alfred A. Knopf, 1974.

———. *Beyond Freedom and Dignity.* New York: Bantam Books, Inc., 1971.

———. *Science and Human Behavior.* New York: The Macmillan Co., 1953.

Stagner, Ross. *Psychology of Personality.* New York: McGraw-Hill Book Co., 1961.

Watson, J. B. *Behaviorism.* New York: W. W. Norton & Co., Inc., 1930.

Wolpe, Joseph. *The Practice of Behavior Therapy.* 2d ed. Elmsford, N.Y.: Pergamon Press, Inc., 1973.

CHAPTER 3

Personality Development: Stages of Growth

Gail Davis, R.N., Ed.D. and Allene Jones, R.N., M.N.

INTRODUCTION

The dynamics of personality development become increasingly complex throughout the life span. This premise is supported by those personality theories previously discussed, even though the theorists may not entirely agree on the mechanics of what actually happens; for example, (1) E. Erikson's psychosocial theory presents the eight stages of man, illustrating primary tasks to be accomplished at each stage; (2) the behaviorists believe that personality and behavior continue to change based on previous conditioning and the present environment; and (3) the humanists support the belief that the individual is basically growth-oriented, unless there are deficiency needs which have not been met.

On the basis of the different theories, an eclectic Model of Positive Personality Development is demonstrated in Figure 3-1. This Model assumes that (1) the individual is an open system constantly affected by genetic and environmental influences, (2) the individual's accomplishments—learning and adaptation—at each stage of life are basic to further development, (3) the mental health status is primarily positive as growth occurs, and (4) each individual grows and develops at his own rate, so that tasks cannot be solely related to chronological age.

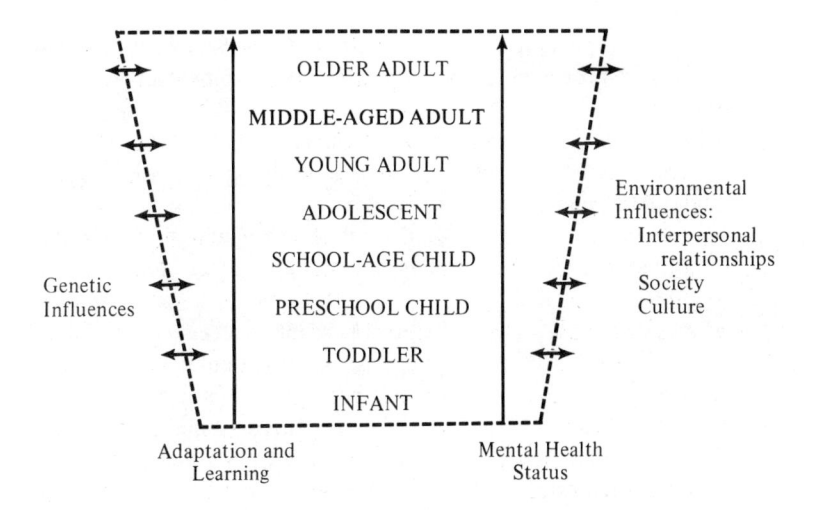

```
                    OLDER ADULT
                  MIDDLE-AGED ADULT
                   YOUNG ADULT
                                              Environmental
                    ADOLESCENT                Influences:
                                                Interpersonal
                  SCHOOL-AGE CHILD               relationships
Genetic                                         Society
Influences       PRESCHOOL CHILD                Culture

                    TODDLER

                     INFANT

      Adaptation and              Mental Health
        Learning                    Status
```

Figure 3-1: Model of Positive Personality Development.

Assumptions:

1. The individual is an open system constantly affected by genetic and environmental influences.
2. The individual's accomplishments—learning and adaptation—at each stage of life are basic to further development.
3. The mental health status is primarily positive as growth occurs.
4. Each individual grows and develops at his own rate, so that tasks cannot be solely related to chronological age.

The positive growth of personality assumes positive mental health status. While there are many different definitions of mental health, the concepts provided by M. Jahoda (1958) in a report to the Joint Commission on Mental Health and Illness are helpful as a basis for assessment. The six concepts provided, along with some of their specific emphases, are listed below:

1. *Attitudes of an individual toward his own self.* Some aspects of the self-concept are (1) accessibility to consciousness, (2) correctness or ability to view self realistically and (3) acceptance of self as realistically viewed.
2. *Growth, development or self-actualization.* One is motivated toward self-actualization with a high degree of investment in liv-

ing. The important areas identified are (1) self-concept, (2) motivational processes and (3) optimum development or achievement.
3. *Integration.* Emphasis is placed on (1) a balance of psychic forces within the individual, (2) a unifying outlook on life and/or (3) resistance to stress.
4. *Autonomy.* In an individual's relationship with his environment, two areas are emphasized—independence and internal regulation of behavior.
5. *Perception of reality.* A healthy perception occurs when what the individual sees corresponds to what is actually there. Two aspects emphasized are (1) that perception is not distorted by one's needs and (2) that there is empathy or social sensitivity.
6. *Environmental mastery.* Mastering one's environment is considered successful if the individual exhibits (1) the ability to love, (2) adequacy in love, work and play, (3) adequacy in interpersonal relations, (4) efficiency in meeting situational requirements, (5) capacity for adaptation and adjustment and (6) efficiency in problem-solving (Jahoda, 1958, pp. 23-64).

These mental health concepts are most applicable to assessment of the adult. They are comprehensive and include the major thoughts of a number of individual personality theorists. For example, the "growth toward self-actualization" concept of the humanists is included along with the "adequacy in love, work and play" stressed by the psychoanalysts.

Certainly any division of the life span into life stages is artificial to some degree. For the purpose of studying some of the important tasks of personality development throughout the life span, the divisional breakdown is helpful in providing a classification system. Table 3-1 presents one type of developmental scheme by comparing the psychosocial, psychosexual and cognitive developmental stages. These three theories deal with divisions by generally specified ages which are identified on the chart. The psychosexual and cognitive theories deal primarily with development through adolescence, while the psychosocial extends through maturity. The cognitive development as presented by Piaget is crucial in personality development, in that it is essential to understand how the individual is perceiving the world around him.

Collective information from all of the personality theories pre-

TABLE 3-1

Comparison of Psychosexual, Psychosocial and
Cognitive Developmental Stages

Age	Cognitive (Piaget)	Psychosocial (Erikson)	Psychosexual (Freud)
0–1 mo	Sensory – Motor Period: I	Trust vs. Mistrust	Oral Stage
2–3 mo	II		
4–6 mo	III		
8–10 mo	IV		
12 mo	V		
18 mo	VI		
2 yr	Pre-Operative Period	Autonomy vs. Shame, Doubt	Anal Stage
4 yr		Initiative vs. Guilt	Phallic Stage
6–8 yr	Concrete Operational Period	Industry vs. Inferiority	Latency Stage
10–12 yr			
Adolescence	Formal Operational Period	Identity vs. Role Confusion	Genital Stage
20–30 (Young Adulthood)		Intimacy vs. Isolation	
40–50 (Adulthood)		Generativity vs. Stagnation	
60–70 (Maturity)		Ego Integrity vs. Despair	

sented in Chapter 2 has been summarized to determine the major developmental tasks throughout the life span (Table 3-2). Each task present has been associated with the life stage at which it *most often* occurs. The eight stages into which the life span is arbitrarily divided are: (1) infant, (2) toddler, (3) pre-school child, (4) school-age child, (5) adolescent, (6) young adult, (7) middle-aged adult and (8) older adult.

While the psychosocial, psychosexual and cognitive theories are based on division of the life span into specific stages, the behavioristic, humanistic and existentialistic theories are not. Each theory, though, contributes to the generalized presentation of personality development in its unique way, as reflected in the task summary.

INFANT

Infancy approximates the first year to eighteen months of life and is equivalent to the oral period as presented by Freud. It is during this stage that the basis for future physiological and emotional growth is formed. To many, the infant appears totally nondiscriminating and defenseless. This is far from the truth, for at birth the infant can hear, smile, see, touch and alter his position. Infancy is not a time for rigid and mechanical handling of the baby, for at this time he possesses great capacity for adapting as a human being.

If basic needs such as love, security, safety, and protection are not met during infancy, certain behavior patterns may be apparent in later life. The infant equates these needs with food, since the taking of food, for him, is synonymous with love, security, safety and protection. In later childhood and adulthood, therefore, one's tension may be relieved through oral gratification such as eating, chewing gum, smoking and drinking.

If the infant is severely deprived of satisfying these basic needs, he may be overwhelmed with attempting to relieve the associated tension and anxiety. This attempt may leave him incapacitated, thus affecting further psychological development. On the other hand, if the basic needs are unconditionally met by caring parents, he tends to grow up to be an optimistic person (Mereness, 1970, p. 12).

A discussion or summary of developmental tasks to be accomplished by the infant is important. The overall task of infancy is to learn to depend on others to satisfy basic needs and wishes with a feeling of trust rather than of mistrust and helplessness. In addi-

TABLE 3-2

Portrait of an Individual's Personality Development Throughout the Life Span

INFANT
(0-12 months)

Development of trust is basic to all later interactions in life.

Oral activity is important as exhibited through sucking and putting objects in the mouth.

Learning occurs as a result of experiences to which an infant is exposed.

Play—exploration and use of own body, touching and feeling objects, enjoying sounds he can make—are important to later development.

TODDLER
(1-3 years)

Development of autonomy is the all-important task and is evident through:
1. learning the expected social norms, i.e., right vs. wrong
2. elimination control
3. talking and expressing himself verbally.

PRESCHOOL CHILD
(3-6 years)

A basic task is the development of initiative which comes from successful encounter with others and his environment.

Identification with the parent of the same sex is important to later development of sex roles.

Development of the conscience becomes more obvious to the child himself and to observers.

The child exhibits increased use of imagination.

SCHOOL-AGE CHILD
(6-12 years)

The development of a sense of industry is exhibited by (1) an ability to get along with members of his peer group, (2) learning to follow rules and regulations, (3) finding success in school as well as in other activities and (4) accepting increasing responsibility.

The interest in learning about his world becomes more intense.

ADOLESCENT
(13-20 years)

Development of individual identity—self-concept, body image, sexual identity, vocational selection and independence from parents—is extremely important to ongoing development.

Adjustment is made to the development of the external sexual organs and secondary sexual characteristics.

Involvement as a member of a peer group aids his individual development.

More sophisticated signs of growth (as meeting the self-esteem needs) toward self-actualization are exhibited.

(Continued)

TABLE 3-2 (Continued)

YOUNG ADULT
(20-35 years)

The development of intimacy is achieved through work and love.

The meaning of love (sexual vs. nonsexual) is learned, and he is able to differentiate between the two.

There is selection of a mate who fulfills sexual and emotional needs.

Work, career and family commitments are successfully combined.

Parenting abilities are developed.

Successful adjustment to acquired family members (children, in-laws, etc.) is made.

MIDDLE-AGED ADULT
(35-65 years)

Development of generativity as evidenced through (1) increased ability to care for and about others and (2) feeling of satisfaction concerning career.

The physiological changes occurring in his own life are accepted.

There is realistic acceptance of his own strengths and weaknesses, and these are put into proper balance.

There is preparation for and acceptance of approaching retirement and/or change in life style.

OLDER ADULT
(Over 65 years)

Integrity of the ego is evidenced by the ability to review his past life realistically and to accept those mistakes and failures made without despair.

There is increasing evidence of growth toward self-actualization.

Successful adaptation to retirement is made with a continuing interest in life.

Adaptation is made to subtle and/or pronounced bodily changes.

He serves as a source of wisdom for younger individuals.

There is increased acceptance of and preparation for death—his own, his spouse's, his friends'.

He successfully learns to live on a reduced income, if necessary, and he adapts to associated changes in life style.

---

tion, there are some specific tasks that the infant should accomplish during this stage of growth and development:
1. Adjustment to extrauterine life during the neonatal period
2. Adjustment to and development of new motor skills
3. Development of beginning verbal skills
4. Recognition of animate and inanimate objects in his environment
5. Beginning ability to see himself as separate from others
6. Development of a desire for love and affection from others

Physical Development

The infant is termed a neonate during the first month of his life. The neonatal period includes the critical transition from the parasitic fetal existence to independent physiological existence (Murray and Zentner, 1975, p. 26). The infant must adjust to living on his own. Not only is the neonatal period an adjustment from the birth process, it also includes the adjustment of vital functions such as respiration, circulation, digestion, temperature regulation and elimination to existence in a new environment (Craig, 1976, p. 141). During the neonatal period the infant spends most of his time sleeping, since one of the major physiological needs is sleep. Other major physiological needs include temperature regulation and milk (Lidz, 1968, p. 96).

Infancy is a time for rapid growth. At birth, the average full-term infant weighs between 5½ and 9½ pounds, with an average of 7½ pounds. The length of the infant ranges from 19 to 21 inches, with the average being 21 inches. Girls are slightly shorter than boys. At the end of the first year, the infant has tripled his birth weight and increased his height by 50 percent. Obviously, the growth of the individual is greater during infancy than at any other stage of life.

Since physical growth is rapid during infancy, some basic principles regarding motor development should be mentioned:

1. Motor responses are undifferentiated and diffuse at birth and become more specific and controlled later, depending on neurological development. The child first moves his whole body; later he reacts with a specific body part.
2. Muscular development is *cephalocaudal, proceeding from head to feet*. Hence, the baby can hold his head and neck erect before he can sit or walk.
3. Muscular control is developed from the proximal axis to the distal extremities; development begins from the central axis of the body and progresses toward the periphery or extremities.
4. In addition, development proceeds from the simple to the complex or from general to specific movements. For example, the child waves his arms long before he is able to control his finger muscles (Murray and Zentner, 1975, pp. 25-26).

These principles concerning motor development are descriptive of the term "developmental sequence" which means that "changes are specific, progressive, and orderly, and eventually lead to maturity" (Murray and Zentner, 1975, p. 25). In addition to physical growth, the infant is growing mentally, emotionally and socially.

Oral Needs

Infancy is often referred to as the oral stage, because the infant's activity is centered around his mouth and its functions. The infant receives pleasure as well as nutrition from sucking if he is talked to, cuddled and smiled at during the feeding.

The infant's skin is quite sensitive to touch, and he receives pleasure from being held close to the parenting one and cuddled. With loving care, the infant feels loved and trusts his environment; he feels safe to explore that environment. A frightened infant tends to refrain from exploring with his hands and mouth; thus, his ability to develop physically and emotionally is decreased.

During infancy, the infant operates on the pleasure principle. He seeks pleasure and avoids pain. His behavior is under the control of the id. As a result of id control, too much should not be expected of the infant. If he is punished for infantile behavior, he learns to mistrust his environment.

The infant should not be subjected to long periods of frustrations such as extended waiting for his feeding. As the ego develops, the infant can tolerate longer periods of frustrations. If the infant is subjected to too much frustration, he may become withdrawn, reluctant to cry and fail to thrive. The reason for these behaviors is that the infant has given up trying to receive nurturing from his environment.

Parenting and Its Importance to the Infant's Development

The parents of infants experience frustrating as well as happy times. Parents must remember that each infant is an individual with his own temperament. Some babies are easy to cuddle, while others are less receptive. Parents must not blame themselves for the infant's "slow to warm up" style. Mothers, especially, should not feel that they have to give all their time to their infants. The time spent with the infant should be relaxed and unhurried. It is not the quantity of care that counts but the quality of care (Lidz, 1968, pp. 93-

155; English and Pearson, 1963, pp. 11-50; Robinson, 1972, pp. 60-62; Kalkman, 1967, pp. 25-31).

TODDLER

Early childhood, or the toddler stage, occurs between 1 or 1½ and 3 years of age, and it is often referred to as the anal, toilet-training or habit-training period. The child's behavior changes considerably during this time.

The period of early childhood is extremely important for several reasons. The toddler usually has quite an impact upon his family. Parents may be threatened by the growing independence of the toddler. Parents learn to cope with the child's frequent stating of "no" and his temper tantrums, as they set reasonable limits on his behavior.

Toilet training is one of the most important tasks of this stage as it initiates self-control. The goal is to help the child learn bladder and bowel control without damaging his personality.

The superego begins to develop during this stage. The child starts to internalize what the parents consider good and bad. The goal is for the child not to leave this stage with an under- or overdeveloped superego.

The basics for self-concept and body image are formed during this period. The child needs to leave this stage liking himself (good me) rather than hating himself (bad me). With love, limits and consistency the toddler leaves this stage with a feeling of autonomy and is ready to accomplish tasks of the preschool stage (Mereness, 1970, pp. 13-14).

Like the infant, the toddler has developmental tasks to be accomplished during this stage of growth and development. The major developmental tasks to be accomplished include:
1. adjusting to the use of newly acquired verbal and motor skills
2. becoming an individual member of his family
3. establishing healthy daily routines including toilet training, good eating habits and others specified as important within his particular environment.

When the child enters the second year of life, his growth rate slows down, and he begins to assume a more adultlike appearance. He continues to be clumsy in movements, because his fine motor control has not developed. He is quite active and seldom seems to tire. The skills of walking, running and climbing are thoroughly enjoyed.

Play

Play is the toddler's work. It is through play that he learns about his world. It also provides a means for the release of anger, aggression and anxiety. Play is also an important aid to the developing socialization of the child.

His play with other children is still solitary and parallel. He is curious about other children but is unable to play cooperatively. The toddler is narcissistic; and parents should not force the child, especially at the beginning of the toddler stage, to play cooperatively. He still has a poor concept of ownership and, therefore, is unable to share. If forced to play cooperatively, he may repress anger and aggressive feelings in order to maintain parental love and acceptance.

Safety Needs

With increased mobility comes the need for safety. The toddler still has to see, taste and touch objects in his environment in order to learn. Obviously, some objects should be kept out of reach of the toddler. Putting dangerous objects out of the child's reach prevents parents from setting unrealistic expectations for the child and also decreases opportunities for needless punishment. On the other hand, all objects cannot be put away, or the child will not be able to set and learn limits.

Cognitive and Emotional Development

The toddler's cognitive development is still limited. He is mainly concerned with the present and has little understanding of the past or future. He is unable to understand the wholeness of things or the why of a simple explanation.

Some of his learning occurs through imitating his parents; therefore, they must be careful of what they say before the toddler, as he usually considers his parents' behavior acceptable. Since his attention span is short, he may only remember part of an explanation of command; thus, he acts on the part he remembers and his resultant behavior seems strange.

Emotionally, the toddler is quite labile—selfish one minute and loving the next. He is unable to control his curious behavior. He is quite demanding and unable to show consistent concern for the rights of others.

The toddler is quite comical in that he frequently engages in behavior that causes adults to laugh at him. He thinks his behavior is pleasing, so he repeats the performance. The laughing thus provides the reward which reinforces the behavior. It is important that parents are aware of what they are doing, so that inappropriate behavior is not reinforced and appropriate behavior is rewarded.

Separation from Parents

The toddler is able to be separated from his parents or parent substitutes for only short periods of time. If he strays some distance, he needs to return at frequent intervals to experience the security provided by his parents. If the child is necessarily separated from the parents for a prolonged length of time, as may happen during hospitalization, he may experience much anxiety. Due to the need for security, approval and protection from his parents, he abandons some of the negativism which typically occurs at this stage.

Toilet Training

Toilet training occurs during this stage of personality development and can be trying for both the parents and the child. Before attempting toilet training, the parents should make sure that the child is physically and psychologically ready. Readiness usually occurs somewhere between 2½ and 3 years.

If toilet training begins prior to physical and psychological readiness, the child may experience considerable anxiety and frustration when he is unable to meet parental expectations. Parents are encouraged to approach toilet training in a relaxed and matter-of-fact manner. Ridicule and references to "dirtiness" are avoided so as to decrease shameful feelings for the child. Following successful toilet training, children often regress under stressful situations such as the birth of a sibling, illness or separation from parents.

Following harsh or punitive toilet training, the child may either suppress his negative feelings or act them out toward the person responsible for the toilet training. Some residual aspects of toilet training are observed in adulthood. For example, an adult who had experienced harsh toilet-training experiences may be meticulous, stingy and stubborn.

Discipline and guidance are essential for toddlers. Limits must be set for the toddler with his immature ego and beginning superego (Murray and Zentner, 1975, pp. 60-76; Lidz, 1968, pp. 176-178; English and Pearson, 1963, pp. 52-72; Kalkman, 1967, pp. 32, 38; Craig, 1976, pp. 214-292).

Discipline of the Toddler

Disciplining the toddler poses problems for parents, when they equate discipline with punishment and control of behavior. Discipline is *"guidance that helps the child learn to understand and care for himself and get along with others"* (Murray and Zentner, 1975, p. 76).

Listed below are some simple rules to help the parent in disciplining the child:
1. Set limits that are reasonable and consistent
2. State limits in a clear and concise manner and in a calm voice
3. Be patient with the child while he is learning limit-setting
4. Provide a place for the child to play that is safe and free of restrictions
5. Consistently reinforce and reward appropriate behavior
6. Avoid overprotecting the child

PRESCHOOL CHILD

The preschool stage is sometimes referred to as later childhood or as the phallic stage of growth and development. It spans from 3 to 6 years of age. This stage is described as the period of the family triangle. This phase of psychosexual development denotes that the erogenous zones now include the genitalia. For the infant and the toddler, respectively, the foci were upon the mouth and the anal area. During this stage the child resolves the Oedipal situation and thereby learns to identify with the parent of the same sex (Mereness, 1970, pp. 14-15).

The preschooler's physical growth slows down, and his daily activities become increasingly routine. He becomes more socialized and is able to join a group for play, as well as follow rules. He is less id oriented, with obvious superego development noted in his ability to be critical of himself and others, when set standards are not followed. He is also able to separate himself from his parents for longer periods of time.

Listed below is a summary of developmental tasks to be accomplished by the preschooler during this stage of growth and development:
1. Establishing healthy patterns of eating, sleeping and exercising
2. Mastering large and small muscle coordination
3. Improving communication skills
4. Conforming to expectations of family and others
5. Learning to let conscience govern his behavior
6. Resolving Oedipal conflict and learning gender identity
7. Beginning to understand himself and his world
8. Expressing emotions more effectively.

Play

During this stage, play is the child's work. He is now able to play cooperatively with other children and can play for hours without seeming to fatigue. During play the child uses fantasy which serves to dissipate anger, anxiety and aggressive feelings. It also helps him to develop his creativity and imagination. Frequently during play, a child is heard verbally abusing his parents or other significant people. Parents should not reprimand the child for his behavior, as this is a healthy way to deal with negative feelings. He may also express loving and warm feelings. The parents should become concerned if the child spends most of his time during free play expressing anger, aggression and hostility.

The safety of the preschooler is a major concern for the parents. The preschooler's increased freedom, due to increased mobility, muscle development, initiative and the ability to imitate adults, frequently gets him into hazardous situations. Clear-cut rules need to be established by the parents to avoid unnecessary injury to the child.

Cognitive Development

Cognitively, the child is developing rapidly. One must remember, however, that the child is in the period of egocentric thinking. He is not being selfish just for the sake of it, but he only has himself as a reference. He thinks that others see his world as he does. He thinks in a concrete manner and is unable to use and understand abstract thinking. If the child is treated with patience and understanding, his ability to think in an abstract and logical manner during the latter part of latency and adolescence increases.

Sibling Rivalry

Sibling rivalry poses a problem for the child in this stage, especially when he is struggling to resolve the Oedipal situation or conflict. The child feels threatened when parents share their love with a new baby. He may feel unloved and compete for the parents' love. The preschooler frequently openly resents the new member of the family. If parents understand the child's behavior, they can be a source of comfort to him (Craig, 1976, pp. 224-292; English and Pearson, 1963, pp. 94-110; Kalkman, 1967, pp. 39-50; Lidz, 1968, pp. 189-234; Murray and Zentner, 1975, pp. 81-119).

Emotional Development

Emotionally, the preschooler is more stable than the toddler. He is usually a source of pleasure to his parents. He continues to enjoy imitating adults, and his ability to tolerate frustration is somewhat limited.

Developing initiative and avoiding excessive guilt are developmental tasks for the preschooler. Developing an overwhelming sense of guilt affects the child emotionally, because it makes him anxious, rigid and frightened.

Resolution of the Oedipal conflict affects the child emotionally. During this stage, children begin to explore their own bodies. They discover pleasurable sensations when the penis and clitoris are manipulated. If the child is made to feel that he is bad for exploring his body, he tends to experience too much guilt.

Children in this age group become aware of the structural differences of the sexes. The girl feels that she has been deprived of her penis (penis envy), and the boy fears losing his penis (castration fear). The little boy's fear of castration can be intensified if his parents threaten to cut off his penis.

Before children learn to identify with the parent of the same sex, which is the resolution of the Oedipal conflict, they tend to identify with the parent of the opposite sex. For example, the little boy may tell his mother how much he loves her, and that he is going to marry her when he grows up. The little girl behaves in a similar manner toward her father. The child's romantic love for the parent of the opposite sex is known as the family triangle or romance.

Why does the child relinquish his romantic love for the parent of the opposite sex? One reason is that parents discourage this type of behavior, because it is not socially acceptable. The second reason is the child's fear of the parent of the same sex. For example, the little boy fears his father because of his size. He fears his father may use punishment (castration), because of his preference for his mother. Through trial and error the little boy concludes that it is less threatening to be like his father, and that this also means he is more likely to receive his mother's love. The boy then begins to identify with his father and learn the male role.

The little girl begins to learn the feminine sex role in a manner similar to that of the boy. However, the process for learning the feminine role is not as clearly understood as the male-oriented process. Freudian theory proposes that a girl blames her mother for not providing her with a body like the boy. She resents her mother for this and turns to her father for affection. The girl's resentment toward her mother poses a problem, because she still needs the love and affection of her mother; thus, she identifies with her mother. The maternal identification is less threatening, and she can then also please her father.

The child who finds it difficult to emulate the parent of the same sex usually experiences communication problems in adult life. Society expects him to behave in one way, and he behaves in another. Individuals who do not achieve gender identity during this stage suffer sexual role confusion, and the foundation for homosexual activity in adult life may be set.

Providing guidance and discipline for the preschooler is a major task for the parents. The child needs permissive discipline rather than overpermissive discipline. Permissive discipline "accepts the childish behavior as normal and recognizes that the child is a person with a right to have all kinds of feelings and wishes that may be expressed directly or symbolically," whereas overpermissive discipline "permits undesirable behavior that can be destructive." Limits are set in a kind and firm manner. Setting limits on behavior should leave the child with a sense of integrity (Murray and Zentner, 1975, p. 110).

The parents are faced with several other important tasks during this stage of life:
1. Preparing the child for school
2. Providing him with sex education when the need arises
3. Teaching religious and moral principles

SCHOOL-AGE CHILD

The period of the school-age child ranges from 6 to 12 years and is sometimes called the juvenile or latency stage. The latency stage is divided into the juvenile and the preadolescent periods. The juvenile period ranges from 6 to 10 years and the preadolescent period from 9 or 10 to 12 years. The juvenile period is characterized by a need for peer relationships. The preadolescent period is "marked by a new capacity to love, when the satisfaction and security of another person of the same sex is as important to the child as his own satisfaction and security" (Murray and Zentner, 1975, p. 123).

This stage of development is termed latency, because sexual drives are somewhat repressed until puberty. The child is interested in pursuing educational interests and forming relationships with a peer group. He begins the emancipation process from his parents by forming intense relationships with his peer group.

Although the child during this stage continues to work on developmental tasks from the previous stage or stages, he is faced with new developmental tasks which include:
1. learning about his world through formal education
2. learning how to compete, compromise and cooperate
3. becoming more responsible for his behavior
4. beginning emancipation from family.

Physical Development

Physically, the child looks more like an adult than the preschooler. Growth is slow and steady until puberty. Usually, up to about age 12, girls are more advanced in growth than boys.

With the advent of prepuberty, physical changes occur in both sexes. The physical changes that occur in the female are somewhat more obvious than those in the male. The changes are due to hormonal influence.

Play and Socialization

Play for the child during this stage is somewhat different from the play observed in the preschooler. Play usually takes place with the child's peer group, and the peer group usually consists of members of the same sex. Boys tend to cling together, as do girls. This stage is sometimes referred to as the normal homosexual stage, because members of the same sex tend to play together.

The gang becomes more significant during the preadolescent period. A "gang" is a group whose membership is learned on the basis of skilled performance of some activity, frequently physical in nature. Its stability is expressed through formal symbols such as passwords or uniforms. Belonging to a gang allows the child to work out social problems and patterns without adult interference. Achieving a task on his own is a boost to the child's ego.

The chum stage is common around the ages nine or ten. A chum is a special friend usually of the same sex and age. A chum relationship is important to the child, because it is his first intense close relationship outside the family. He also has someone who is more understanding and accepting of his behavior.

Play is an important aspect of socialization at this stage, since it promotes the child's independence, developing roles, respect for others and problem-solving ability and also provides opportunities to compete, compromise and cooperate.

Safety Needs

Protecting the child from injury is still a major concern for parents. Although the child is further advanced physically and psychologically than he was during the preschool stage, he still has difficulty in seeing danger in a situation. It is not wise to overcaution or protect the child, since this limits or decreases his ability to mature. Since a great deal of the child's learning is taking place through imitation, the parent can demonstrate safety techniques needed for work and play.

Cognitive Development

Cognitively, the child is in the concrete operations period of development. He is usually able to learn factual information but is typically able to use little abstract thinking until the latter part of this stage. The child is so busy learning about the world that the inability to do abstract thinking does not seem to bother him, unless he is punished or ridiculed by parents or other significant people.

Emotional Development

Emotionally, the school-age child is relatively stable compared to the preschooler. The child is now in Erikson's industry versus inferiority stage of development. He is usually happy if allowed to learn new tasks, solve problems and assume a responsible role in his daily activities. However, if he is not allowed to assume such an industrious role, he feels defeated, gives up trying and may experience difficulty in learning. Feelings of inferiority are sometimes coped with by behaving in a socially unacceptable manner or by withdrawing. Overall, the school-age period is an exciting time in the child's life, although it is not free of crisis. The child having completed this stage is now ready for adolescence (Craig, 1976, pp. 295-360; English and Pearson, 1963, pp. 171-188; Kalkman, 1967, pp. 51-58; Lidz, 1968, pp. 264-295; Murray and Zentner, 1975, pp. 122-152).

ADOLESCENT

Identity

Identity is crucial in the development of the adolescent. He is moving from the world of the child to the world of the adult, and this means that he must establish *who* he is. When all facets of identity—self-concept, body image, sexual identity, vocation or career, independence from parents—are considered, one can easily see why adolescence is often a time of turbulence for the individual.

In addition to the tasks to be accomplished, numerous factors influence how the adolescent will respond and grow. Such factors include (1) achievement of prior developmental tasks, (2) family, peer and societal influences, and (3) how he generally perceives the world around him.

Self-Concept

In order to develop a positive self-concept, it is essential that the adolescent recognize himself as a unique person with individual feelings and capabilities, and that he experience some success in what is important to him as a person. His "ideal self," what he would like to be, should be close to the "real self." For this to occur, his goals must be closely related to his abilities.

The self is not a given capacity, but one that must be achieved; the adolescent becomes acutely aware of this. The psychoanalysts believe that the ego is already set on a fairly certain course at this point; but, however well-developed it is, the ego continues to develop through growth-oriented activities.

For the first time in his existence, the person is beginning to look critically at himself as a separate entity—apart from parents, siblings, peers, teachers and friends. To determine how much he is like others and how much he wants to be like others becomes important. The "others" also become important; for example, who does he want to be like, if anyone, and why?

Important achievements of personality development prior to adolescence include:
1. perception of oneself as adequate
2. constructive relationship with parents
3. ability to get along with peers
4. acceptance of increasing responsibility.

The individual who has not made these prior achievements may be more prone to cope with the pressures and identity crisis of adolescence by turning to drugs, alcohol and/or delinquency. These crutches may convey a false feeling of adequacy, and, as a result, one's identity development is only delayed.

Body Image

Body image refers to the perception one has of his own body and physical abilities. This is usually a changing perception rather than a static one. Associated with adolescence are physical changes of height, weight and body build and the appearance of the secondary sex characteristics. Whether the adolescent and/or his parents interpret these changes as being normal or abnormal is extremely influential in how the changes are incorporated into the person's body image.

The existent differences in the growth patterns of males and females may have an influence on the individual concept developed. The growth spurt occurs earlier for girls, so in early adolescence they are generally taller and heavier than boys of the same age. By late adolescence, the average height of boys exceeds that of girls. Boys at this age often feel much pressure, because society tends to favor the taller male. They realize, too, that this is their "last chance"—their last growth in height. One of the major problems experienced by both boys and girls at this time of rapid growth is awkwardness. If the awkwardness is emphasized by themselves or others around them, it may be incorporated into the body image.

A major factor in the developing body image of the adolescent is the growth of the sexual organs and development of secondary sex characteristics. Since the male sex organs are external, boys become very conscious of their size, comparing themselves to others. Boys also become more conscious of the development of secondary sex characteristics—voice change and growth of body hair. Girls are more aware of their changing body shapes, especially as the breasts develop. Hormonal changes are occurring for both sexes, creating new feelings of sexual interest.

The rapid growth and the sexual changes need to be understood and viewed as normal by the individual. Lack of understanding, in combination with many varying connotations given to the broad area of "sex" by society, can be extremely confusing to the adolescent. It is important that he understands and accepts these changes, if they are to be positively incorporated into his body image.

Sexual Identity

The sexual identity one develops is biologically, sociologically and psychologically influenced. The social role is learned during childhood through identification with the parent of the same sex, cultural role assignments and peer interactions. These prior experiences provide the person with continuous feedback for the sociological development of the role. This existing role structure provides a framework for continuing development.

Human sexuality is influenced by genetic differences, although it is difficult to separate entirely the genetic from the sociological and psychological influences. Some generalities which exemplify this at adolescence are: (1) males are more muscular and athletic, while females prefer less active and less strenuous activities and (2) males are more aggressive in their relationships with others, while females show more interest in helping relationships such as working with underprivileged persons. How much this kind of role development is genetically or socially influenced is difficult to determine.

The biological sexual changes are occurring at progressively younger ages. The onset may be from 7 or 8 to 17 or 18 years, with the termination being from 15 or 16 up to 24 or 25 years. The order in which these changes appear for males and females is outlined by Sutterley and Donnelly (1973, p. 142):

Male
1. Growth of penis and testes
2. Appearance of straight, pigmented pubic hair
3. Voice changes
4. Ejaculation
5. Kinky pubic hair develops
6. Maximum growth spurt
7. Growth of axillary hair
8. Further voice changes
9. Beard growth

Female
1. Breasts enlarge
2. Appearance of straight, pigmented pubic hair
3. Maximum growth spurt
4. Kinky pubic hair develops
5. First menses
6. Growth of axillary hair

The adolescent must accept and adapt to these changes. He may receive very little assistance or education from parents or society which will help this acceptance to be a positive one. Some exploration and experimentation is necessary. At puberty and during early adolescence, experimentation may involve sexual play and comparison of bodily changes with peers of the same sex. By late adolescence, more likely the sexual interaction becomes heterosexual. For males, the peak age of sexual activity is usually 17 or 18 years.

Within the accepted mores of American society, the timing of these biological changes can place a great deal of stress upon the individual. Since the development of a positive sexual identity is extremely important at this time, it merits professional concern. The adolescent needs someone with whom he can intelligently explore his feelings and discuss situations which he is encountering.

The average age of both males and females at the time of marriage is becoming progressively lower. There is also a higher incidence of divorce among couples who married at a younger age. The fact that the person is marrying before he has had a full opportunity to develop his self-concept, including sexual identity, seems at least partially to explain this higher divorce rate.

In order to develop a positive sexual identity, the individual needs to gain an understanding of sexual love and responsibility. Although this may not be entirely developed until much later, the adolescent can begin to develop some conception of the ramifications involved. Masters and Johnson (1970, p. 15) explain this kind of maturity:

> .... sexual responsibility has a twofold implication in today's world. Primarily, we are responsible only for ourselves in our sexual commitments, for full communication of our sexual wants, and, subsequently, for physical expression of our sexual drives. Also, we are committed to remaining fully attuned to partner communication and to the cooperation necessary to enable one's partner to satisfy his or her sexual needs. Secondarily, our sexual responsibility extends not only to full obligation for pregnancy, but to adequate control of conception.

The adolescent, in working toward positive sexual identity, needs to come to grips with what, for him, are acceptable outlets for his sexual needs. Masturbation, especially in males, has long been a form of positive sexual outlet if used without associated feelings of guilt and anxiety. Psychoanalysts have placed emphasis on the sublimation of the sex drive into various kinds of creative activities, such as drawing or writing diaries, poems and stories.

Vocation or Career

In selecting a vocation, an adequate self-concept is important in making the right decision. The vocation selected will hopefully be one which is realistic for the abilities and interests of the person. Positive motivation for self-growth may be evidenced through the selection of work or additional educational preparation for work, which is stimulating and forces him to make the most of his abilities. Setting standards too high, on the other hand, can be defeating.

The adolescent is able to conceptualize at an abstract level; e.g., referred to by Piaget as the "formal operational period." This ability to perform more challenging intellectual tasks might offer new ideas to the individual about career opportunities—careers requiring more analytical thought.

Idealism is another factor which might influence vocational choice. Adolescent idealism might lead to questioning of some of the basic structures within society; this, in turn, might lead the person to philosophy, education, political science, etc. Often, idealism also leads to the altruistic occupations such as nursing, medicine, social work and psychology.

Independence from Parents

If he is to develop into a mature adult with realistic interpretations of his own abilities, the adolescent must develop independence from his parents. Existent problems during this time usually relate to the fact that there are some areas, such as financial support and discipline, in which parental intervention is required.

The kind of parent-child relationship which has existed through childhood is important in determining what the outcomes will be. If the relationship was a constructive one during earlier years, the parents will be more likely to grow with and permit growth for the adolescent. Such a relationship must be built on respect and trust. If, however, the relationship has been characterized by hostility or excessive dependence, growth during adolescence may be inhibited.

As the adolescent achieves more freedom from his parents, he identifies more strongly with a peer group. This association can have profound influence upon his development, because he is sensitive to and desirous of peer approval. It is important to positive development, therefore, that the peer group be one which helps provide for constructive outlets. If the peer group is one whose values are in opposition to society, then antisocial personality organization will be likely to develop. It is often the person with an already poorly integrated personality, who is more vulnerable to membership in such groups.

YOUNG ADULT

If positive development has characterized adolescence, the person enters young adulthood with some sense of who he is. The struggle for establishing one's identity is by no means over, but a good base for continuing development has been established.

There are several major tasks to be accomplished by the young adult; these tasks deal primarily with the firm establishment of intimacy, family and work. E. Erikson classifies this as the stage of "Intimacy versus Isolation"; he gives a positive explanation of this as follows:

> Sexual intimacy is only part of what I have in mind, for it is obvious that sexual intimacies often precede the capacity to develop a true and mutual psychosocial intimacy with another person, be it in friendship, in erotic encounters, or in joint inspiration. The youth who is not sure of his identity shies away from interpersonal intimacy or throws himself into acts of intimacy which are "promiscuous," without true fusion or self-abandon.
>
> Where a youth does not accomplish such intimate relationships with others—and, I would add, with his own inner resources—in late adolescence or early adulthood, he may settle for highly stereotyped interpersonal relations and come to retain a deep *sense of isolation* (Erikson, 1968, pp. 135-36).

Physiologically, an individual has generally achieved adulthood by age 18. Society, however, is continuing to delay further the begining of adulthood for a large segment of the population. A college education, often with additional graduate preparation, is becoming more essential. Many are also becoming more involved with sociological, political and ecological problems of society; this involvement is probably due to more widely used methods of communication and increased awareness through education. In looking at these factors, it becomes evident that the transition from adolescence to adulthood is probably faster for the individual who does not attend college, who marries younger and assumes family responsibilities earlier. It is not known which approach is more desirable in terms of the long-range effects on personality development, since there are so many variables involved. Divorce rates are the one type of data collected which might give some indication, and these data show that earlier marriages more often end in divorce than do later marriages.

Intimacy

Whereas the adolescent has been concerned with establishing a sexual identity, the young adult is ready to move into a stabilizing relationship. Once secure with himself, he can establish open, close relationships with other individuals. This is not restricted only to sexual relationships; it may be found through work and close friendships. This kind of intimacy is characterized by honesty and openness of feelings; it involves the functioning of the "real self." For a relationship to be a truly intimate one, it must also support and allow for the growth of the persons involved. Through development of an intimate relationship with a selected mate, one is also able to determine the meaning of sexual and non-sexual love and to differentiate between the two.

A relationship which is growth-oriented and person-centered is described by C. Rogers (1977, pp. 50-51):

> The partners tend to develop more trust in each other as they are more real with each other. Being more real, they take more risks in being open, and thus enhance their growth as persons. As they communicate more deeply, they are likely to discover, and to wish to develop, more interests that they can do or share.

Rogers (p. 51) also states: *"Roles, and role expectations, tend to drop away and are replaced by the person, choosing her own way of behaving."* With this kind of relationship, then, it is more likely that the traditional male and female roles will change.

Family

Adaptation to the various aspects of family life—marriage, in-laws, parenthood—may present some crises for the young adult. Resolution of these crises is important for the individual's developopment, as well as to the development of all those involved. If intimacy, as previously described, has been achieved or is growing between the couple, they are more prepared for parenthood.

The birth of a child makes certain demands on the already existing relationship. If the parents are prepared for the fact that this will happen, they will be better able to cope. In addition to the added stress of the responsibility of caring for an infant, there may also be a difficult role change for either or both parents. The mother, accustomed to working and in the process of establishing her own career, may give up her work. Many young mothers, though, are now making the choice to combine the roles of parenthood and career. Whichever decision is made, it is important that it be a comfortable one for the couple, and especially for the mother, if growth is to remain positive. Child care is also the father's responsibility, and his involvement is important in a number of ways: (1) sharing this responsibility can keep all members of the family in a closer relationship, (2) the father is less likely to become jealous of the infant for demanding too much of the mother's time and (3) equalizing the time spent in child care allows more time for the parents to develop and pursue common interests. If a comfortable arrangement for parenting is worked out in the early stages, if the parents understand themselves and their own relationship, and if they have some understanding of the growth and development of children, their chances for being successful in the parenting role are greater.

Another facet of family life is adjustment to in-laws and other extended family members. Two major factors are important to successful adaptation: (1) the individual's acceptance of the spouse's parents as they are and (2) willingness of the parents to let go of their child. A crucial point in the relationship may come with the birth of a child, especially if the grandparents disapprove or interfere with the parents' childrearing practice.

Work

The vocation (or lack of it in some cases) selected by the young adult soon becomes a part of his self-concept. He and others form a socialized view of him as "the plumber," "the salesman," "the lawyer," etc. The associated level of economic stability is also an influential factor. The person enters early adulthood as a student or as a beginner in his work. By the end of this period, he is usually well established in his chosen vocation; he has set his goals and is well on his way to accomplishing them.

Selection of a vocation should receive serious consideration during one's development, for it is a far bigger decision than many realize. Basically, the vocational decision should be made in relation to several factors: (1) Is there personal interest and motivation? (2) Is it suitable to individual abilities? (3) Are the potential goals to be achieved such that they will be individually gratifying? (4) Is the prospective financial reward one that will be acceptable in relation to desired life style? Answering such questions as these in initial selection of a vocation will help to eliminate some unhappiness later. Too often, selection is made for such reasons as following in father's footsteps or pleasing one's parents.

Young women may even fail to recognize that they need to consider and answer these career-related decisions regarding the planning for their future lives. In American society, many girls are socialized to the belief that establishing a marriage and family is their only real option. This may meet their esteem needs during the very early phase of adulthood; but toward the end of early adulthood, many factors may cause them to question their assumed role. By this time the children are in school, the husband may be involved in his work to a greater extent than ever before, and she may realize that her self-growth has not been as great as that of her husband, who has been involved in a greater variety of activities. Often, then, at the end of this period, the woman is just beginning seriously to select a vocation in addition to her roles of wife and mother.

Both men and women are often concerned at this point about what they are doing with their lives. One's work is certainly a big part in ascertaining self-worth. Most of all, the work needs to provide satisfaction—satisfaction found in the enjoyment of the type of work, in feeling pleased with the outcomes of the work, and in being able successfully to balance work with family life. If this kind of satisfaction is achieved, then one's development is most likely positive at this point.

MIDDLE-AGED ADULT

Middle age has not been studied and reviewed as much as the other age groups; therefore, the expectations are not as well understood. There are certainly continuing tasks of personality development to be accomplished by the person at this stage. The self-concept is continuing to grow; for example, the middle-aged person is concerned with his use of self in achieving his desired goals. There is also a change in the perspective with which one views oneself, as shown by this statement of a middle-aged woman:

> It is as if I'm looking at a three-way mirror. In one mirror I see part of myself in my mother who is growing old, and part of her in me. In the other mirror, I see part of myself in my daughter. I have had some dramatic insights, just from looking in those mirrors... It is a set of revelations that I suppose can only come when you are in the middle of three generations (Neugarten, 1964, p. 383).

Erikson identifies the major task to be accomplished at this stage as *generativity*, a term which "encompasses the evolutionary development which has made man the teaching and instituting as well as the learning animal" (Erikson, 1963, p. 266). This concept includes the productivity and creativity which one applies to reaching his self-identified goals, as well as to the guidance which he provides for the development of the next generation. It means "feeling a voluntary obligation to care for others in the broadest sense" (Sheehy, 1977, p. 405). The alternative to generativity is stagnation, which develops if the individual directs most of his concern to himself.

The humanistic theories would also support the need of the individual to become involved in the supportiveness and growth of others. In Maslow's hierarchy of needs, for example, "the love and belongingness" need precedes "self-esteem." The fact that one has satisfied this need does not mean that it disappears or the person no longer needs to give or receive love. In fact, Maslow (1962, p. 39) states:

> ...clinical study of healthier people, who have been love-need-satiated, show that although they need less to *receive* love, they are more able to *give* love. In this sense, they are *more* loving people.

It would seem, therefore, that the more loving individual described by Maslow is a person who is free to be involved in completing the task of generativity.

For the purpose of discussing personality development during middle age, the areas of family, work and physiological changes seem to be appropriate divisions. These are major areas which continue to provide a challenge to the further growth of the individual. *Self-evaluation* is a characteristic activity at this stage, as is evidenced in one's growth throughout all of these areas.

Family

The family includes primarily the relationships one has with his spouse and children, although in some instances there may be close involvement with parents and extended family members. The adjustments necessary for one as a family member have changed in recent years due to a number of factors: (1) the changing role of women in society, (2) the increased mobilization within society, (3) more studies about and increased openness in the discussion of human sexuality and (4) increasing emphasis on higher education.

At mid-life, an individual begins to look critically at himself, and the family is an important aspect of this self-evaluation. Whether or not a relationship between spouses can survive this critical examination depends to a great extent on the growth and maturity attained thus far by each.

The change in the woman's social role may become an issue, since this is often when the woman evaluates where she is in her life and decides for the first time to become more independent of her husband. This is generally a time when the husband is very involved in his work, and he may depend on his wife to provide much of the stability for the family functioning. His involvement leaves her with more time to think seriously about her own life.

As she experiences more value in herself and her own life, the husband may begin to feel less valued. In gaining some independence, she may have less time to provide the kind of support for her husband to which he has become accustomed. The role change, thus, can require countless adaptations for both.

While the woman, at age 35-40, is taking inventory of her life situation and making decisions concerning it, the man is plunging deeper into his work. The male often has set work-related goals. At age 40-45 he may either accomplish these goals or realize that he is not going to. It is at this point that he begins to reassess who he is and what his role is in relation to his family. The fact that his "life assessment" generally comes later, after age 40, is a potential problem for couples of approximately the same age. Much depends on the awareness and understanding which each spouse has of himself and his partner. Openness of communication between them is a key factor.

This self-evaluation may also lead to concern with losing one's sexuality. Women are more prone to experience this in their later 30s; for men, this occurs more often in the 40s. To prove that sexuality is not diminishing, the individual may seek out sexual partners other than his mate. This is a stress which, when not understood, makes the family ties extremely vulnerable to separation.

For those couples whose relationships survive this period of testing and examination, a closer relationship will probably continue to develop. Sheehy (1977, p. 506) states:

> Studies record a dramatic climb in satisfaction with marriage in the mid-forties for those couples who have survived the passage into midlife together. What this finding reflects is not that our mate miraculously improves but that tolerance can become spontaneous once we stop displacing our inner contradictions on our spouse. The steep rise of contentment levels off after 50 at a higher plateau.

Another major change occurring in the family during middle age is the departure of children. This is a change which requires adaptation; and, if parents have prepared themselves for the anticipated change, they will be able to deal with it more constructively. For those who are able to anticipate this as a time when they will be free to pursue more of their own interests, the jolt may not be as great. The better integrated the personality, the better are the chances for successful adaptation. Again, this is often a time of self-evaluation, especially for the mother whose primary task has been childrearing. Women who have allowed themselves little involvement in interests or activities other than family are more likely to experience identity problems.

The primary factors which provide for growth of the individual and of the family during this period are (1) willingness of each family member to express himself freely and (2) willingness of each member to be himself and permit others to be themselves. Carl Rogers (1961, p. 328) summarizes these beliefs as follows:

> ... a therapy which results in the individual becoming more fully and more deeply himself, results also in his finding greater satisfaction in realistic family relationships which likewise promote the same end—that of facilitating each member of the family in the process of discovering, and becoming, himself.

Work

The type of work that was started by the young adult generally continues into middle age, especially if the selection was given adequate consideration initially. Hopefully, work provides pleasure for the individual, but the type of pleasure provided may vary greatly, including (1) making progress toward meeting self-set goals, (2) meeting one's need to be productive and creative, (3) gaining recognition and/or admiration of others and (4) fulfilling a compulsion to work. While the last, compulsion to work, is not always desirable, it may meet the individual's need (a deficiency need) by allaying guilt feelings. Eventually, though, its effects may be apparent in his personality and relationships with others—family, coworkers, etc.

The first three pleasures of work listed provide positive forces for individual growth, if they do not become all-consuming. Middle age is the time of self-evaluation, and this evaluation does include one's work. The person who has been highly successful may now become bored with success, wondering what other rewards are possible. On the other hand, the person who is still striving to meet his goals may become frustrated. This frustration can be valuable if it leads to constructive reassessment of goals and self-evaluation.

Toward the latter part of middle age, one needs to begin anticipating and planning for retirement. Planning for, rather than denial of, approaching retirement, is a positive move, though many may not have the necessary energy, interest and motivation to make this move. In anticipating future needs, one needs to consider developing an avocation which is of real interest, developing and maintaining friendships and planning for financial security. If these tasks are accomplished, at least in part, positive growth at this stage is facilitated.

Physiological Changes

The effects of physiological changes on the personality are probably almost as great at this stage as in adolescence. Some of the more obvious changes include the greying hair, increased wrinkles, decreased levels of vision and hearing, loss of height and changes in body shape.

One's adaptation is strongly influenced by how he perceives these changes. Our society's emphasis on youth and looking young may make the acceptance of these changes difficult for the middle-aged person. Some may actually attempt to cope by adapting the interests, values, dress, etc., of a much younger person. This is positive adaptation only inasmuch as it is consistent behavior for the individual and does not present a drastic change in life style.

The female menopause (cessation of menstrual activity) and climacterium (cessation of the reproductive period) are among the most discussed physiological changes during this stage. As the ovaries stop functioning, menstruation ceases. Eventually, then, the ability to reproduce is lost. The decreasing production of estrogen, usually beginning in the mid-thirties, is responsible for many of the subtle and pronounced changes which occur. Certainly, it is believed that estrogen loss is related to the well-known "hot flashes." Its relationship to the depression and other emotional problems sometimes occurring is not as well understood. It is quite possible that emotional problems occurring at this time are more related to one's past personality development than to hormonal changes, though the two are probably interrelated (Sherman, 1971, pp. 236-237).

One's emotional reaction to the menopause may be representative of her personality development. If the woman perceives menopause as a loss of femininity, she may actually experience the grieving process; this may be accompanied by depression. If, however, her self-concept at this point is positive and she understands the physiology of what is taking place, she should be less likely to experience severe emotional problems. There have been certain psychological changes related to the menopause, probably triggered by the changing hormonal balance and the on-going adjustments to change in life style. Some of these commonly noted changes include: (1) emotional instability—rapid changes in mood, (2) nervousness and anxiety, (3) insomnia, (4) fatigue and (5) depression (Galloway, 1975, p. 1007).

Increasingly more debate exists as to whether a "male menopause" exists. It cannot exist in terms of the strict definition of menopause; however, men also experience physical and psychological changes. The hormonal changes in the male are more gradual, beginning around age 18 when testosterone production is at its peak. A more pronounced change occurs, though, "beginning between the ages of 40 to 55" (Sheehy, 1977, p. 456).

The symptoms exhibited by the male are very similar to those experienced by the female. Again, the psychological symptoms are probably related to a number of events occurring at this time of life, e.g., his self-evaluation related to his work, family and life, generally, and the physical and psychological changes. Much of the man's adaptation will be related, as with the woman, to his past personality development. His existing self-concept is probably the most important factor in determining how he will cope with the physical and psychological changes and disruptions.

Since there has been little understanding and discussion of these changes occurring in the male, it is important to his adjustment that the person understand that what he is experiencing is a "normal" phenomenon. The symptoms most often associated with the male climacteric are summarized by Sheehy (1977, pp. 458-459):

> Morning fatigue, lassitude, and vague pains are the most common. Nervousness, irritability, depressive phases, crying spells, insomnia, memory lapses, apprehensiveness, and frustration are the cerebral symptoms.
> Diminished sexual potency and loss of self-confidence are particularly subject to the reciprocal effect of his situation at home and at work.
> And then there may be any one of a mixed bag of circulating signs: dizzy spells, hot flashes, chills, sweating, headaches, numbness and tingling, cold hands and feet, plus an increased pulse rate and heart palpitations . . . .

In addition to these, Sheehy (1977, p. 459) states that the symptoms which are "most bothersome" are the pronounced mood swings. These can be very damaging to one's interpersonal relationships in all aspects of life, since these changes in mood may, at the time of decline, involve depression, pessimism and/or extreme loss of temper.

One of the most talked about and least understood of the changes affecting the middle-aged person is that related to sexual functioning. Many tales exist concerning the loss of sexual functioning during middle age; however, as this area is being exposed to more study, these tales are not necessarily proven true. The story of the middle-aged man seeking sexual relations and sometimes marriage with a younger woman, in order to prove his sexual prowess to himself and others, may often be true. Such occurrences, though, may also be related to a number of factors, e.g., general evaluation of where he is in life, lack of understanding of the male climacteric and fear of losing his "maleness."

There are concrete physiological changes, psychological changes and growth needs affecting sexual changes. The more these are understood by the individual, the more likely it is that he can use this understanding to make positive adaptation in his own life. Certainly, physiological sexual functioning is only one aspect of a personally satisfying sexual relationship. This is intertwined with personality, growth or deficiency needs and a personal value system. As one understands more about all of these aspects of his life, he will be more likely to establish a relationship with another that is satisfying and growth-producing for both. The middle-aged person, given the necessary understanding along with his experience and maturity, should be better able to establish such a relationship than the younger adult.

Women actually experience few physiological changes which affect sexual functioning. As estrogen production slows, atrophic vaginitis tends to occur; the vagina becomes dry due to atrophy of the mucous membrane. As a result, sexual intercourse may be painful. In most instances, lubrication can be maintained or corrected through regular intercourse or application of estrogen creams.

Likewise, men do not experience physical changes which need interfere greatly with sexual activity. The fear of these changes may be inhibitors which are as great or greater than the changes themselves. In middle age, the male's testosterone production continues to decrease and his female hormone level remains stable or increases slightly. Physically, his body becomes more similar to that of the female during the latter part of middle age. Many men experience impotence; however, Masters and Johnson (1970) propose that most often impotence is psychological rather than physiological in origin. Penile erection may not be obtained as quickly as in the past, and the man may place too much emphasis on this occurrence, feeling that he is losing his manhood. Actually, a change in lovemaking techniques, primarily prolonging the physical intimacy with his mate, may be all that is needed to solve the problem. This may even lead to a stronger relationship between them.

There are many other physiological changes in middle age, including cardiovascular changes, increasing impairment of sensory function and osteoporosis. These changes, too, may severely alter one's life style and body image. These changes can lead to a variety of health problems; for example, the incidence of myocardial infarction is significantly increased. Although the many acute and chronic physical disorders which present themselves most often during middle age will not be discussed here, the nurse needs to be aware of the ways in which the effects of these disorders can alter personality development.

OLDER ADULT

Studies have indicated that personality remains stable and consistent through adulthood and that the "stable" personality can continue its adaptation to life. B. L. Neugarten and associates (1964, p. 198) summarize these findings as follows:

> In a sense, the self becomes institutionalized with the passage of time. Not only do certain personality processes become stabilized and provide continuity, but the individual builds around him a network of social relationships which he comes to depend on for emotional support and responsiveness and which maintain him in many subtle ways. . . .
> . . . Behavior in a normal old person is more consistent and more predictable than in a younger one . . . the personality structure stands more clearly revealed in an old than in a younger person.

The humanists have described the older adult as more often reaching self-actualization. This is growth in a positive sense. Certainly one learns more about himself through experience, if he remains open to his experiences. The learning through continued life experiences is an important aspect of "becoming," or growth towards self-actualization. It is primarily, then, the older person who has experienced enough of life to reach this end in the process of "becoming."

These views supporting positive personality development of old age are consistent with the major task of this stage—Ego Integrity—as identified by Erikson. Negative development at this stage is exhibited through despair. Erikson (1963, p. 269) describes despair as "the feeling that the time is now short, too short for the attempt to start another life and to try out alternate roads to integrity." Ego integrity refers to the ability of one to identify with mankind. He is accepting of his life and of the fact that his life and his human integrity are only a part of the vast expanse of humanness or civilization.

Such understanding allows the individual to accept eventual death, not fear it (Erikson, 1963, p. 268).

There are some continuing tasks of personality development to be completed by the older adult. In our society, these are influenced by some social factors, such as loss of income, retirement from work and loss of role and/or status. The major developmental tasks are related to (1) changes in life style—role changes, retirement, loss of income, (2) physical and psychological changes and (3) bereavement and acceptance of death.

Changes in Life Style

Changes in life style are probably more pronounced for the older adult than for any other group. Major changes may be experienced due to retirement, loss of income and changes in family structure.

Retirement and loss of income usually are interrelated. Not only may the person feel that he is losing his usefulness to society, but he may also be reduced to a much lower income level than that to which he has been accustomed. This plight is described by Senator Charles Percy in his book, *Growing Old in the Country of the Young* (1974, p. 19):

> What does it mean to be over sixty-five today in our country? For too many men and women who have worked hard all their lives and saved for their retirement, it means lack of sufficient money to enjoy those later years. Most of these men and women worked hard until age or disability forced them to stop. A huge number of elderly Americans become poor *only after they become old*.

Changes in family structure may involve the death of the spouse and/or loss of the parental role. These felt losses may only further aggravate the feeling of uselessness.

Both socioeconomic status and marital status are related to mental illness. A positive relationship exists between *low* socioeconomic status and mental illness. This is true of all age groups, including the older adult. In addition, single older adults exhibit a higher rate of mental illness than do older married persons (Palmore, 1973, pp. 44-45).

Maslow's hierarchy of needs gives some basis for understanding what may happen to the older adult affected by social problems. The person who is experiencing problems of income may be most concerned with how he is going to take care of his physiological needs—food, shelter, clothing. If these most basic needs are unmet, the individual is rarely concerned with anything else. An individual's very basic physiological needs may be met, but if he has experienced loss of family members, job and/or friends, he may be concerned with satisfying the need of "love and belonging." In these terms, the loss of self-esteem which too often occurs seems explainable.

How one adapts at this stage of the life span may depend significantly on several factors: (1) past personality development, (2) assistance from concerned individuals and groups and (3) health status. The prior adjustments made are extremely important; for example, preparation for retirement by developing an avocation during middle age. The personality structure will remain fairly constant, unless the adverse pressures provided by the environment and/or one's health status are too great.

Concerned individuals and groups can be an important factor in assisting the older person to maintain and even improve his personality structure. Family members need to be aware of what is occurring; their concern can be shown in any number of ways—monetary, physiological and/or emotional support. Community action groups can also help provide needed resources. Some examples of existing problems are (1) foster grandparent programs which allow the individual to provide the grandparent role for children in nursery schools, hospitals, etc., (2) meals-on-wheels, which serves nutritious meals at a minimal fee to the older person in his home, (3) transportation services for the elderly to do their shopping, visit the doctor's office, etc. and (4) legal aid services. Such services as these may allow the individual freedom from worry about basic things and the opportunity to pursue those things which will allow for continued growth. It is essential that this support from family or groups be provided in such a way as not to lower the recipient's self-esteem.

Physical and Psychological Changes

Whereas physical and psychological changes at the preceding stage of life often have been perceived as negative, at this stage they are more often perceived as a normal occurrence and possibly even as a challenge. This is exemplified by the 94-year-old woman who repeatedly answers inquiries concerning her health status by saying, "Well, I don't always feel so good, but you don't expect to when you're as old as I am." This answer may help to explain why she exhibits such a positive life style at age 94.

The physical and psychological aspects of aging are closely related. The common factor relating physical and psychological growth is stress. How the individual learns to cope with and adapt to stress is an important part of his total development. The coping mechanisms and patterns of dealing with stress are well developed in old age, and these determine, to a large extent, the total health status (including personality) of the individual.

Some of the physiological changes occurring in the older adult include:

1. Cardiovascular changes leading to elevated blood pressure, arteriosclerosis, and reduced circulatory blood flow
2. Reduction in the kidney's tubular function affecting kidney function
3. Reduced elasticity of the lungs and reduced capacity to cough and deep breathe, leading to more respiratory complications
4. Musculoskeletal changes leading to decreased physical stature, strength and endurance
5. Central nervous system changes, including loss of brain cells and decreased reaction time, leading to slower response under stress
6. Sensory changes, especially hearing and vision, leading to gradual loss of hearing (often the high frequency sounds) and vision

There seem to be commonly occurring intellectual changes directly related to some of the physiological aspects of aging. These changes are difficult to measure because of the large number of variables involved—education, health status, socioeconomic status. It is reported that Piaget has observed that older persons tend to regress from "formal" to "concrete operations" which are more typical of school-age children (Kimmel, 1974, p. 377). A decrease in memory seems to be more common among older adults, though it is certainly not characteristic of all. This is not entirely understood, as exemplified by the following explanation:

> There are several theories about memory loss: that memories are lost

through *disuse;* that memories are lost through the *interference* of other memories in the large store of memories that is accumulated with age; and that *neurochemical* change or loss of cells in the CNS is responsible for memory loss. Currently, the interference theory in combination with neurochemical factors seems to be favored; that is the amount of stored information increases with age while the neural changes . . . lead to slower and less efficient processing of the stored information with age (Kimmel, 1974, pp. 379-380).

Some of the psychological problems which are more closely associated with the older adult than with any other stage are also related to physical changes, as arteriosclerosis and organic brain syndromes. (For discussion on the organic syndrome, see Chapter 13). Those psychological problems with no known physiological relationship are referred to as functional disorders. Those functional disorders which are more common among the older age group include depression, anxiety neurosis, paranoia and psychochondriacal neurosis.

It is known that the incidence of mental illness is greater in the older adult. This is partially explained by the rising occurrence of depression and organic brain disorders. It is encouraging to note that many of these conditions are acute, or reversible. Even a great number of the organic conditions are reversible, since they are caused by malnutrition, congestive heart failure, drug reactions and infections (Butler and Lewis, 1973, p. 50). It is quite possible that the increased isolation of the elderly is also a causative factor in mental illness.

Certainly mental illness affects the individual's personality development. Psychosis, such as senile psychosis, markedly disrupts one's relationships with others; thus, personality development regresses. With the neuroses, personality integration is not profoundly affected. In fact, in many instances, the neurotic symptoms have existed prior to this stage of development. They may become more pronounced at this time due to increasing anxiety. The neurotic behavior may provide a means of coping with various kinds of anxiety.

Acceptance of Death

The individual's beginning concern with and acceptance of death usually begins during middle age. Gradually, as more of one's contemporaries are lost through death, the acceptance of death becomes a reality. This seems to be a necessary adjustment in order to maintain an adequate personality. This adjustment is in keeping with the concept of ego integrity as discussed by Erikson.

R. N. Butler (1968, p. 487) hypothesizes that the older adult experiences a life review. This life review includes increased reminiscence and bringing unresolved conflicts back into consciousness. As past experiences are reconsidered, one seems to be able to integrate these more fully into his total personality. In this sense, the reminiscences of the old serve a very constructive purpose.

Another theory which has received much attention is that of "disengagement" as it relates to successful aging. Disengagement, as it was originally presented by Cumming and Henry (1961) indicated that there was a decrease in social interaction and in one's ego investment in social roles with aging. This process of decreasing one's investment in living was seen as an aid in making positive adaptation to one's own approaching death. This theory, however, has been disputed by those who believe that one's investment in living only changes as he replaces lost roles and activities with new ones. Later studies have also shown that the person's satisfaction with life often increases with aging. There may be a compromise between the opposing theories; e.g., either approach may represent positive adjustment, depending upon the individual's personality structure (Kimmel, 1974, pp. 314-317).

E. Kubler-Ross has significantly contributed to understanding the process of dying through her studies with dying patients. She identifies five stages in the dying process: (1) denial and isolation, (2) anger, (3) bargaining, (4) depression and (5) acceptance (Kubler-Ross, 1969). Although these stages were identified from actual work with dying patients, these same stages may occur in a less pronounced way over a longer period of time during the aging process. Many persons experience a "mid-life crisis," sparked by the realization that half of the life span has been used up. The initial reaction of denial may account for the individual's searching for change which often occurs at this time. Gradually, by the end of middle age or the beginning of old age, the individual usually comes to a stage of acceptance.

BIBLIOGRAPHY

Butler, R.N. "The Life Review: An Interpretation of Reminiscence in the Aged," in *Middle Age and Aging*. Edited by B.L. Neugarten. Chicago: The University of Chicago Press, 1968.

Butler, R. N., and Lewis, M.I. *Aging and Mental Health.* St. Louis: The C.V. Mosby Co., 1973.
Craig, Grace. *Human Development.* Englewood Cliffs, N.J.: Prentice-Hall, Inc., 1976.
Cumming, E., and Henry, W.E. *Growing Old: The Process of Disengagement.* New York: Basic Books, Inc., 1961.
English O. Spurgeon, and Pearson, G.: *Emotional Problems of Everyday Living.* New York: W.W. Norton & Co., Inc., 1963.
Erikson, E.H. *Childhood and Society.* 2d ed. New York: W.W. Norton & Co., Inc., 1963.
———. *Identity: Youth and Crisis.* New York: W.W. Norton & Co., Inc., 1968.
Galloway, D. "The Change of Life," *American Journal of Nursing.* LXXV, No. 6 (June, 1975), 1006-1011.
Jahoda, M. *Current Concepts of Positive Mental Health.* New York: Basic Books, Inc., 1958.
Kalkman, Marion. *Psychiatric Nursing.* New York: McGraw-Hill Book Co., 1967.
Kimmel D.C. *Adulthood and Aging.* New York: John Wiley & Sons, Inc., 1974.
Kubler-Ross, E. *On Death and Dying.* New York: The Macmillan Co., 1969.
Lidz, Theodore. *The Person: His Development Throughout the Life Cycle.* New York: Basic Books, Inc., 1968.
Maslow, A.H. *Toward a Psychology of Being.* New York: D. Van Nostrand Co., Inc. 1962.
Masters, W.H., and Johnson V.E. *The Pleasure Bond: A New Look at Sexuality and Commitment.* Boston: Little, Brown & Co., 1970.
Mereness, Dorothy. *Essentials of Psychiatric Nursing.* St. Louis: The C.V. Mosby Co., 1970.
Murray R., and Zentner, J. *Nursing Assessment and Health Promotion Through the Life Span.* Englewood Cliffs, N.J.: Prentice-Hall, Inc., 1975.
Neugarten, B.L. *Personality in Middle and Late Life.* New York: Atherton Press, Inc., 1964.
Palmore, E.B. "Social Factors in Mental Illness of the Aged," in *Mental Illness in Later Life.* Edited by E.W. Busse and E. Pfeiffer. Washington, D.C.: American Psychiatric Association, 1973.
Percy, C.H. *Growing Old in the Country of the Young.* New York: McGraw-Hill Book Co., 1974.
Robinson, Lisa. *Psychiatric Nursing as a Human Experience.* Philadelphia: W.B. Saunders Co., 1972.
Rogers, C.R. *On Becoming a Person.* Boston, Houghton Mifflin Co., 1961.

_____.*On Personal Power*. New York: Delacorte Press, 1977.
Sheehy, Gail. *Passages: Predictable Crises of Adult Life*. New York: Bantam Books, Inc., 1977.
Sherman, J.A. *On the Psychology of Women: Survey of Empirical Studies*. Springfield, Ill.: Charles C Thomas, Publisher, 1971.
Sutterley, D.C., and Donnelly, G.F. *Perspectives in Human Development: Nursing Throughout the Life Cycle*. Philadelphia: J.B. Lippincott Co., 1973.

PART II. The Nursing Process in Psychiatry

CHAPTER 4

Therapeutic Communication

Jeanette Lancaster, R.N., Ph.D.

INTRODUCTION

Hey, You!
Look at me!
Listen to me!
Do you really see or hear?
Sometimes the sound is silence
And the look I see is separateness.
I want to communicate but don't know how to reach out.
So I may slap, hit or retort with a dirty word.
I'm really trying to say. . .
Could you like me, accept me?
Could I trust you?
It's risky business,
This reaching out, because I may get hurt
And I am afraid of that. . .
I guess I am afraid of you, too.
But somehow I need you.
And just maybe, you need me?
Hey, you!
Can you hear me?
I am just trying to find. . .me.
Do you have time to reach out?
To listen?
To help me see
and be. . .me!!

(Poem on p. 97 reprinted with permission from the Tarrant County, Texas Mental Health Association.)

How well a nurse can determine the correct intervention for a nursing care problem depends largely on her communication skills, her ability to listen to the overt as well as the covert information. Subtle needs being expressed by the patient affect the planning and implementation of nursing care. Communication is central to the nursing process in assessing and understanding the patient and his family as well as planning and implementing nursing measures.

The difference between therapeutic communication and that which occurs in ordinary conversation lies in the motivation of the participants. The nurse engaged in therapeutic communication tries to motivate the patient without misusing her power to achieve personal advantage (Ruesch, 1961). The goal of therapeutic communication is to increase the patient's ability to function in social settings.

Both participants in an interaction inject conscious and unconscious purposes related to individual goals, needs and cultural expectations. Moreover, the meaning of communication is affected by individual differences, attitudes, expectations and the ongoing situation.

According to Ruesch (1961), communication embraces all modes of behavior consciously or unconsciously employed by an individual to affect another. It includes not only spoken and written words, but also gestures, body movements, somatic signals and symbolism. An individual's nonverbal communication is considered a more accurate gauge of his true feelings than what he actually says, since he has far less control over his nonverbal reactions than over his verbalizations.

Nonverbal communication is the individual's first interactional experience (Applbaum, 1973). Four general areas of nonverbal communication are identified: personal space and proxemics, physical activity, visual interaction and vocalization.

Personal space or proxemics refers to the distance or area each person maintains between himself and the person with whom he is interacting. Trespassing into another's personal space boundaries elicits defensive behavior. The person, feeling his territory has been invaded, backs away or terminates the conversation.

Physical activity refers to the body movements of the communicator which provide clues as to the actual intent of the verbal message. A person's movements reflect his unconscious feelings and attitudes.

Visual interaction is increased when a person is listening, as opposed to when he is speaking. When both participants in the conversation are interested, there is generally a high degree of eye contact. If a person is unable to maintain eye contact, it is important to determine the cause. He may be embarrassed by the interaction, feel anxious, guilty or physically unfit. There tends to be increased eye contact if the participants like one another.

Vocalization refers to vocal tone and vocal stress as well as to pauses or hesitations. Vocal cues can agree with or contradict verbal cues. For example, if a person says, "You look nice," in a tense, flat, clipped tone the listener receives an incongruent or confused message.

PROCESS OF COMMUNICATION

One way to view communication is to consider it a process consisting of specific elements: sending, receiving, message, signals, setting and feedback. The clear sending of a communication depends on the degree of congruence between the message sent and the nonverbal message simultaneously communicated. The greater the incongruence between what a person is thinking and feeling (which may be observed in the nonverbal message) and what he actually says, the more likely is the receiver to hear an ambiguous message. The risk in sending congruent messages is that the sender will reveal himself as he actually is.

Messages may be verbal, nonverbal, written or spoken as well as implied but not spoken. The signals may be direct or overt as well as covert, indirect, subtle and disguised. The sending of a message in no way guarantees that it is received, much less received by the intended recipient. Figure 4-1 portrays one model for sending a message.

SENDER —— MESSAGE —— RECEIVER

Figure 4-1

A variety of factors affects how a message is sent, as well as how and by whom it is received. The words used, the tone of voice, facial expression, setting, expectations of both sender and receiver, as well as the relationship existing between them, all determine how a message is communicated. For example, a compliment from a person with whom one has a competitive relationship may be received with suspicion and doubt as to its sincerity.

Feedback is essential if the communication is to be completed. What A says to B must be received with B providing A clues as to the message he heard, and A either recognizing that his message was received as he meant it to be, or attempting to resend the message which B received in a distorted manner. Figure 4-2 depicts a more complex explanation of message sending and receipt than that of Figure 4-1.

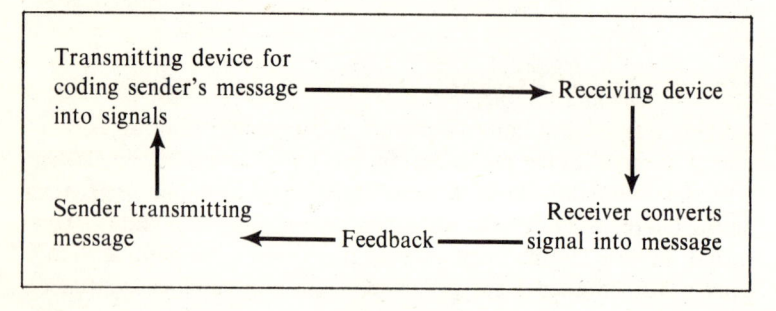

Figure 4-2

In order to receive a message accurately, the receiver must be actively involved in the communication process. His receiving ability is greatly decreased if he is simultaneously listening to the sender and counting the squares in the ceiling tile or is otherwise distracted. Thomas Gordon (1961) says that the most severe test of one's ability to listen and receive a message eventuates when an individual forces himself to put into his own words the meaning of the sender's message and "feeds back" the words he hears for verification from the sender or for subsequent correction.

VERBAL AND NONVERBAL COMMUNICATION

Communication takes place on two levels: verbal and nonverbal. The verbal level refers to the spoken word and involves the physiological processes required for speech production and reception. In considering communication, one often thinks of the spoken word, which actually represents only a small portion of human communication. It is estimated that in normal communications between two people, one-third of the meaning is transmitted on a verbal level and nearly two-thirds on a nonverbal level. Nonverbal communication takes place whenever two strangers meet. Each sizes the other up and assesses the other as a person (Brill, 1973). Nonverbal communication is continuous with or without verbal accompaniments. It is the principal means by which attitudes and feelings are conveyed. A patient is less apt to talk with a nurse who stands beside a chair looking around the room, than to the one who sits near him and maintains eye contact during the conversation.

The more congruency between the verbal and nonverbal message the greater the likelihood that the message will be correctly received. If the nurse asks patient A, "How are you today?" and he responds with a warm smile, "Fine, I am going home today," the congruency between verbal and nonverbal levels of communication is high. On the other hand, if the nurse asks patient B the same question and he responds, eyes downcast, in a slow, low tone of voice, "Fine, I am going home today," there is marked incongruence between the verbal and nonverbal message. An analysis of the nurse-patient communication might reveal the following information:

Data	Thoughts	Feelings	Principles
N. "How are you today?"	I wonder how Mr. B. is feeling today.	Curious Interested Concerned	Asking questions can lead to clarification
P. "Fine, I am going home today."	I am so afraid to go home; who will take care of me?	Fear Anxiety Insecurity	Fear of unknown, untried situation leads to increased anxiety

The nurse now has two completely different responses from patient B. The overt response is that he is fine, while the covert response communicates fear and anxiety. In a situation where the covert response seems clear, the nurse's next gambit would be to focus on the signs she is picking up and provide this perception as feedback to Mr. B. She might say, "Mr. B, you don't look as if you feel fine. You seem worried about something." Mr. B might experience tremendous relief at the nurse's invitation for him to express himself honestly or he might angrily respond, "I told you I am fine so leave me alone." Mr. B's second response would indicate that he is threatened by his own feelings and fears expressing them. The nurse might leave the room telling Mr. B she will return in a short while. By leaving, she gives him an opportunity to examine his feelings; returning soon, she communicates a caring attitude and receptivity to his true message.

Incongruent messages provide perplexing situations for the nurse. Which level should she respond to? The decision about the level of nursing response depends on the nurse's relationship to the patient as well as the nurse's ability to listen to true, "raw" feelings. If the patient trusts the nurse, he is more likely to feel comfortable in expressing painful feelings. Occasionally, a patient's feelings are so near the surface that he expresses them freely upon slight interest by any nurse. The nurse's communication, both verbal and nonverbal, largely determines whether the patient will express his true feelings. If the nurse asks, "How are you, Mr. B?" as she walks out of the room, he is not likely to respond in depth about how he is actually feeling.

An individual's inner feelings are displayed in his nonverbal communication by the way he sits, what he does with his hands and legs, the expression on his face and the little sounds he makes such as clicking or smacking noises. Emotionally disturbed individuals are particularly sensitive to the behavior of the nurse and generally detect any anxiety on the part of the nurse. Thus the nurse must be aware of her level of anxiety as well as that of the patient.

Information is also communicated by a person's appearance. His physique, posture, body odor, manner of dress, level of tension, facial expression, tone of voice, use of gestures and amount of eye contact convey a great deal of information to the observer. For example, the person who smells bad, has food smeared on his clothes or sits in a slumped position may be so anxious that his mechanisms for coping have become regressive. Expression of self through actions is learned before speech is developed. Under stress, an individual often reverts to early preverbal communication. Since verbalizations are easier to control consciously than is body language, an individual may communicate more about himself in his actions than in his words.

Tone of voice can range from a carefully noncommittal monotone, possibly representing control of feelings such as anger, to loud expressions of anger or happiness. Deliberately speaking in a barely audible tone may be a person's way of communicating anger and gaining control of the situation.

Further, a person's movements and gestures are indicators of feelings. For example, one who bites his nails, moves restlessly in his chair, swings his leg or foot continuously or repeatedly cracks his knuckles is doubtless experiencing a high level of anxiety.

Communication of moods and emotions is more important than communication of facts; often it is not what is said but how it is said that conveys the true message. The mother who says to the three-year-old, "I do love you," yet never looks directly at him and rarely touches him or smiles at him, communicates a message of indifference or rejection rather than one of love and acceptance.

The uniform of the nurse, a form of nonverbal communication, often suggests a protective function rather than a threatening one. The uniform may provide security to the nurse, for it readily conveys her identity and power in the hospital hierarchy. The nursing uniform assists patients to identify personnel and may ease the orientation to a new setting.

The name by which a patient is addressed is a further form of communication. To call a person by his first name without being asked to do so is often insulting and condescending. Also, to call a person by his last name without the prefix Mr., Miss or Mrs. can suggest relegation to inferior status. The basic rule is to call a patient Mr., Miss or Mrs. and his last name. Psychiatric illness is generally damaging to self-esteem and dignity; the nursing role is to enhance self-esteem and dignity in each nursing care action.

TOOLS OF COMMUNICATION

Murray and Zentner (1975) identify five tools of communication: language, observation and perception, silence and listening. Knowledge of these tools is essential for successful application of the nursing process.

Language

Language is basic to communication. Listening facilitates the higher-order cognitive processes of thinking, reasoning and generalizing. Words have different meanings to different people.

Consider how personalized the words are in the following statements: "I don't have *many* friends" (How many does the person mean? What does the word, friend, imply?); "I feel bad today" (What does he mean by bad—ill or naughty?).

Word meanings vary from one cultural group to another as well as within the sub-components of a cultural group. For example, words have different meanings to differing age groups. Adolescents frequently adopt a peculiar vocabulary. When an adolescent says, "That is a tough outfit," he does not mean that the fabric is coarse but rather that the outfit has great eye-appeal; the words "far-out" do not refer to a lengthy distance in miles but rather to a truly contemporary and praiseworthy item, whether it be a sound, clothing or other item.

Language forms change over time and in response to social developments and events. Problems in communication arise when individuals fail to watch for signs that they are misinterpreting what they hear. If the nurse consistently misses the meaning of the patient's words, he may decide it is not worth his time and energy to continue orienting her to his language style.

Words are used both to express and to camouflage feelings. When a person says he is fine, he may mean he is functioning at an adequate level; or, secondly, he may be responding in what he assumes is the acceptable manner to such a casual question as, "How are you?" Thirdly, the patient may feel terrible but be hesitant to say so, either because he is not comfortable in communicating with a particular nurse or is unsure if the nurse wants to hear the truth.

Touch, as a form of nonverbal language is a powerful technique. Touch is an early form of communication. An infant initially learns a great deal about the mothering one by the way he is touched. An infant feels safe if the mothering person holds him securely and close to her body, so he can feel warmth and not fear being dropped.

Cultural differences are apparent in regard to touch. In American culture a taboo often exists regarding touching other adults. It is acceptable to touch children; yet touching adults may seem "unnatural." Touch can alter a relationship in either a positive or negative direction. The nurse keenly attuned to the impact of touch notes each patient's reaction. Does the patient stiffen or smile broadly when the nurse puts her hand on his shoulder? How does the nurse react when a patient or staff member touches her? Each one's reaction to touch depends on the interpretation of the gesture, cultural background, level of social maturity and the appropriateness of the touching gesture both to the relationship and the setting.

Observation and Perception

Observation and perception comprise two more tools of communication. Observation is an active process referring to the noting of a fact or event, whereas perception refers to the "process by which we select, organize, and interpret sensory stimulation into a meaningful and coherent picture of the world" (Hamachek, 1971, p.33). Observation seldom occurs without the attachment of personalized perceptions. What each one observes about another depends on the observer's frame of reference and value system. Have you ever looked at a picture with a friend and, in discussing it, found that you each see different pictorial aspects?

The following factors are identified as primary influence in what each one observes:

1. Physical, mental and emotional states and needs of the person
2. Cultural, social and philosophical background
3. Number and functioning ability of the senses involved
4. Past experiences associated with the present situation
5. Meaning of the observed event to the self
6. Interests, preoccupations, preconceptions and motivational level
7. Knowledge of or familiarity with the situation being observed
8. Practice in purposeful observation
9. Environmental conditions and distractions
10. Availability of technical devices
11. Presence, attitudes and reactions of others; for even if observations and perceptions are accurate, if they do not agree with group consensus, the person is likely to conform to the group (Murray and Zentner, 1975, p. 52).

Consider the following perceptual differences which might occur at dinner time in a psychiatric unit. The nurse, who has not eaten since breakfast, brings a well-appointed dinner tray to Mr. Jones, who has just been informed by his physician that he will have electroconvulsive therapy at 8 o'clock the following morning. Mr. Jones receives this information with great fear and foreboding which he fails to communicate to his physician. His stomach seems tied in knots, and he begins to feel nauseated. When the nurse says, "Mr. Jones, here is your dinner," and he responds, "I'm not hungry," a perceptual gap occurs if the nurse goes on to say, "Oh, it looks good; eat it and you will feel better." Unless the nurse responds to Mr. Jones' nonverbal cues, the interaction will terminate with no effective communication occurring.

Not only do an individual's basic needs and values affect his perceptions, but his view of self is instrumental in observing and perceiving. The view a man holds of himself affects his perceptions. Consider Mrs. Bills, an attractive 35-year-old woman who recently lost more than 50 pounds, yet continues to view herself as an obese, unattractive person. Upon discharge from the hospital, job planning may be influenced by her self-view. The nurse may help Mrs. Bills problem-solve to determine which type of employment will suit her abilities and needs. Mrs. Bills says, "I would prefer factory work to working in a department store." When the nurse asks Mrs. Bills to list the advantages and disadvantages of each type of work she replies, "I am so ugly the world should be spared from seeing me." The nursing response should help Mrs. Bills clarify what would be the disadvantage of everyone seeing her. It may be that she cannot give up her negative self-view at this time, and the nursing action would be to accept her decision and continue working in ways to validate her self-worth. Often a technique such as asking a person to speak about qualities he likes about himself for two minutes will provide clues both for the speaker and listener as to the person's self-perception and provide a starting point for communication. For many, two minutes of positive self-remarks seem like an eternity, whereas two minutes of negative self-characteristics can be accomplished with less difficulty.

What does the process of observation encompass? Observation seems such a spontaneous process that one seldom considers the components. For any observation to take place, a stimulus must be present. Something or someone must capture the attention of the observer. As mentioned, meaning is attached to the stimulus consistent with the observer's perceptual abilities. If the stimulus is new, unfamiliar or in some way antagonistic to the observer's expectations or preferences, he may have difficulty understanding the message. In the next step, the individual focuses attention and limits his perceptual field. For example, if the nurse is talking with a patient whose verbal and nonverbal messages are incongruent, she may focus attention on his frown rather than the pleasant words. By limiting the perceptual field, extraneous stimuli are excluded, and the observer's full attention can focus on the most relevant observational aspect.

Three characteristics define observation. First, it is purposeful either in a general or specific manner. The nurse's observation in performing a psychological assessment is purposeful in contrast to aimless examination and questioning. Secondly, effective observation is planned. The nurse thinks carefully about what she observes. Some observations occur spontaneously, although once a situation catches the nurse's attention and she narrows her perceptual field, she will begin to evaluate critically what she is observing. The nurse may be walking down the corridor of a psychiatric unit and smell a peculiar odor. She begins to observe more carefully in specific areas to locate the source of the odor. She immediately plans a course of action. If the odor smells like smoke from a fire, she may call for other staff to assist her, whereas if it smells like marijuana smoke she will look in the bathroom and closets of the rooms where the smell is most intense.

Objectivity, the third characteristic of observation, refers to truth and lack of bias rather than to emotional coldness and aloofness. Experience is a great teacher of observational ability regarding objectivity. As one notes the observational areas in which he seems blind, objectivity increases. Co-workers assist in developing objectivity by helping an individual see what he at first misses in a situation.

Silence

Silence is a potent communication tool. If silence is to facilitate communication, the nurse must recognize the types of silence. At times silence impedes communication and needs to be interrupted, whereas at other times it is a facilitator of communication. The following types of silence are identified:

1. Thoughtful or contemplative silence occurs when the person is thinking through a situation or trying to sort out information so as to respond. This is a productive silence and should not be interrupted unless it is prolonged. In terminating a silence, the

nurse needs to be aware if she is interrupting the silence to meet her needs or those of the patient.
2. Nonproductive silences occur when the patient is bored. If the nurse detects signs of boredom such as an averted glance and overt disinterest, she needs to interrupt the silence and attempt to determine the cause of the stalemate.
3. Silence may occur when the patient is fearful and unable or unwilling to venture into communication. The nurse might interrupt the silence by asking the patient what he is feeling at that moment. The patient may be experiencing anger, which he is reluctant to express for fear of alienating the person with whom he is communicating. He may also have had previous interactions with the person during which he felt intimidated. The nurse's presence may provide support, and if the patient feels accepted, he may feel free to express himself.

Listening

Listening is the fifth tool of communication. It is rarely an innate endowment but more often a patiently learned skill. Carl Rogers, in describing some of the satisfactions he has received from many years of working with human beings says, "When I can really hear someone, it puts me in touch with him" (1969, p. 222). He also says, "When I have been listened to and when I have been heard, I am able to reperceive my world in a new way and to go on" (Rogers, 1969, p. 224). Thus listening, a way of communicating "I care about," fosters the nurse-patient relationship.

Listening consists of more than just hearing. It is an active process requiring the nurse's complete attention and considerable psychic energy. An ideal situation in which to practice effective listening is with a patient who has numerous complaints. Often a patient's complaints are merely a camouflage for feelings of a more personal nature such as fear, loneliness, insecurity or helplessness. Before filling a request, the nurse tries to determine what the patient is experiencing when he complains or makes numerous requests. Is he really asking for a glass of water, or is he lonely? Is he in need of medication for pain, or is he afraid that no one will voluntarily pay attention to him? Is his room really too warm or is he asking to be noticed, to be cared for, as one with human suffering and needs?

Often the nurse responds to the overt demands of the patient and ignores the covert pleas. Not to hear what he is really saying and asking for is like giving aspirin for a broken leg. Unless the broken leg is set and put in a cast, the injury is unlikely to heal. Likewise patient's needs, though not specifically stated, are unlikely to be met unless careful listening occurs.

MODES OF COMMUNICATION

Bormann (1969) categorizes individuals according to their ability and typical mode of interacting. He describes source-oriented persons as being preoccupied with themselves during the conversation. This type of person feels insecure in relationships and worries about how he is coming across. Typical source-oriented behavior includes a loud voice, exaggerated gestures, lack of eye contact and frequent topic changes. In providing nursing care to a source-oriented person, gradually change his psychological environment by keeping him informed of what is going on around him and what he can expect to happen to him, providing opportunities for him to express himself and keeping him informed of his progress. Each of these interventions serves to reduce the psychological threat. Once he views the environment as less threatening, his conversation will become more personal, verbal and descriptive.

The message-oriented person has a strong task orientation. He is too busy merely to sit around and talk. He cannot take time to be concerned with the feelings and reactions of others. Frequently, the task or procedure-oriented nurse fits into this category.

Typical of the third mode of communication is the receiver-oriented person who has a strong commitment to help people grow as human beings. This person recognizes the importance of trust and is able to listen to others, thus facilitating their trusting him. The receiver-oriented person utilizes a variety of communication techniques to encourage the other person to keep talking.

Although conversation with a patient may be initiated by the nurse, it is important that the patient have some control of the conversation. The nurse avoids, when possible, asking direct questions and tries to ask open-ended questions so the patient cannot answer by saying either "yes" or "no." The verbal activity of the nurse is at a minimum, with the patient doing much of the talking.

The first conversation the nurse initiates with a patient in a psychiatric area may be uncomfortable for both participants. In the initial greeting, the nurse finds her personalized style of interaction, although it is best not to be overly cheerful or deadly solemn. It may be helpful to introduce a neutral topic. When the nurse first meets a patient, her relationship with him is not so clearly defined that she can immediately pursue interpersonal topics. Indeed, it may be seen as a sign of poor mental health if the patient pours out his problems immediately after meeting the nurse.

ASPECTS OF CONVERSATION

The behavior of each participant in a conversation depends largely on his growth and developmental input. Rarely does a person think consciously about everything he says. Much speech is spontaneous. Moreover, not every message is received with the same intent as the sender anticipated. The Johari Window Concept (Figure 4-3) provides a framework for looking at interactions (Chicago Board of Education).

| | PERSON ||
	Known to Self	Not Known to Self
Known to Others	I Area of Free Activity	II Blind Area
Not Known to Others	III Area Avoided or Hidden	IV Area of Unknown

Figure 4-3

Area I refers to that which each of us is willing to display openly and which observers can perceive. This area includes, in addition to manifest behavior, known thought, ideas, beliefs, values, motives and feelings.

Area II represents that which others see in us but of which we are unaware. This includes a person's mannerisms or characteristic way of speaking.

Area III represents behavior which is known to each person. The individual has conscious control of whether or not he will display this aspect of himself. This includes actions which may not be appropriate to different groups in which the individual has contact. In essence, he matches his behavior to the trends and expectations of the group with which he is interacting.

Area IV includes behavior of which the individual is unaware. This behavior may be seen when in the presence of a strong leader, or when the person is unable consciously to control how he behaves.

In an unfamiliar group, Area I is generally small with limited free and spontaneous interaction, until trust and some sense of safety are obtained. The operational definition of finding meaning in relationships in a new or ambiguous group is as follows: New situation—anxiety—seeking help from expert on task and role definition—perception of a refusal to help—increase in anxiety and dependency (Chicago Board of Education).

TECHNIQUES THAT FACILITATE COMMUNICATION

Few individuals have an innate ability to say the right thing at the right time on a consistent basis. For the majority of people, effective communication is a learned process. It is learned through study, self-awareness, collaboration with others and experience. The nurse uses a variety of techniques to keep the interaction with a patient moving, knowing that any technique overused loses its effectiveness. Communication techniques assist the nurse in keeping the patient actively involved in the interaction. Therapeutic communication facilitates the formation of an effective nurse-patient relationship and fulfills the purposes of the nursing process.

Therapeutic communication involves both nurse and patient in the planning of nursing interventions. It permits mutuality in nurse-patient interaction. A variety of techniques is available for the nurse to use in communication. Techniques alone do not guarantee communication; the attitude of the nurse is of crucial importance. Attitude is conveyed in each verbal comment and nonverbal gesture or movement. When the nurse tells the patient either by words or by thoughtful, caring actions that he is important to her, she enhances his self-view. Congruency between verbal and nonverbal communication determines how effective communication techniques are. If the nurse says, "I have time to sit with you," and during periods of silence gazes around the room, jumps up to arrange items on the bedside table or continuously swings her leg, the patient detects an incongruent message.

The following techniques, used appropriately, serve to facilitate communication:

1. *Asking direct questions:* This technique may be useful in completing an assessment of the patient but is certainly not the only communication technique available. Direct questions do not tend to facilitate maximum participation and often lead to dead ends in the conversation. For example, "Mr. Jones, do you have any children?" may evoke the reply, "Yes," thereby ending this segment of conversation. A more facilitative nursing response might have been, "Mr. Jones, tell me about your family." In the second response, the patient is more apt to elaborate than when asked a direct question. Often students ask innumerable direct questions to allay personal anxiety. In asking questions, it is important to remember that "how" asks for process; "why" asks for reasons, causes, explanations or conclusions; "which" asks for a choice or decision; "who," for the name of a person; "where," for the name of a place; "what," for the name of a thing; and "when," for a time sequence.

2. *Asking open-ended questions:* This technique is helpful in assessing what a patient thinks and how he feels. Asking open-ended questions provides the patient with a relaxed framework within which to respond. Broad, open-ended comments allow the patient to decide the direction of the interaction. They also convey the message, "I believe you can help yourself." Questions such as "Where would you like to begin today?" allow a person flexibility of focus. Questioning may revolve around the analysis of a recent situation, which has left the individual with ambivalent or negative feelings.

3. *The reflective response:* This communication technique encourages elaboration, conveying to the person that both his words and feeling tone are heard. In the reflective response, the nurse paraphrases the feelings she hears. For example, "Mr. Smith, it sounds like you're really angry at . . ." In the reflective response, the word *you* should be emphasized.

The reflective response helps the person to explore his thoughts and feelings about a situation. The listener thereby facilitates communication for the speaker. The following interaction demonstrates the reflective response:

Client: My teachers don't understand me. They tell my father that I am withdrawn and sit around daydreaming all day.
Nurse: You feel that your teachers don't understand you?
Client: Right, they have a mold for the ideal student and I don't fit the mold.

The nurse's response may be tangential to what the patient is actually expressing; this occurs when the nurse is not skilled in communication, is anxious or has not given the patient her undivided attention. When the nurse frequently "misses" what the patient is trying to communicate, she cuts him off from the understanding he needs and may not know how to ask for.

4. *Small talk and the introduction of neutral topics* may be used at the beginning of a conversation to put both nurse and patient at ease. This technique must be neither overused nor used in times of high emotion. A patient, upset over a home visit, is in no mood to discuss the patients' social outing for the week. The timing at which each technique is used facilitates communication. Careful assessment of each interaction provides information on the appropriateness of the technique as well as the timing.

5. *Confrontation* can either facilitate or block communication. In facilitating communication, confrontation refers to "laying the cards on the table and looking at them as they are." Confrontation must be followed by problem-solving, whereby the patient makes a concrete plan for future action. For example, Jane is an obese 26-year-old woman adept at sneaking extra food when eating in the hospital cafeteria. She has been restricted to eating on the unit in order to limit her caloric intake. Jane protests this action and says the people who say she sneaks food are lying. The nurse confronts Jane with the 5-pound weight gain the past week and the two slices of cake found in her purse. The nurse goes on to plan with Jane a way for her to eat in the cafeteria and not eat more than her allotted food. This may initially require that the nurse sit with her. It may be that Jane feels lonely and alienated at meals and overeats to compensate for the empty feeling. Perhaps the choice of food on her diet

is not appealing. Success on the diet may follow a conference with the dietary staff to arrange choices or a different food selection for Jane. In problem-solving, Jane should participate in deciding which approach might work for her. If the nurse makes the plan with Jane reluctantly agreeing, the probability of success is limited.

6. *Seeking clarification* helps both nurse and patient understand what is being communicated. It is an attempt to understand what is being communicated by feeding back to the sender the message which was heard. Examples of the clarifying response include, "I am not sure I understand what you mean" or "Would you explain that again?" The nurse thus conveys that she is listening and wants to understand the patient's message but needs further assistance to do so. If the patient talks about seeing red dots on the walls, the nurse might respond, "Can you tell me more about what you see?" or "What is happening with you right now?" or "What are you feeling now?" Once the patient discusses his perceptions, it is useful for the nurse to present reality such as, "There are no red dots on the wall; it must be frightening to see things that others don't see." Clarification is useful when patients speak in global or unclear terms. Patients often use global pronouns that must be clarified. When the patient refers to he, they, we or other vague and non-specific referents, the nurse needs to clarify who "they" are. At times the patient may be referring to imaginary persons or things, and this must be determined. It is not essential to understand everything the patient says as long as one honestly lets him realize one's doubt about his meaning.

7. *Restating* occurs when the nurse puts the patient's message into her own words. The patient might say, "I can't eat. I just sit at the table staring at my food." The nurse would restate something like, "You are having a lot of difficulty eating now." This approach brings out related aspects that one may previously have missed. It is another way of saying, "I am listening to you." Restatement also allows the person to validate that the nurse has understood him. An example of restatement is:

Patient: My father is not happy with me because I skipped school a few times. He says I am withdrawn and he cannot handle me anymore.
Nurse: He says he cannot handle you?

Patient: Right, that all I do is sit around, and I never get involved with other people.

8. *Placing an event in the correct order* helps the patient examine what happened in relation to other events. It is helpful to discuss the event in a sequence of actions, thoughts and then feelings. Most people find it easier to speak about what happened than to speak of thoughts and feelings. Thoughts are often easier to discuss than feelings. A trusting relationship must exist before two individuals can discuss feelings. Questions such as, "What led up to . . .?", "When did this happen?" and "What were you doing when this happened?" reconstruct the event. Focusing next on "What did you think when . . . happened?" and moving on to "What feeling can you identify in relation to . . .?" or "It sounds like you were really angry at . . ." help to describe the situation.

Following a reconstruction of the event and identification of thoughts and feelings, the next step is to problem-solve and help the patient examine available alternatives for action should a similar situation occur, as well as to describe other courses of action which were available to him when he acted in a less productive manner.

9. *Encouraging comparisons* of both similarities and differences helps the patient relate situations to each other. Statements such as, "How was this like . . .?" or "What was the biggest difference between . . .?" help to relate situations one to another.

10. *Acknowledging* communicates to the patient that you heard him, and that you are an active participant in the conversation. Examples of acknowledging comments include, "Yes" and "I hear what you're saying."

11. *Door-openers* are invitations for the patient to say more. This technique is particularly effective when the patient stops speaking in the middle of a statement or conversation, when it seems indicated for him to continue. Invitations to say more include, "Tell me about it," "I'd be interested in what you have to say" or "Go on."

12. *Focusing on specifics* is useful for patients who speak in global terms due to high levels of anxiety. For example, a patient says, "Everyone hates me at school. All the teachers yell at me." It is use-

ful for the nurse to ask the patient to tell her about the last time a teacher yelled at him. The nurse helps the patient focus on the time sequence such as the last time, one time, the worst time or the best time something happened.

13. *Voicing doubt* helps patients separate fantasy from reality. For example, when a patient says, "I was in the Miss America Pageant last week," and the nurse responds, "You would really like to be in the pageant?" or "You were in the hospital last week, but I imagine you would like very much to be in the pageant," the nurse is focusing on reality by casting doubt on the patient's assertion. Her approach is also ego-preserving in that the patient is neither censured, ridiculed nor contradicted. In voicing doubt, the purpose is to present alternate ways of thinking about the subject, not to attempt to convince the patient of the error in his thinking by engaging in an argument. Arguing with a patient only provokes resistance and strengthens his point of view. The important message to communicate is that not everyone sees the situation as he does, nor do all draw the same conclusions. By expressing doubt, one may reinforce some doubtful inklings the patient has but hesitates to consider. Statements such as, "That is hard for me to believe," or "Did it really happen just as you describe it?" serve to voice doubt.

14. *Verbalizing the implied* or what the patient has hinted at or made subtle references to faciliitates communication. For example, if the patient says, "I bet it would be fun to go swimming at the community pool," the nurse might respond, "Have you asked the doctor to allow you to go swimming?" thus conveying that the patient's wish has a basis in reality; that he might be able to go swimming, but that he has to take the initiative in seeking permission.

15. *Summarizing:* Toward the conclusion of an interaction, it is helpful to summarize with the patient the main points of the conversation. Summarizing provides closure and helps both nurse and patient recall the most relevant points of the discussion. The summary may lead to a plan for the next interaction. An instance in which the nurse summarizes an interaction would be:

Nurse: Today we talked about several of the problems you have when you work full-time. What do you see as the most important area for us to discuss tomorrow?

Patient: I really want to look at ways to organize my time at work so I don't get so flustered.

BLOCKS TO COMMUNICATION

The failure to facilitate communication occurs when the environment is distracting, the receiver has a limited capacity for receipt of information or when the behavioral approach or technique used is ineffective.

Distractions in the environment hamper communication, such as when loud music, other people speaking nearby or machinery interfere with the sending or receiving of a message. In addition, the temperature of the room may prove distracting if the patient or nurse feels uncomfortable due to temperature extremes.

Limitations of the receiver's capacity to communicate occur when there is an impairment in the ability to see, hear or comprehend all incoming stimuli. If the sender is talking too rapidly for the receiver to comprehend, if two people are talking at once or if the patient is hearing an imaginary voice, communication is not effective.

The manner in which the nurse approaches an interaction affects the patient's receptivity. When the nurse appears stiff and stilted and uses unfamiliar language, the patient may not respond warmly. Frequently, students as well as graduate nurses try too hard to be like the role models they respect and desire to emulate. Rarely can one person assume the style of another and appear genuine. Students must develop a personalized style based on principles of behavior, using language in their typical vocabulary. A beginning student in psychiatric nursing is invariably spotted when she asks, "What do you think about that?" or "How did that make you feel?" Both therapeutic and social relationships are affected by the overuse of newly learned phrases and jargon.

Internal distractions are more difficult to control than external distractions, since the sender may be unaware of their presence. The sender's nonverbal behavior may provide clues to feelings of increasing anxiety such as when he fidgets in his chair, twirls a strand of hair or continuously cracks his knuckles.

Communication is also hampered when the nurse brings judgmental feelings to the clinical setting and is unaware of the existence of these feelings. A student must be aware of the biases and feelings she brings to the setting and accept them with the recognition that it is her right to have beliefs and opinions. Somewhere in life, most individuals adopt the assumption that they "should" like everyone else. This assumption proves a handicap in the psychiatric setting, for not all patients prove likeable to each nurse. Some remind students of either liked or disliked persons known in the past.

Judgmental statements include "that's good," "that's bad," "you should" and "why don't you?" These statements convey that the nurse's values, opinions and beliefs are more important than the patient's. They are conditional in that the covert message is, "I will accept you if . . ." Judgmental messages foster a negative self-view, in that the patient is spoken down to, not treated as an equal.

A further block to communication occurs when the student experiences ambivalence. This refers to simultaneous positive and negative feelings toward an object, person or action. The difficulty arises when the nurse denies the negative component of the ambivalence due to guilt feelings at entertaining unkind feelings toward a patient. A common belief in the helping professions is that it is not acceptable to find some patients disagreeable. A nurse does herself a disservice when she censures negative feelings, for she denies herself the privilege of an honest feeling. When anger is not dealt with directly, it comes through in covert ways such as the overly sweet smile, the slightly loud slam of the door or the delay in responding to a patient's request.

Ambivalence is a normal, universal feeling. Doubtless the student who loves his parents dearly can recall moments of great anger. In dealing with ambivalence, it is helpful to sort out whether feelings of dislike are for the person or his behavior. Each of us may care about a person, yet be angered by his behavior.

Reassurance occurs when the nurse jumps ahead of the patient and replies with a cliche which serves to block further therapeutic communication. Common examples of reassurance include, "Nothing can be that bad" or "Everything will be all right." The nurse, in using such cliches, communicates to the patient that what he has to say is unimportant. Patients are actually reassured when they are helped to use their own skills to work with problems that seem overwhelming at the outset. By definition, reassurance means to restore confidence, and this can be achieved only when the nurse knows that her reassurances are factual. It involves assuring the patient that the situation with which he is struggling does have a solution. Also, in moments of great anxiety, reassurance comes from being not alone.

Rejecting a patient's point of view is a major communication block occurring when a person reacts to an emotionally charged statement by evaluating it from his own point of view. An example of this occurs when a patient says, "This is the worst hospital in the city. Not one nurse here cares if the patients get better or not, and the doctors hope we won't get better because they make their money off our being sick." The communication block occurs when the nurse replies, "Mr. J, this is a fine hospital, and we do our best for all of our patients." The nurse's defensive response indicates that she is listening only to the overt message. What might have been Mr. J's response had the nurse said, "Mr. J, it sounds like you are worried that you are not getting better?" If the nurse can listen with understanding (empathy) and try to hear the feelings being covertly expressed, she has a greater opportunity to communicate effectively. An exercise for effective listening is when in a heated discussion, before presenting one's point of view, stop and try to understand and summarize the other person's thoughts aloud.

The myth in nursing that "a good nurse is a busy nurse" often blocks communication. In developing the ability to communicate effectively, it is imperative that messages be accurately received; to receive messages the nurse must listen. In the role of listener, the nurse, often sitting at the patient's bedside, may appear passive and "not working." When a nurse perceives her role as task-oriented, she is "too busy" to take time to listen. Patients are not encouraged to express needs and feelings to the nurse who appears to be on a "100-yard dash" through her day's activities. Just as listening is essential to the development of the nurse-patient relationship, failure to listen prevents relationship formation. Failure to listen represents an inability of the nurse to direct her attention outside herself and place the needs of the patient above her own needs. Failure to listen is further noted when the nurse cuts the patient off before he finishes speaking, asks a question without waiting for an answer or fails to hear the implied or covert message. Not listening implies that "I am not concerned with you. You are of little value to me."

The nurse who is unable to wait or to tolerate silence may feel that when she is not doing something (either a nursing care activity or speaking), she is wasting time. Her first impulse in talking with the patient who responds slowly may be to fill in the conversation gaps with questions. One student noted in talking with a nearly catatonic adolescent that the patient would allow two- to three-minute pauses between the nurse's questions and her response. The student found it impossible to wait for the patient to answer and went on to ask a second question. When the patient responded, it was to answer the first question. Difficult as it may be, waiting often pays off in that it conveys to the patient that the nurse is genuinely interested.

Learning to sit with a silent person is a difficult lesson. Initially, the student may only be able to sit in silence for two to three minutes; she may need to leave the room as her anxiety level increases. In an interview setting, silence may be hostile or rejecting, secure or accepting. In an interpersonal relationship, what is not said may be as meaningful as what is actually said. It is necessary to "listen between the lines." When does a patient stop talking? What was said immediately before the silence? What is one's characteristic way of handling silence? Can one tolerate silence enough to wait until the patient speaks again?

Giving advice or trying to persuade the patient may block communication. For example, when a nurse says "If I were you ... ," she is trying to impose her values and choices on another. The nurse is not the patient; she has never dealt with his problem situations and has limited information about what has been effective for him in the past. A further drawback to giving advice is that it encourages dependency. The nurse may meet her needs when she fosters dependency in the patient; extensive dependency upon another adult is rarely growth-producing for the patient. Also when the nurse gives advice to the patient, she assumes part of the responsibility for the patient's actions. For example, if the patient is angry with his wife, the nurse might respond with, "If I were you I would tell her how angry I feel; be forceful and honest when you talk with your wife." The patient subsequently goes out on pass and says to his wife, "I am furious with you, and I would like to bash you right between the eyes." The wife, upon hearing the patient's words as well as the undisguised anger motivating them, dashes out of the house to spend the entire day with her mother. When the patient returns to the hospital, he immediately finds the nurse and yells, "It is all your fault; you told me to tell my wife how angry I was and now look what happened."

Sermonettes, used frequently when the patient says something which collides with the nurse's value system, block communication.

For example, if the patient talks about the great feelings he experiences when he steals citizen band radios to support his drug habit, the nurse may respond with a judgmental statement. Upon hearing a patient say, "Those fat, middle-class dudes don't need their CB's as much as I need my grass," the nurse might deliver a mini-sermon on the consequences of stealing, respect for the property of others and the detrimental effects of marijuana. This interaction is likely to be laced with several shoulds and oughts, both serving to turn off the listener from further listening.

Disagreeing or criticizing often occurs when the student has difficulty keeping her values out of the interaction. For example, when the patient says, "I am the world's best baseball player," and the nurse replies, "I disagree; you missed three balls in the first ten minutes of the last game," the nurse's needs are generally being met at the expense of the patient. A more facilitative approach to protect the patient's self-image would be to focus on his obvious skill if he is an adequate player, or to voice doubt if he is a weak player. The nurse might say, "You do hit the balls well" or "You really try to play a good game."

Patients may ask questions which cause the nursing student to feel uncomfortable. The subsequent ill-at-ease feelings of the student, if not identified and dealt with, impair communication. Frequently, patients are more similar to students than they are different; they may be near the same age, from the same community or remind the student of a close friend or relative. A patient may also ask questions of a personal nature. The student's first response is often to look for a mode of escape and subsequently avoid the patient. It is well to remember that when a patient asks a question, the student does not always have to answer. It is essential, though, to let the patient know that he has been heard by saying, for example, "I heard what you said, but I would prefer not discussing my own family situation." At times the patient asks personal questions, because he knows no other way to begin a conversation. Some patients are much like children in their recognition that acceptable and expected questions may elicit minimal responses, whereas questions of a less acceptable nature are sure to get the listener's full attention.

It is not uncommon for patients to ask for the student's telephone number and address. In deciding upon a response to such a request, one must consider how much free time she is willing to devote to a patient. What will the student's response be if a patient calls on a Saturday night just as she is preparing to go on a date? For a patient to call a student and be rejected is yet another blow to a generally low self-image. Once the student decides how she will handle requests for addresses and telephone numbers, it is helpful to explore with the patient his reason for wanting the information. For example, the patient might ask, "Where do you live?"

Student: I live in a dormitory.
Patient: What is your telephone number?
Student: What would you do with my number if I gave it to you?
Patient: I would call you.
Student: What purpose would calling me have? (Or how would calling me be helpful to you?)
Patient: Sometimes I get really lonely, especially in the evenings.
Student: What is it about the evenings that causes you to feel lonely?
Patient: I am scared of being alone, and sometimes there is no one else at home with me at night.
Student: Would you like to think of ways to deal with this fear and loneliness?

By pursuing with the patient his purpose in calling her, the student discovers a deeper issue than the patient's actually wanting to talk with the student.

CRITERIA FOR EVALUATING NURSE-PATIENT COMMUNICATION

Five criteria are used for evaluating nurse-patient communication: effectiveness, appropriateness, adequacy, efficiency and flexibility (Sundeen, *et al.,* 1976). Effectiveness determines how completely the communication met the goals of the interaction. It is not easy to evaluate effectiveness at the time of the interaction. A person may seem to be responding positively to a situation when, in actuality, he is confused or frightened about the content of the interaction. In determining effectiveness, it is helpful to watch carefully for both verbal and nonverbal cues to message reception.

In determining communication effectiveness, the interactional outcome is measured against the designated goals. Communication is facilitated when the nurse is informed about the topic of discussion, is flexible and able to talk about the client's priority and is sensitive to cues generated in the interaction. The following student-client interaction provides an opportunity to assess the lack of effectiveness of the communication:

Miss Jones, a student nurse, was assigned to meet weekly with a 9-year-old boy recently placed in a home for dependent and neglected children. Joey and his brothers, ages 5 and 7, were being given up permanently by a mother who had neglected and abused them for years. Eventually the boys would be placed for adoption. Each child was assigned a sponsor family in the community who regularly invited him to their home. In Joey's case, after two visits to Mr. and Mrs. Smith's home, the couple decided to begin adoption procedures. Both Mr. and Mrs. Smith had been previously married. Mrs. Smith had a 6-year-old daughter, and Mr. Smith had a 7-year-old daughter and a 9-year-old son.

As Miss Jones began meeting with Joey, she was also able to visit Mrs. Smith to discuss any concerns regarding being a sponsor family. During the first home visit, Mrs. Smith mentioned how much she hoped to adopt Joey. The student, forgetting that the Smith's were both a sponsor family and a tentative adoptive family, asked if they planned to adopt Joey. Mrs. Smith immediately asked if another family was under study for the adoption. When the student replied that she knew a family was under study but did not know who they were, Mrs. Smith said they had applied but now wondered if the agency had two families under consideration.

When the student left that day, she thought the issue of who was applying to adopt Joey was settled, since she had carefully explained to Mrs. Smith that she obviously had been confused herself. The following day, Miss Jones met with Joey, who also asked if the Smiths were going to adopt him. The student responded that she really was not sure.

Little did Miss Jones know that immediately after she left the Smith's home, Mrs. Smith called the agency. She was worried that the agency staff were misleading her by telling her they only studied one family at a time for each child. On the week-end after the confusion, Joey visited the Smiths and had several nightmares. Mrs. Smith became increasingly upset, feeling that she was doing something wrong or that Joey did not like her family. She also wondered if the agency was being truthful in that they rarely placed children with families having a history of divorce.

Eventually, the entire misunderstanding was clarified, and Mrs.

Smith learned that Joey's brother had been placed for adoption the day prior to the week-end beset with nightmares. Joey was not reacting to the Smith family but was grieving for the loss of a cherished source of support.

In assessing the situation as to the effectiveness of the communication appropriateness is considered first. Appropriateness refers to the relevancy of the communication in meeting the desired outcomes (Davis, 1963). The student's lack of information caused the communication to lack appropriateness. Her goal in making the home visit was to offer support to the sponsor family, since bringing a child into an established family system can upset the equilibrium. Instead of providing support, the communication disrupted the equilibrium.

The adequacy of the communication refers to the amount of communication used to reach the goal. In this case, an excessive amount of time was spent by the student, agency staff and nursing instructor in clarifying the communication to decrease Mrs. Smith's anxiety.

If communication is to be efficient, simple and concise language is used. In this case, the student's lack of information prevented her from efficiently communicating in that her comments were preceded by, "I don't really know," or "I'm not sure."

In the initial student patient interaction, flexibility was evidenced when the student acknowledged her uncertainty as to the validity of her impression. Mrs. Smith was unable to deal with the flexibility due to her high level of anxiety. Later, when the instructor accompanied Miss Jones on a home visit, the situation was analyzed, and each could identify ways in which the communication had become confused.

PRINCIPLES

1. Clarification leads to increased communication.
2. Reflection of feelings increases communication.
3. "How" questions ask for process.
4. "Why" questions ask for reasons, causes, explanations or conclusions.
5. "Why" questions often elicit a defensive rssponse, as the individual being questioned may be threatened by the question.

6. Encouraging description of thoughts and feelings increases recall.
7. Successful interviewing depends upon attitudes of acceptance, objectivity, kindness and warmth.
8. A comfortable environment is conducive to successful interviewing.
9. Interviewing is more effective when geared to the interviewee's age and mental and physical capabilities.
10. The greater the congruence between the sender's verbal message and the simultaneously sent nonverbal message, the more likely the receiver is to pick up an accurate message.

SUMMARY

Communication influences all aspects of the nursing process. Without effective communication, an accurate assessment becomes impossible, thereby debilitating all further stages of the nursing process. Communication is more than attending to the actual words; it is listening to the spoken as well as unspoken, implied message. Communication means listening for congruence between what is said, the way in which it is said and the subtle factors conveying added information.

An important aspect of communication includes observation. How does the speaker look, what gestures does he demonstrate, is his affect appropriate to the content he is describing? Communication transcends the spoken word and includes actions such as touching, grimacing, smiling, crying and silence.

While some individuals seem to possess an innate ability to communicate effectively, others find the study and practice of communication techniques to be beneficial. A variety of techniques can be utilized to facilitate communication. Moreover, an awareness of commonly observed blocks to communication tends to remind the nurse of ineffective technology.

BIBLIOGRAPHY

Applbaum, Ronald, et al. *Fundamental Concepts in Human Communication.* San Francisco: Canfield Press, 1973.

Bormann, Ernest, et al. *Interpersonal Communication in the Modern Organization.* Englewood Cliffs, N.J.: Prentice-Hall, 1969.

Brill, Naomi. *Working with People: The Helping Process.* New York: J.B. Lippincott Co., 1973.

Chicago Board of Education. Johari Window. In-Service Training Component. Department of Human Relations. Chicago, Illinois: Chicago Board of Education.

Davis, Anne. "The Skills of Communication," *American Journal of Nursing,* LXIII, No. 1 (January, 1963), 66-70.

Gordon, Thomas. "The Risks in Effective Communication," *National Training Laboratory Human Relations Training News,* IV, No. 4 (1961).

Hamachek, D. *Encounters with The Self.* New York: Holt, Rinehart and Winston, Inc., 1971.

"Hey You." Growing Up Ain't Easy. Mental Health Assoc. of Tarrant County, Texas.

Murray, Ruth and Zentner, Judith. *Nursing Concepts for Health Promotion.* Englewood Cliffs, N.J.: Prentice-Hall, Inc., 1975.

Rogers, C.R. *Freedom To Learn.* Columbus, Ohio: Charles E. Merrill, 1969.

Ruesch, Jurgen. *Therapeutic Communication.* New York: W.W. Norton Co., 1961.

Sundeen, S. et al. *Nurse-Client Interaction: Implementing the Nursing Process.* St. Louis: C.V. Mosby Co., 1976.

CHAPTER 5

Aspects of the Nurse-Patient Relationship

Jeanette Lancaster, R.N., Ph.D.

INTRODUCTION

The nurse-patient relationship refers to three sequential phases occurring in the implementation of the nursing process. These phases—orientation, working and termination—may not be clearly differentiated one from another, although selected tasks are appropriate to each phase.

The nurse-patient relationship is facilitated in either a structured one-to-one interaction or in a fluid, spontaneous format. In this chapter the term *interview* refers to any nurse-patient interaction, whether it occurs at a specific designated time or in response to an immediate patient need. Certain clinical settings readily lend themselves to a structured nurse-patient relationship, whereas others having a rapid patient turnover or daily bombardment with students do not provide intensive one-to-one relationships. When several groups of students have clinical experience on one unit weekly, the overstimulation to patients may be such that structured interview situations with more than one student group are contra-indicated.

In settings where structured interviews are not appropriate, principles of interviewing are applied to informal interactions. In actual practice, much of nursing intervention relates to spontaneous or fluid group interaction with the nurse responding to a patient or group of patients at the moment of need, in contrast to a mutually predetermined time.

Prior to the initial interaction, the student or graduate nurse needs to assess her reaction to the situation she anticipates encountering. She may have access to information about the patient before she meets him, or her reaction may be colored by the patient's age, race, sex or diagnostic label. Identification of preconceived notions facilitates self-awareness and hastens the nurse-patient relationship. Some students arrive on the psychiatric unit nearly immobilized with anticipatory anxiety toward this strange, unknown area of nursing.

To facilitate adjustment to the psychiatric clinical area, it is necessary to study a number of concepts comprising the framework for the nurse-patient relationship. Nursing, as both an art and a science, is founded on behavioral principles. The effective nurse recognizes that to provide competent nursing care, she must be more than a kind, well-meaning person. Certainly these characteristics are essential when coupled with a broad conceptual basis related to the dynamics of human behavior and the process of providing supportive services.

In providing nursing care, it is first essential to differentiate between the social and professional or therapeutic role. In a therapeutic relationship, the nurse assumes responsibility for the consequences of her behavior, works toward increased self-awareness and discriminates between facilitative and non-facilitative approaches for interaction with patients. Both nurse and patient enter the therapeutic relationship as strangers not friends. The nurse, early in her work in psychiatry, develops the ability to differentiate between her needs and those of the patient. Other staff members prove valuable in helping the nurse discriminate between whose needs are being met. Frequently, nursing care becomes "nurse-centered," that is, designed to meet the needs and convenience of the nurse rather than the patient. When a nurse ignores a patient's request because she does not want to interrupt what she is doing, her action is considered to be "nurse-centered nursing"; when she puts a patient in a seclusion room because, "I am tired of hearing him yell," her action is again nurse-centered. In contrast, when the nurse listens to a patient's request and refuses to meet the demand or request because it is contraindicated for the patient, or when the nurse places a patient in seclusion because he is overstimulated by the loud ward atmosphere, the care is "patient centered." Nursing practice is based on assessment of the needs of the patient at any given moment.

The nurse-patient relationship is professional, although the nurse is often sociable and friendly. In a social relationship, the needs of both nurse and patient are met, whereas a professional relationship focuses on the needs of the patient. A social relationship develops spontaneously, while a therapeutic relationship is planned to meet the patient's assessed needs.

In a social relationship, each participant expects to be respected and liked by the other person with the freedom of expression limited by accepted protocol. In contrast, in the therapeutic professional relationship, the patient is free to express thoughts and feelings which may not be socially desirable. The nurse accepts the patient as he is and begins planning interventions consistent with the patient's current level of functioning.

In the therapeutic situation, consistency and dependability are imperative. If the nurse says she will return in an hour, she must return or inform the patient immediately, either personally or by message, that she has been detained.

Social conversation is limited in the therapeutic relationship, and the nurse refrains from using cliches and reassuring the patient. Moreover, confidentiality, rigidly maintained in the therapeutic relationship, varies in the social relationship.

In a therapeutic relationship, the nurse is responsible for her behavior. She continually examines what she says and how she acts to assess the impact of her behavior on the patient. Thoughtless, impulsive or angry comments have no place in the therapeutic relationship. In the social relationship, some degree of rashness in communication and behavior may be tolerated.

CONFIDENTIALITY

Confidentiality is strictly maintained in all therapeutic relationships. The basic guideline regarding confidentiality is that all information about himself belongs to the patient, not to the staff or students; thus, if personal information is given to individuals not affiliated with the hospital or agency, it is an act of the patient, not of a member of the staff. Confidentiality implies not sharing privileged information with individuals outside the hospital setting, as well as not discussing one patient with another.

Caution is urged in discussing patients in any setting outside the clinical area. Often students mention the names of patients in cafeterias and other public areas not realizing they can be overheard. Respecting a patient's right for confidentiality is no easy task for the nursing student. Often, students have tremendous emotional reactions to patients or clinical occurrences and seek to discuss the event. Clinical events must be discussed in appropriate areas, maintaining the patient's right to privacy by not mentioning his name or sufficient descriptive information to identify him. Confidentiality also includes not mentioning the patient's name or identifying descriptive information in written work, as the work might fall into the hands of persons not involved in the clinical supervision.

On occasion, students meet friends and acquaintances who are patients in the psychiatric area. When this occurs, the student discusses confidentiality with the friend and assures him that his right for privacy will be maintained. Patients often fantasize that the student will tell mutual friends the full extent of their hospitalization and emotional problems.

On occasion, when a patient may ask that a nurse keep certain information confidential from other members of the staff, the nurse informs the patient that she cannot promise this. She has an obligation to share information that might harm the patient or others or that might describe actions the patient intends to take which would conflict with his treatment plan.

INVOLVEMENT

Involvement refers to "caring deeply about what is happening and what might happen to a person, then doing something with and for that person" (Goldsborough, 1969, p. 66). The nurse is involved with the patient as one caring human relating to another. The patient is not seen as a specimen or disease entity, and the nurse does not turn to a specific page in a book of care plans to decide how to relate to him. Each patient is unique with individualized needs and goals.

In the past, nurses have been urged to maintain an aloof, professional demeanor and to remain uninvolved with patients. This approach seems ineffective in that the majority of mentally disturbed persons suffer from difficulties in relationships. Involvement is essential in assessing and planning care. The nurse-patient relationship provides a rich medium for a patient to learn new communication skills.

Involvement begins on the day of admission. Initially, the nurse talks with the patient about non-threatening topics such as current events, social problems or his special interests. While these topics may not seem directly relevant to the therapeutic relationship, they provide an avenue for the patient to see the nurse as a person. The nursing role in most patient interactions is that of a listener. The nurse should not burden the patient with long discourses on her point of view. Each person has narcissistic tendencies; when an individual becomes overwhelmed with stress and requires hospitalization, his psychic energy is largely bound up within himself. Thus, patients have minimal interest in hearing detailed information about the nurse and her opinions. Involvement implies that the nurse creates an atmosphere where a patient can freely discuss his feelings; accepts him as a person with every right to self-expression; and actively seeks to understand the patient's perspective.

Objectivity is implicit in involvement. As the nurse begins genuinely to care for a patient, she may have difficulty differentiating between a therapeutic professional relationship and a social relationship. Her ability to see the patient as a unique individual whose needs are separate from her own may be decreased. She may think that the patient is helpless without her support and encouragement, or that she is the only nurse able to recognize his needs and provide nursing measures. At this point, an instructor or supervisor can help the nurse to examine her own needs so as to discover what need of the nurse is being met by her "rescuing" feelings toward the patient.

EMPATHY

Empathy is the "ability to enter into the life of another person, to accurately perceive his current feelings and their meanings" (Kalish, 1973, p. 1548). Empathy is an essential component of the nursing process, for it is only through the ability to empathize with a patient that the nurse is able to recognize covert, subtle needs. In the nurse-patient relationship "to empathize means to share and experience the feelings of the patient" (Ehmann, 1971, p. 76). Empathy deals with the current feelings of the patient, not what he felt yesterday or last week.

According to Ehmann (1971), "empathy occurs in response to cues, verbal or nonverbal, sent by another person, and we are seldom aware of our assimilation of the cues" (p. 72). Through empathy we abandon ourselves temporarily and walk as though in the other's shoes. Empathy enables each of us to understand another, to hear his needs, feel his pain, and gain a deeper understanding of him.

Empathy is described by Harry Stack Sullivan (1954) as one of the first modes an infant has for relating to another. Initially, an infant perceives the tension and anxiety in the mothering one; he feels with the mothering one and experiences the anxiety she experiences.

Kalish (1973), in differentiating between empathy and sympathy, says that "in empathy the helper borrows his patient's feelings in order to freely understand them, but he is always aware of his own separateness. He realizes that the feelings of the patient are not his own" (p. 1548). In contrast, sympathy denotes a process whereby the helper loses his self-identity and incorporates the patient's feelings and situation as though it were his own. Carl Rogers (1958) describes the difference between empathy and sympathy when he notes that empathy is the ability "to sense the client's private world as if it were your own but without ever losing the 'as if' quality" (p. 99). If the nurse incorporates entirely the patient's feelings, she ceases to be of help in that she is likely to become as immobilized with the situation as the patient.

Moreover, in empathy, the patient retains responsibility for securing relief for his situation. The nurse communicates by word and/or attitude: "I hear your feeling of helplessness; I will work with you to problem-solve this situation." In sympathy, the nurse assumes some of the responsibility for solving the patient's problems. She says, in essence, "I hear your feeling; you are so unable to help yourself I will do for you what you cannot do for yourself." Or put another way, empathy is to feel *with* the person, and sympathy is to feel *for* him.

In communicating empathy, it is important to validate for the patient what was heard. If the nurse says, "I know how you feel," the patient has no idea of the perception of the situation. A more facilitative response might be, "I hear your feeling of pain" or "You seem ambivalent about your decision to go back to work."

Depending on the patient's verbal style, the nurse might use the word uncertain instead of ambivalent. As mentioned in Chapter 4, communication must be in the personalized style of the sender. In communicating empathy, use words that are a part of one's vocabulary to avoid sounding stilted and parrot-like. Not only must the words used be suited to one's style of speaking, but they must also be suited to the patient's level of comprehension. If a patient cannot understand the language of the nurse, he does not experience the empathic understanding the nurse is trying to communicate. In utilizing language meaningful to the patient the nurse does so without appearing artificial or unnatural. If the patient's language style is foreign to the nurse, her attempts to adopt the style seem stilted. For example, adolescents often use terms in ways contrary to the nurse's usage. If adopting the adolescent's style seems unnatural, it is better to use one's own words.

The nurse not only attempts to respond in a manner similar to that of the patient but also tries to match her feeling tone to the patient's. If the patient is speaking with anger, the nurse's response conveys the same tone. The nurse does not share the patient's feelings but borrows them to convey her understanding.

Kalish (1973) summarizes the value of empathetic communication by saying that it helps the patient overcome a feeling of loneliness or isolation in the world with his own problems; "that the nurse's willingness and desire to understand how the patient feels about his world implies that his point of view is of value" and "that empathic understanding places the focus of evaluation within the patient rather than within the helper" (p. 1552).

Empathy and acceptance go hand-in-hand in that the nurse does not offer advice, suggestions or make evaluative statements regarding what the patient says. Instead, she attempts to understand and accept the patient's feelings as she hears them being expressed. To listen for understanding is an active process requiring considerable energy. It is also a skill developed through practice.

ACCEPTANCE

Acceptance is a term casually used in the service-oriented professions, often with limited recognition given to the difficulties experienced in operationalizing the concept. Acceptance is more than being kind and agreeable to others. Acceptance represents a process or action forming an integral component of the nurse-patient relationship. The process involves self-awareness for the nurse, as well as recognition of possible value conflicts with patients. To be able to say, "I can accept you as you are, different as you are from me," is often a complex and agonizing task. Each one wants to impose his values and beliefs on others. Nurses are often characterized by egocentrism, the belief that one's point of view or way of doing something is the only or best way.

A non-judgmental, accepting attitude does not imply indifference to or rejection of value systems. It means, instead, that the nurse allows the patient the right to subscribe to his own set of beliefs without feeling "put down."

The first step in acceptance is to recognize judgmental feelings. This takes courage, honesty and the ability to tolerate the pain of self-examination. Secondly, the nurse must accept her own judgmental feelings and examine where each one came from. When a certain feeling surfaces, it is important to consider who and what comes spontaneously to mind. Each nurse must recognize that she has opinions, beliefs and values which need not change; similarly, she cannot expect the patient to change his value orientation so as to be consistent with hers.

Acceptance of another communicates recognition of the individual's intrinsic human worth. Each person is worthwhile, even though at times his behavior conflicts with acceptable standards for behaving. Acceptance does not imply permissiveness but rather indicates the ability to discriminate between the person and his actions. Acceptance means conveying to a patient: "You are an adequate, worthwhile person, although at the present time your behavior is not acceptable."

A graduate student's relationship with Miss Jackson operationalizes the principles implied in the concept of acceptance:

The client, Miss Jackson, is a 25-year-old mother of six illegitimate children under the age of 7. John, the oldest boy, was adopted by his maternal grandparents. The family unit consists of Miss Jackson, 5- and 4-year-old sons, a 3-year-old daughter and 14-month-old twin girls.

After four visits to Miss Jackson's dilapidated building in an otherwise neat, lower-class black neighborhood, I finally found her at home. To my surprise she was an attractive, pleasant person. I had expected her to resent my visits, since she never was at home at the three other prearranged times. Inside her apartment, amid worn but clean furniture, I met the two boys, both appearing clean and well nourished. The 3-year-old girl, an adorable, petite child, was clearly the apple of her mother's eye. In sharp contrast, the twins were undersized, dirty and had runny noses and food-smeared faces. The three older children seemed to perform in accordance with growth and developmental expectations, whereas the twins were retarded in motor development skills. One twin could crawl and sit alone, while the other could perform neither of these tasks. It really bothered me that neither Miss Jackson nor the three older children paid the slightest attention to the twins. It was as if they just did not exist.

Having met the family, I began an assessment. It was now abundantly clear that acceptance of this family situation would be difficult. Already I was angry at Miss Jackson for avoiding our first four meetings. With great patience and soul-searching, I recognized that she may have been anxious about the visit and thus avoided me. Perhaps she thought I might criticize her for not being more interested in the twins. I also realized that accepting the family's attitude toward the twins would prove difficult, for I believed that adults should provide responsible care for their children.

Prior to my second visit with Miss Jackson, I reviewed the phases of the nurse-patient relationship. My primary goals following the family assessment were to convey acceptance, open channels of communication, develop trust and plan nursing intervention.

Upon arriving for my second visit, I was immediately aware that the television was blaring so loudly that verbal communication would be difficult. Never was the principle that unmet expectations leads to increased anxiety so clearly demonstrated. I wondered how I was ever going to carry out my goal of communicating with Miss Jackson, if the television was so loud that she and I could not hear each other speak. Also, I was uncomfortable about having almost to knock the door down to gain entry into the apartment. Perhaps if I had been less anxious, I would have suggested that she lower the television volume. The second visit seemed so different from the first. Looking back, I wonder if Miss Jackson felt that she shared too much with me during the first visit. She may have been attempting to avoid investing any energy in our relationship. The loud television volume may have been her way of saying, "I don't want to get to know you or to allow you to know me." She looked tired, and her responses to my questions lacked spontaneity or enthusiasm. She merely answered the questions without offering additional information. As I prepared to leave that day, she said that she hoped we would be able to keep our appointment the next time. The explanation was that she was looking for a job and might be working by then. I wondered if she really hoped to be home, or if she was saying that she would make an effort to avoid our next meeting. Too often, we forget that many people feel threatened by close relationships and consequently avoid becoming involved with others.

Miss Jackson was home on the third visit. She had enrolled in a nurse's aide training program. The boys were attending a day care center, and the three girls were being cared for by a neighbor. During this visit, I noticed she seemed to have positive feelings toward the three older children. She constantly combed her older daughter's hair and smiled at the boys. When she made references to the twins, her tone of voice conveyed both disinterest and dislike. She said that she had asked her grandmother, who lived several hundred miles away, to take the twins. The grandmother had apparently replied that she would keep the twins, if Miss Jackson would deliver them. Miss Jackson was unable to find anyone who would take the twins to the grandmother's home so, as she said, "I am stuck with them." She said that she would not mind having the twins leave, because the smaller twin would not respond to her at all. As she went on to say that it "really doesn't matter" if they respond to her or not, I became increasingly uncomfortable. I could not imagine a mother showing such indifference to her children. I suspect I conveyed my feelings of alarm by my nonverbal behavior—by my facial expression as well as my tone of voice.

How disturbing it was to me, as my weekly visits with Miss Jackson progressed, to realize that she was never behaving as I expected her to behave. My expectations for her behavior were based on what I thought I would do under the same circumstances. I would have cared if my child failed to smile or laugh or enjoy my company. At that time, I could not understand how she could appear indifferent to whether her children responded to her or not. From my frame of reference, having one 15-month-old child, I could understand her overwhelming responsibility and her desire to give her children to relatives, but I could not understand a lack of concern. At this point, I knew that something was wrong, but I could not identify the problem. I felt an uneasiness I could not identify. Now I recognize that it was due to a "head-on collision" between her behavior and my expectations—her values and my values.

It took a few additional confrontations between my system of values and hers to increase my anxiety and anger to the point of immobilization. The turning point in our relationship, leading from the introductory to the working phase, occurred after a series of incidents forced me to grapple with my feelings toward Miss Jackson. My reaction to her responses to the twins was the first incident necessitating examination of the nurse-patient relationship in terms of the concept of acceptance. The following chain of events provided additional stimuli.

When I arrived for my sixth visit, I observed that Miss Jackson had purchased a new console color television, as well as new living room furniture complete with custom-made plastic covers. My first thought was, "How could she spend her welfare money so foolishly?" I was completely disgusted with Miss Jackson for behaving in a manner so inconsistent with what I considered appropriate. Recognizing my anger, I decided to examine my feelings toward her expenditure of money before I said anything. Even though I refrained from verbally confronting Miss Jackson with my disgust, I suspect my nonverbal behavior conveyed anger. Miss Jackson was restless during this visit, doubtless due to her perceiving my anger and disapproval. I did manage to say that the furniture was pretty, but almost in the same breath I asked how she was going to pay for the furniture. Just as I began to work through my feelings regarding the furniture, I observed that Miss Jackson used disposable diapers. How could one individual waste so much money? Disposable diapers seemed a convenient luxury item. I assumed she used disposable diapers because she was not aware a laundromat was less expensive. When I suggested that Miss Jackson use a laundromat she replied, "I have a washer and dryer, but they are not connected." Miss Jackson went on to explain that she had previously used a diaper service. By this time I was so angry with her for spending money the way she did, that I refrained from commenting any more about the diapers. Moreover, I recognized that I was not only failing to accept Miss Jackson as an individual of worth but also was judging against my personal standards and finding her guilty of extravagance. If our relationship was ever to progress to the working state, I had to examine and change my disdainful feelings toward her way of life.

At the time of my visits, Miss Jackson was an attractive, young black woman who, at the age of 25, was forced to assume the responsibility for five preschool children. She had been reared in a stable, upwardly mobile black family where both of her parents worked to raise their socioeconomic level. On the occasions when I met Miss Jackson's siblings, I noted that each was attractive, well dressed and had only one or two children. Her way of life was inconsistent with the values of her family as well as with my values.

Values, developed over a lengthy period of time, are not changed overnight. Changing my feelings of disdain for Miss Jackson's way of life to feelings of acceptance and understanding was no easy process. In trying to understand Miss Jackson's attitude toward furniture, I recognized that she could never hope to save enough money to pay for the furniture, as I would have done. I considered the possibility that she may as well enjoy the items while she paid for them, for there was little likelihood that she could buy the furniture any other way. I had been encouraging Miss Jackson to take her twins to the pediatric clinic at a nearby hospital for immunizations; she forgot to call or said she did not have time. At last one day she said, "Guess I had time to call—what I need is a vacation from these twins." She went on to say the twins "bugged her." I asked her to tell me one thing about the twins that bugged her. Miss Jackson's reply was, "Their just being here—from the time I knew they were twins, I didn't want them. I really wanted to leave them at the hospital." She had previously asked the welfare department to send a worker out to talk about placing the children in a foster home or for adoption. Each time she left home prior to the arrival. She said she felt guilty for not being able to love them or even give them an adequate amount of care. As I saw her struggling with guilt and ambivalence toward her children, I began to feel warmly toward her. I assessed Miss Jackson as incapable of providing adequate care for the twins. She kept them in a playpen situated in a dark corner of the dining room. Both twins sat quietly for long intervals. Miss Jackson locked the twins in the bedroom, so she could sleep during the day. To me the twins seemed to be environmentally retarded. They had no opportunities for the needed growth and developmental experiences, and this frightened me.

As I increasingly understood Miss Jackson, I recognized the importance of acceptance. Ujhely (1967) defines acceptance as "taking another person at face value without feeling the need to change him so as to fit him better into one's own frame of reference." I had been so far from accepting Miss Jackson during the initial phase of our relationship, that I condemned her for being different from me.

Upon my assuming a non-judgmental attitude toward Miss Jackson, we began to communicate and move from the initial phase of the relationship to the working phase.

The task for the working phase of the nurse-patient relationship is to establish goals and work toward accomplishing these goals. I formulated both short-term and long-term goals. Goals were based on supporting Miss Jackson's strengths in attempting to care for herself and three of her children, her ability to problem-solve and her lack of gross psychopathology.

My short-term goal was to hold one or both twins while I talked with Miss Jackson. After a few visits during which I held one twin, she held the other. A long-term goal was to support Miss Jackson in placing the twins in a foster home, until she could either work through her animosity toward them or make a decision to give them up permanently. A further long-term goal was to communicate my observations and evaluations regarding Miss Jackson's inability to care for her twins to the community services center. As my work with Miss Jackson drew to an end, I encouraged her to work with the neighborhood aide, who would visit her after my semester ended.

ANXIETY

Anxiety is present in all patients; those in an acute care setting awaiting surgery or those in hospitals for the emotionally disturbed experience anxiety. According to Rollo May (1950), "anxiety is an apprehension cued off by some threat to the values which the individual holds essential to his existence as a personality."

Students anticipating the first day in a new clinical setting can identify the feeling of anxiety. Frequently, an entire group of students spends most of the first day on a psychiatric unit walking around in one large clump. They exemplify the principles that fear of the unknown leads to increased anxiety and that anxiety is contagious. This anxiety felt on the first day of the clinical experience should be remembered, for it will assist the student in empathizing with the patient who says, "I was so afraid the first day I came to the hospital. I did not know where anything was or who any of the people were."

A number of characteristics pertain to anxiety:

1. Anxiety is an energy and as such cannot be directly observed. The only observation is that which is inferred due to the behavioral effects of anxiety.
2. Anxiety is an emotion without a specific object. It is perceived in relation to a diffuse apprehension.
3. Anxiety is a subjective experience. It is generally felt first in the abdomen as a feeling of great uneasiness.
4. Anxiety is a reaction or apprehension unrelated to any specific object, but it always occurs as a result of an interpersonal process. The reaction one feels at the supermarket when starting to pay the cashier and, all of a sudden you wonder if you left your wallet at home, is fear. The object of the uneasy feeling is easily noted, and the feeling is a direct result of fear of embarrassment. Anxiety occurs when you approach a new situation and feel vaguely uncomfortable but cannot really describe the situation eliciting the reaction.
5. Anxiety is caused by a threat to the security of an individual. Two general categories of anxiety-precipitating events include:
    A. Threat to biological integrity.
    B. Threat to the self-system. The self-system refers to the beliefs and values a person holds about himself. It includes his perception of "me." There are three categories of threats to the self-system or self-concept of a person:
    1. an interruption of expectations. (For example, the student who expected an A on his first nursing exam may experience a threat to his self-system when his paper is returned and his score is a B. He may be unable to see himself as a B student in that he has always conceived of himself as being capable of making a high score and, to him, a B may not seem very high.)
    2. an interference with prestige needs. (For example, when the patients in a therapeutic community have recently elected a unit president who believes he has done a fine job, yet the patient group asks that a called election take place to find a new president. The other patients say they

are displeased with the laxity with which the president approached his task. The current president, thinking he had done a fine job, is acutely threatened by the loss of his status.)
    3. a threat which interferes with the individual's existence as he perceives it. (For example, a mother may feel that her role and very existence as a person are threatened when her last child moves out of the home. Her concept of self may be bound up with the needs and accomplishments of her children. When the children no longer need her on a day-to-day basis, her existence and feelings of being worthwhile and useful are shattered.)
6. A spectrum of signs and symptoms is commonly associated with anxiety. Few of the symptoms are foreign to the student, in that each individual experiences anxiety and has a defined reaction pattern. Frequently experienced symptoms include the following systems:
   A. Respiratory System—labored breathing, sighing, dizziness, giddiness and lightheadedness due to hyperventilation.
   B. Motor System—rapid movements which may seem uncoordinated; blinking, smacking lips, swinging legs, crossing and uncrossing legs, pacing and wringing hands.
   C. Cardiovascular System—rapid pulse, increased blood pressure, clammy hands, flushing, blushing, increased perspiration.
   D. Gastrointestinal System—abdominal pain, nausea, vomiting, anorexia, dry mouth, diarrhea.
   E. Genitourinary System—urinary frequency.
   F. Mental functioning—feeling of helplessness, impending doom, inability to pay attention, poor concentration, irritability.
7. As anxiety increases, an individual's observational skills are affected (Burd and Marshall, 1963).
   A. Stage #1 anxiety is recognized by the quickened powers of observation and the increased ability to comprehend.
   B. Stage #2 anxiety is observed when the individual begins to have involvement with the ability to comprehend. He cannot comprehend all incoming information, thus his responses are inadequate.

C. Stage #3 anxiety occurs when there is a marked decrease in observational powers, and the ability to hear is decreased. At this point, the individual focuses on one detail and hears only what he wants to hear. His perception is limited to one focal point. He now experiences tunnel vision rather than peripheral vision.
D. Stage #4 anxiety is evidenced when panic ensues. At this point, the individual can do nothing; he is immobilized and feels helpless and hopeless. An individual cannot remain alive at this level of anxiety for more than a brief amount of time.
8. Anxiety is operationalized as follows:
    A. An expectation or need is held by the individual.
    B. The expectation is not met (the individual feels tension and powerlessness).
    C. Tension leads to anxiety.
    D. Relief behavior occurs when:
        1. the anxiety is somatized
        2. anger is experienced
        3. the individual withdraws and internalizes anxiety
        4. problem-solving skills are employed, and the individual learns new ways of coping with increased amounts of anxiety.

TRUST

Trust is a further component of the nurse-patient relationship, for without the capacity to trust, a patient feels isolated, lonely and anxious. Trust develops from early mother-child interactions, forming the prototype for one's future relationships. A person who learns trust at an early growth and developmental stage can transfer this feeling toward later relationships. For many individuals seeking psychiatric treatment, the ability to trust did not develop in childhood; instead the home atmosphere was permeated with anxiety and mistrust.

Individuals not having trusting relationships as children later doubt the reliability of significant people in their environment, since they were unable to rely on parents or other significant persons in early developmental stages. When significant people repeatedly fail to meet a child's needs, he views the world around him as being cold and unfeeling or hostile and dangerous. He mistrusts the sincerity and intent of others and scrutinizes each relationship for signs of mistrust.

Psychiatric nursing seeks to provide opportunities for patients to learn to trust others and to experience the warmth and security of a trusting relationship. Several factors within the nurse-patient relationship promote trust. First, it is essential that what the nurse says be consistent with her actions. It is necessary to think through clearly what is to be said in advance of speaking. Competency in physical skills promotes trust. Often nurses in psychiatric areas lose skill in performing treatment tasks such as catheterizing, inserting a Levin tube or starting an intravenous solution due to lack of practice. Each nurse needs to identify a method of refreshing her skills periodically. If the nursing staff in general is not proficient with skills, two or three nurses could be responsible for all treatments.

A further means by which the nurse can increase the patient's ability to trust is by being consistent and dependable in her action, and by doing what she says she will do. If she says, "I will be back in ten minutes with your medication," then her actions must be consistent with her verbal message. To return in 30 minutes with no intervening communication to the patient regarding the delay, implies that since the nurse cannot be counted on for this, her dependability in other situations is questionable.

Honesty and trust go hand in hand as a foundation for the nurse-patient relationship. Often, a nurse is tempted to guess at the answer to a patient's question rather than simply to explain that she does not know the answer. The patient learns distrust if he is provided with inaccurate information; the likelihood is great that he will, at some point, learn the correct answer.

Consistency between verbal and nonverbal behavior facilitates the development of trust. Lack of consistency between what is said and a person's actions, gestures, tone of voice or facial expression communicates an unclear, ambiguous message; the patient is wary of the nurse who seems to mean something other than what she says. Few patients feel secure enough to clarify, if the nurse seems to be giving a double message.

Patients often go to great lengths to determine if nurses can be trusted. Mr. Barton was such a patient, who devoted considerable time and energy to testing the nursing staff of the psychiatric unit of a large medical center to determine who could be trusted. The following nurse-patient relationship depicts the development of trust:

>Mr. Barton, a 56-year-old non-practicing physician, had been in and out of University Hospital several times. Although many of the staff knew Mr. Barton from past admissions, few spent time with him. They treated him almost as though he were part of the surroundings. When a staff member tried to talk with him, he seemed to withdraw into a protective shell like a threatened turtle. He conversed with staff about topics alien to him as a person, that is, intellectual topics revealing little personal involvement.
>
>I recognized that Mr. Barton used intellectualizing as a distancing maneuver. By causing staff members to feel uncomfortable when they talked with him, he did not have to fear involvement. I interpreted this behavior as a facade to protect his vulnerable feelings. He actually thought himself unworthy and unneeded. It seemed that his condescending attitude helped him hide a low self-image, acquired over 25 years of intermittent psychiatric hospitalizations. Spending time each day with Mr. Barton, I sought to enhance his self-esteem by asking him to tell me about the activities he enjoyed. We spent hours exploring things he liked to do: fishing, sailing and woodworking. Seldom did we focus for long on his feelings. Rarely would he mention how hard his being in and out of the hospital all those years had been on his family. One day he said, "My wife has had her hands full raising our three children." My initial response was to ask where he saw himself in relation to his family. We then touched on how useless he felt, when he was unable to live up to his own expectations.
>
>As I deliberately attempted to intervene in his feelings of low self-esteem, I recognized that he was beginning to drop his facade a little. My persistence in coming back to talk with him conveyed that I did care enough to get to know him.
>
>In the early stage of our relationship, I made an effort to talk with Mr. Barton daily. After a few weeks, he waited near the nursing station at the beginning of the day to ask when we could meet. I offered him some say in when we met by asking the time most convenient for him. His taking part in making this type of decision conveyed: "You are worthwhile enough to have some input into decisions that affect you." Little did I know he was stringently testing therapeutic skills. After our relationship was cemented, and I had passed his test, Mr. Barton shared with me details of his testing procedure.
>
>One day as we were talking, Mr. Barton commented on his evaluation of the nursing staff. He thought I might want to know what he

had learned about the staff. Like a child who had just made a new friend, he told me that I had passed his test with "flying colors." For Mr. Barton, I was a new friend, in that my unsuspecting actions had conveyed that I cared for him.

He said that being consistently prompt for our talks had been important to him. The biggest hurdle in the test had occurred earlier that day, when I was giving him some medication. He reminded me that I had handed him a cup of medication, which he put on a nearby table, saying that he would take it later. He approvingly pointed out that I had sat down with him and said that I would stay with him, until he was ready to take the medication.

He went on to list nurses who had handed him medication and had not watched him closely to see if he actually swallowed it. He had given considerable thought to ways of hoarding medication, and he elaborated on how long he could hold medication in the side of his mouth. How sad and lonely he must have felt, when the nurses did not care enough to make sure he took his medication.

Hospitalized on a locked unit, he had done considerable testing of staff regarding the "keeping of the keys." He described one nurse having difficulty opening the outside door. He had offered to help, and when the nurse gave him the keys, he opened the door. He pointed out how easily he could have run out the door, keys in hand. He also mentioned the times he had helped the nurses open the door to the unit's kitchen. He said that when he and a nurse would leave the kitchen, he would always hold the door and let the nurse leave first. This gave him an opportunity to shut the door after the nurse and remain in the kitchen, thus having access to the kitchen tools and utensils.

It was apparent that at least two issues were raised by Mr. Barton's behavior. First, he had experienced all the impulses he described, such as hoarding his medication, leaving the hospital and barricading himself in the kitchen.

Secondly, he did not trust people without thoroughly testing their concern for him. The nursing staff had not acted in ways which helped him develop trust. His suspiciousness and fear of relationships were reinforced in the hospital.

Patients who suspect staff of not being trustworthy frequently attempt to verify their suspicions by "comparing notes," going from one staff person to another asking the same question so as to compare responses. Mr. Barton used a slightly different tactic. He had developed his own measurement tool for a person whom he could trust. He went from one nurse to another determining with each encounter who would measure up to his standard of a "trustworthy nurse."

It is unlikely that Mr. Barton is unique in his need to test carefully before he invests trust in a person. Nursing care, based on the needs of the patient, should measure up to his unique test.

RESPONSIBILITY

Responsibility from the nurse's standpoint has been discussed, in that the professional nurse is responsible or accountable for her actions. Responsibility, defined as the state of being accountable for one's actions, also refers to the patient. When an individual enters a health care setting, he is often stripped of all vestiges of responsibility and accountability. A previously autonomous individual becomes dependent on agency staff for a variety of functions he normally would perform for himself. In some instances the patient is physically or psychologically unable to be responsible for meeting his needs. His ego functions, ability to make decisions, judgments and memory may be impaired. Initially, the nurse may provide ego support and allow a patient to be dependent, until he is able to move into a more independent role.

In far more instances, hospital personnel allow and often encourage dependency beyond that which is useful for the patient. The myth that patients must be "cared for" enhances dependency. The patient arrives at the psychiatric hospital expecting to be cared for. Simultaneously, the nurse may labor under the misconception that her function is to "take care of" the patient. Thus, the patient becomes dependent on the nurse for meeting needs he could meet in an autonomous manner. An early milestone in growth and development is the need for autonomy. Erikson (1950) says that at about age 2, each child grapples with the pull for autonomy to avoid feelings of shame and doubt regarding his abilities. Autonomy, referring to being self-directed, is closely related to responsibility. To abdicate responsibility leads to doubting one's ability to handle a similar situation in the future.

The nursing process is a problem-solving approach, with the implicit assumption that both nurse and patient can solve the presenting problem. Each time a nurse does for a patient that which he can do for himself, she diminishes his autonomy by assuming some of the responsibility rightfully belonging to him. Nursing has traditionally been characterized as a nurturing activity, and many nurses feel that they are providing patient care when they "do for" the patient. Learning to "do with" the patient may prove difficult at first.

The nursing role, while excluding doing for a patient what he is capable of doing for himself, implies that the nurse provides an environment in which the patient can meet his own needs. In order for patients to learn and practice more facilitative environmental interfaces, resources must be provided for successful experiences. Standard VII of the Standards of Psychiatric-Mental Health Nursing Practice published by ANA Congress for Nursing Practice (1973), speaks to the nursing responsibility of providing a therapeutic environment.

STANDARD VII

The environment is structured to establish and maintain a therapeutic milieu.

Rationale

Any environment is composed of both human and non-human resources, which may work for or against the person's well-being. The nurse works with people in a variety of environmental settings, e.g., hospital, home, etc. The milieu is structured and/or altered, so that it serves the client's best interests as an inherent part of the overall therapeutic plan.

Assessment Factors

1. The effects of environmental forces on individuals are observed, analyzed and interpreted.
2. Psychological, physiological, social, economic and cultural concepts are understood and utilized in developing and maintaining a therapeutic milieu.
3. Communications within the environment are congruent with therapeutic goals.
4. All available resources in the environment are utilized, when appropriate, in the therapeutic efforts.
5. Nursing participation and its effectiveness in establishing and maintaining a therapeutic milieu are evaluated.

Not only is it the nurse's responsibility to provide a therapeutic environment but also to assist the patient in participating in activities which can enhance his ability to function in society. Standard V of the ANA Standards of Psychiatric-Mental Health Nursing Practice (Congress for Nursing Practice, 1973) describes the nursing role in facilitating activities of daily living.

STANDARD V

The activities of daily living are utilized in a goal-directed way in work with clients.

Rationale

A major portion of one's daily life is spent in some form of activity related to health and well-being. An individual's developmental and intellectual level, emotional state and physical limitations may be reflected in these activities. Therefore, nursing has a unique opportunity to assess and intervene in these processes in order to encourage constructive changes in the client's behavior, so that each person may realize his full potential for growth.

Assessment Factors

1. An appraisal is made of the client's capacities to participate in activities of daily living based on needs, strengths and levels of functioning.
2. Clients are encouraged toward independence and self-direction by various skills such as motivating, limit setting, persuading, guiding and comforting.
3. Each person's rights are appreciated and respected.
4. Methods of communicating are devised which assure consistency in approach.

William Glasser presents a theoretical framework for working with mentally ill persons known as Reality Therapy. "The crux of the theory, personal responsibility for one's own behavior, is equated with mental health" (Glasser and Zunin, 1973, p. 287). In Reality Therapy, each person is assisted in "understanding, defining, and clarifying: his immediate and long term goals" (Glasser and Zunin, 1973, p. 288). The individual is helped to look at alternatives and encouraged to consider the consequences of each set of alternatives. The assumption is that the patient, not the helper, lives with the consequences of his actions; thus he must choose the alternatives promising the most tolerable consequences. If a patient asks, "Do you think I should divorce my husband?" the nurse would be remiss to provide a "yes" or "no" answer. The patient must live with the loneliness of divorce, the happiness of freedom or the misery of an unsatisfactory marriage.

A patient is most likely to experience success when he assumes responsibility for his decisions and actions. Nursing intervention serves to raise questions, suggest additional areas of consideration and provide a forum for examining alternatives and consequences.

AGGRESSION

Aggression must be understood by the nurse implementing the nursing process in the psychiatric area. Frustration develops in response to a blocked or thwarted goal. If the frustration is not dissipated, it leads to aggression, a basic drive demanding an avenue for expression. If no avenue is readily available, the energy is directed inwardly and leads to feelings of guilt, anger or depression. Anxiety is employed as a mechanism of the ego, with the proper expression of aggression serving as a reinforcement of the healthy aspects of the ego (Brooks, 1967).

Patients seeking psychiatric care generally have not learned to express aggression appropriately. Many are afraid that they will hurt or otherwise overwhelm the person toward whom their aggression is directed, if they unleash their pent-up feelings. Few have learned to express anger at the moment of its onset and toward the person to whom the anger is actually directed. It is often easier to express aggression toward an object than a person, in that the fear of retaliation is decreased. Aggression needs to be released outwardly; if aggression is internalized, the patient feels increasing discomfort and calls into operation defense mechanisms such as sublimation or projection to dissipate the stored aggression energy. Outward expression often leads to a feeling of relief and diminished tension. The crucial issue relates to the way aggression is outwardly dissipated, with some forms of expression having serious repercussions by infringing on the rights and comforts of others.

The hospital provides an arena where patients can learn alternative modes of expressing aggression. Modes of being aggressive are learned at early developmental stages from observations and encounters with significant role models. In the hospital, the staff becomes the role model. When the nurse responds to a patient's comments with sarcasm, she demonstrates an indirect way of expressing aggression which may not prove effective when the patient leaves the hospital. In addition to serving as role models, the nursing staff helps assess with the patient modes for direct dissipation of angry feelings. For some, carving, working on leather, macrame or engaging in sports serve as constructive forms of aggressive release. It is helpful if the mode selected is one the patient can use when he leaves the hospital. A word of caution is needed about competitive sports. Competition "implies moving ahead of or overcoming others" (Brooks, 1967 p. 254). A withdrawn patient is unable to muster the energy for competitive activities. Also, at times, the staff becomes oblivious to its therapeutic role and demonstrates competitiveness at the expense of the patient. Numerous activities are available for patients unable to participate in competitive games such as volleyball, baseball or bowling. Non-competitive activities include swimming, daily exercise, dancing and various crafts.

The primary nursing goals are to provide an environment in which the patient can test new methods of releasing aggression, to serve as a role model and be actively involved in teaching the patient new modes of expression. Teaching involves observing the patient express himself in his new ways. It also involves clearly defining the limits for the expression of aggression. The patient needs to know that property and people are not to be attacked; that verbal expression of anger, as well as a variety of active modes of expression is acceptable. Patients, often immobilized by anger due to an overwhelming fear of devasting a person or object, have a tremendous need to learn new ways of handling aggression by verbalization.

Implicit in the nurse's teaching role with the patient demonstrating aggressive behavior is the need for astute observation. Observation, an essential component of the nursing process, provides cues to signs of mounting tension. The patient may exhibit an increase in motor activity by pacing, wringing his hands, clenching his fists or tightening his jaw muscles. His face may clearly express anger or he may appear "glazed" and seem not to see what is happening around him. The patient with mounting aggression is removed from the group to his room or another private area. The overtly aggressive person often becomes calmer, if one person remains with him. Remaining with him communicates that he is accepted as a person, while removing him from ward stimulation indicates that his behavior is currently unacceptable.

The handling of aggression in a productive manner contrasts with violence in the hospital setting. Attempts are made to decrease the aggressive outbursts before violence occurs. Violence occurs in response to a patient's feelings of helplessness or impotence in the face of a threat (Penningroth, 1975). The fact that a person requires admission to a psychiatric hospital confirms his worst fears about inability to control his behavior. Upon arrival at the hospital, the patient is assigned to the lowest ranks on the hospital hierarchy. His belongings are checked; some are taken, especially sharp or valuable items. He is given a book of rules and immediately told what to do and when he is expected to do it. Most patients respond to the threat of loss of control in a situation with either fight, flight or freezing into immobility. Flight may be difficult, in that the hospital unit may be locked; thus the only place to retreat is a bedroom which he may share with another for the first time in his life.

Providing a patient with choices allows some control over his environment. Asking him to participate in unit activities and allowing him some initiative serve to dissipate anger and decrease the tendency toward aggression expressed in violent ways. Patients are most apt to strike out when they feel trapped and cornered; thus, providing choices and options decreases the trapped feeling.

The first time a patient is outwardly aggressive is often frightening, and staff members may want to run away or respond in a similarly hostile fashion. Neither of these approaches benefits the patient. In contrast, a facilitative approach is to help the patient identify what is frightening him or threatening his feeling of security. The patient needs acceptance and support; he is generally as frightened of some aspect of his internal or external environment as the nurse is frightened by his actions. It is important to avoid reacting to a patient's hostility and aggression as though it were personally directed toward the nurse (Carter, 1976). By remaining calm, one assures the patient that one is in control of the situation. The presence of the nurse and her quiet, calm demeanor convey that she can provide needed support for controlling the behavior. The nurse, in assessing the patient's aggression, decides if she needs assistance in helping the patient regain control. At times, two or three additional staff persons need to be close by and alert to the nurse's possible need for assistance. Avoid presenting a threatening approach, as the patient will react to threats with accelerated aggression. The staff serves to provide ego-control at a time when the patient's own internal controls are proving ineffective. Moreover, the patient's self-esteem is vulnerable when he utilizes aggression to compensate for his insecurity and fear. Avoid demeaning the patient by shaming him for his behavior or by allowing him to behave in a manner which will embarrass or humiliate him later should he hear about the situation.

If the patient demonstrates aggression toward the staff or other patients in an acceptable manner, it is important to reinforce such expression and not squelch his attempts. On one occasion, Mr. J. said, "I hate this hospital and want to punch that - - - doctor out." When the nurse replied, "Oh! Mr. J., that is an unkind thing for you to say—your doctor is one of the finest physicians in town and is trying to help you," she encouraged Mr. J. to repress his expression of anger, and her words likely engendered guilt. In contrast, had the nurse replied, "Mr. J. you are really angry at Dr. Y. What would you like to say to him to tell him how you feel right now?" she would have facilitated the expression of anger and assisted him in practicing an acceptable expression of feelings. Ultimately, it would be useful for Mr. J. to verbalize his anger to Dr. Y. As the nurse supports a patient in communicating honestly and directly to another, she is aware that the reaction of the other person cannot be predicted. For example, Mr. J. might tell Dr. Y. that he is angry with him, and the doctor, tired and disgruntled, might respond so as to "put Mr. J. down." The nurse must be available to support the patient, in case the other person responds in a manner distressing to the patient.

SHAME

Experiences eliciting feelings of shame are often sudden and unavoidable. An incident may appear inconsequential to all but the person involved, who feels self-conscious and considers himself a failure. Shame reactions range from mild embarrassment to almost overwhelming humiliation. The subjective feeling related to shame involves a sudden awareness of anxiety, a sense of painful self-consciousness and a wish to escape or hide.

Shame arises from conflict between the ego and the ego ideal, that is, between the way a person actually perceives himself as contrasted to his idealized self. Shame can be growth-producing or retarding. It can serve either as an incentive helping an individual attain a higher level of functioning or can elicit an overwhelming reaction characterized by self-derogation, hopelessness and withdrawal. In the later instance, the individual can identify nothing good about himself.

A variety of general nursing actions is available for dealing with shame-provoking situations:

1. Avoid causing shame by maintaining the dignity and self-esteem of the individual such as by knocking on the door before entering a patient's room, by calling him by his given name, unless asked to do otherwise, and by omitting all demeaning remarks.
2. Give anticipatory help in situations where shame is likely to occur. If the patient needs to request something from the patient group, allow him an opportunity to practice, such as by role playing, in anticipation of expressing himself in front of a group.
3. Encourage the patient and his family to share shameful situations and deal with them constructively. Help them examine the reason for shame—What causes the patient to feel inadequate? How does he think he fell short of his expectations?
4. Minimize the need for shame in the nursing situation. For example, if the patient sets a difficult goal for himself, works toward the goal and fails, the nurse helps him decide if the goal is desirable and attainable. If the patient decides to try for the goal again, the nurse helps him identify the steps in goal-attainment. If the patient decides not to try for the goal, the nurse helps him examine his alternatives and decide what he does want for himself.

HUMOR

Humor is a controversial component of the nurse-patient relationship. In the past, nursing students were taught not to laugh with patients but rather to communicate a serious air in each interaction. As one patient aptly said, "If I tell a joke and nobody laughs, then I know I am crazy." Humor has its place in the nurse-patient relationship, in that the nurse and patient may laugh with each other; but rarely does the nurse laugh *at* the patient. Humor, a form of communication both nurse and patient bring with them to the treatment setting, serves to establish a warm interpersonal relationship; to relieve anxiety, tension and stress; and to release anger, hostility and aggression in a socially acceptable way. Humor also serves to avoid or deny feelings too painful and too stressful to deal with at the time.

Now that several behavioral concepts have been discussed which serve as a foundation for the nurse-patient relationship, the stages or phases of the relationship can be delineated.

ORIENTATION PHASE

In the first or orientation phase of the interview, the student explains to the patient who she is, why she is there and how long she will be there. Often, both nurse and patient are anxious when they first meet. It may be helpful for the student to put her own feelings into words such as, "Sometimes it is hard for strangers to get started talking." Student and patient can then discuss the difficulties in initiating a relationship and how hard it is to know just what to say to a stranger. Often patients are surprised to learn that students are just as uncomfortable and anxious during the first few interactions as they are. During the orientation phase, the nursing assessment begins. The nurse begins to examine both her own and the patient's communication style, the level of anxiety of each and the relationship between overt and covert messages, gleaning some awareness of the patient's presenting problem.

In the structured interview, the length should generally not exceed an hour. The time will depend on the patient's ability to tolerate a conversation. The acutely anxious patient may only be able to talk for ten to fifteen minutes at a time. He may not be able to sit for the interaction, but rather he and the nurse may interact while they walk or engage in some activity to decrease his anxiety.

The environment in which the interview takes place is important. It should provide privacy and freedom from interruptions. Patients rarely want to discuss interpersonal issues in a busy hospital lobby or the corridor of a psychiatric hospital. In fact, the nurse must assist the patient in refraining from discussing private issues in a public setting. The patient may have diminished ego control and not recognize the inappropriateness of speaking about private topics in a public area. As he gains ego control, he may remember his past verbalizations or be reminded of them and subsequently feel embarrassed around the people who heard him. This is not to imply that all nurse-patient interactions need occur in a private setting. Some meaningful interactions occur in a small group setting in the hall, lounge or patient rooms of a psychiatric hospital. The nurse attempts to protect the patient from discussing subjects which are unsuitable to the setting or group of listeners. For example, on a patient's first day at the hospital, it may be inadvisable for him to discuss intimate, interpersonal issues with the entire patient population. Later, as he becomes comfortable with several patients, it may be acceptable for him to discuss any topic causing him concern. At this point he knows the patients and has some information as to whom he can trust.

Frequently, students are hesitant to enter a patient's room. The hesitancy may be due to fear of the patient or a feeling of inadequacy as to the appropriate verbal approach. Often, students feel that they are guests in the hospital setting and should not enter a room unless specifically invited to do so by the patient. Many think that the patient needs privacy and their presence in his room invades his private territory. The patient retains the right to ask the student to leave his room. Refraining from asking direct questions or pursuing topics toward which considerable feelings are attached may facilitate communication in the first meeting.

WORKING PHASE

Once the orientation is over and the patient begins to relax and trust the nurse, the working phase begins. The goals for the relationship are established in the working phase, as the assessment continues and a plan for care is developed. Goals are mutually decided upon by both nurse and patient. On occasion, it is helpful for the nurse and patient to establish a contract describing the parameters and aims of their relationship. The contract serves to structure the relationship and provide a focal point for future evaluation of progress.

A nursing student working with an 8-year-old girl, M.J., in a children's home found how useful a contract could be. She and M.J.

were to meet weekly for seven weeks with an overall goal of providing an opportunity for M.J. to acknowledge her feelings related to being in the children's home. During the first three meetings, M.J. wanted to play and spoke minimally. The instructor suggested that the student try negotiating a contract with the child. M.J. responded enthusiastically to this idea and said that in the four remaining meetings she would discuss school, her friends and what went on in the home, but she adamantly proclaimed that she would not discuss her parents. The student's goal had been to talk about the family situation and the feelings associated with M.J.'s being placed in the children's home. M.J. said that it upset her to talk about her family. During the remaining four sessions, M.J. freely discussed situations which made her feel happy as well as sad, and, in general, responded enthusiastically to the student's visits. What she communicated in the contract was that seven weeks was insufficient time to pursue topics of intense feelings. She was unwilling to plunge into interpersonal discussions without more intensive involvement than this relationship could provide.

The nurse-patient relationship is the essence of nursing. In all nurse-patient relationships, the patient's problems and the nurse's interventions to assist the patient in solving his problems comprise the relationship. Support is given to the productive parts of the personality, reinforcing behavior and coping techniques which the patient uses effectively. New techniques are taught throughout the hospitalization to replace maladaptive ones. The nurse recognizes that each patient handles his behavior as well as he is able at a given time. Similarly, if the patient is withdrawn and sits curled up in a chair in the corner of the dayroom in a near fetal position, the nurse assesses the presenting problem and works toward planning intervention. In planning intervention, it is imperative to recall that change takes place slowly. A patient does not develop his emotional problems overnight, nor will basic personality change occur overnight. Some of the patient's behavior may be difficult to accept due to inappropriateness to the time or setting, inconvenience to others or conflict with beliefs and values of the nurse. For example, on an outing into the community when a patient behaves in such a manner as to call attention to his inability to function, both other patients and the staff members present may feel uncomfortable. When feelings of anxiety arise due to inappropriate patient behavior, the nurse assesses immediately what is causing her reaction and which needs of the patient are being met by the presenting behavior.

Consider the following example: An adolescent patient was hospitalized for several months after graduation from high school. Academically a weak student in high school, he planned to enroll in a community college the next term rather than in a senior university. He seemed to experience considerable feelings of inadequacy in that his father, a graduate of an Ivy League University, was president of a local bank. Whenever the patient group went on a community outing, Joe assumed the role of employee rather than consumer. On one occasion the patient group attended a movie, and Joe began talking with several in-coming patrons and soon was collecting tickets as though he worked at the theater. The next day Joe was excitedly telling everyone how he had been hired by the theater and would start his new job as soon as he left the hospital. The nursing approach was to recognize that Joe's inability to function outside the hospital caused considerable loss of self-esteem. The incongruence between his ideal self and his actual self was great, thereby causing anxiety and pressure to be a productive person. To him being productive meant employment. The nurse consistently communicated to Joe that although he was not employed at the theater, he might like to work there. Sometimes the nurse can allow the patient to have in fantasy what is not possible at the present in reality.

If a patient's self-respect is to be enhanced, it is important to provide a place where he can keep his belongings, as well as where he can obtain some privacy. For some, the communal nature of hospital living provides a unique and potentially stressful situation. Individuals accustomed to a tranquil and predictable environment find the public nature of hospital living taxing. Often it helps a patient to feel comfortable in the hospital if he brings one or two items from home such as a familiar picture or clock to personalize his room.

A therapeutic environment also provides opportunities for patients to express problems and conflicts within the limits of safety and group living. If a patient behaves in a manner contrary to group living, such as stealing from other patients' wallets, the issue is dealt with by the staff and patient group with an emphasis on identifying the need the patient is seeking to meet by his actions and examining more acceptable ways of meeting his needs. Moreover, if a patient is given tranquilizers or confined to a seclusion room each time he seeks to express anger, little learning takes place. Instead, the environment should tolerate some anger with limits set if the patient infringes on the rights of others. Limits should be clearly and concisely communicated. At some point, each patient needs to work with one staff member or a patient and staff group to examine what provoked his behavior and consider alternative methods of handling the same or similar situation in the future.

A particularly difficult situation arises when a medical staff member enters the psychiatric unit as a patient. Frequently, the person will identify himself by his profession and have considerable difficulty assuming the patient role. Generally, the patient is threatening to the nursing staff on at least two levels. First, the staff may think that the patient knows more than they do. Second, the patient may pose a threat in that staff covertly identify with him and think, "This could happen to me, too."

The first step in relating to a patient who is a member of the health profession is to recognize your personal feelings. Do you feel afraid, intimidated, embarrassed or angry that this person is not coping effectively? The patient needs every opportunity to be treated as a patient if he is to learn more effective ways of coping. If the patient resists becoming a participant in the therapy program, this should be discussed with him openly and a plan generated to allow him maximum utilization of the hospital resources.

Another difficulty which may arise is when a male patient asks a female student for a date. If the student responds, "My instructor will not let me date patients" or "I'm sorry, that is against hospital policy," she is merely avoiding the issue. Comments of this type serve to block discussion of what may be the real issue behind the patient's request. He may be asking if the student sees him as a desirable person, and would other women see him in a similar manner. The appropriate response might be to reply to the covert message of, "Am I OK as a male?" with a comment such as, "Do you sometimes worry that women will not go out with you, when you leave the hospital?" The next step might be to ask him to describe a situation in which he asked someone for a date. What did he say? What was the other person's response? Next, help him look at what went wrong in his past dating experiences. Did he select women who indicated no interest in him, or was he able to note covert cues that the women might also be interested in him? Role-playing can be used at this point to help the patient practice asking for a date. The Gestalt approach of talking to an empty chair representing a real person might also prove facilitative. In the Gestalt approach, the patient initially lets the chair represent the prospective date; he asks her for a date, then changes positions and responds to his request as he thinks the other person might respond to him. By using this approach, the patient practices communication and also examines possible responses to him.

TERMINATION PHASE

Termination is the final phase of the nurse-patient relationship. Early separation experiences for both nurse and patient affect how each will respond to the ending of the relationship. Phillips (1968) lists six reasons for students to utilize termination as a final therapeutic component of the nurse-patient relationship:

1. Termination is a phase of the therapeutic nurse-patient relationship and without it the relationship remains incomplete.
2. Feelings are aroused in both patient and student regarding the experience they have had; when these feelings are recognized and shared, the patient learns that it is acceptable to feel sadness and loss when someone he cares about leaves.
3. The patient is a partner in the relationship and has a right to see the nurse's needs and feelings regarding their time together and the ensuing separation.
4. Termination with the student may be the first successful separation experience for the patient.
5. Termination can be a learning experience; the patient can learn that he is important to at least one person.
6. By sharing the termination experience with the patient, the nurse proves that she cares for him.

In planning nursing actions directed toward termination, the nurse consistently reinforces the healthy aspects of the patient's personality and continues to identify the feelings attached to the relationship. Both nurse and patient need to summarize the events of the relationship, which may be done by exchanging memories of what was significant to each. The evaluation phase of the nursing process occurs during termination. As the nurse and patient summarize the significant occurrences in their past interactions, they evaluate the effectiveness of the relationship.

Several questions can be asked to evaluate the effectiveness of the nurse-patient relationship.

1. What goals have been reached?
2. What have I done for the patient? If in any way I have reinforced guilt, or inadequacy, or my interactions have led the patient to employ deeper defense mechanisms, then I have not helped.
3. Have I helped the patient function on a higher level? If I have helped him use problem-solving skills to cope more effectively with the problems confronting him today, then I have rendered therapeutic nursing care.
4. Have I helped the patient use greater emotional control, when such control is desirable? If I have assisted him to speak with someone about his angry feelings rather than slamming doors, striking out or withdrawing and feeling sad and lonely, then I have helped him.
5. Have I helped the patient work through a problem today, so that he can learn from it and deal more effectively in the future if a similar situation should arise?
6. Have I helped the patient generalize some of his newly learned behavior to similar or other situations?
7. What have I learned from this relationship?

Although the student prepares for termination from the first meeting with the patient, both student and patient may experience feelings of loss. Common reactions include denial that the relationship really meant anything; anger toward the one who is leaving, which may be disguised by compliments toward the nurse and other staff, or by the patient actually rejecting the nurse by being angry, for fear that she will reject him by leaving; regressive behavior such as recurrence of prior symptoms or increased dependency; or withdrawal as evidenced by missing meetings or by only communicating on a superficial basis.

In dealing with termination, the student carefully considers her policy regarding future contact with the patient. The rule of thumb is that there will be no planned meetings either for social or therapeutic purposes. Exceptions may be made depending on the student's learning needs and the school policy. If chance encounters in the community are a possibility, the student should explain that any interchange would be social and very brief.

PRINCIPLES

1. Unmet expectations lead to increased anxiety.
2. Fear of the unknown leads to increased anxiety.
3. Anxiety is contagious.
4. Anxiety is caused by a threat to one's security.
5. Threat of loss of control leads to flight, fight or freezing into immobility.
6. Fear of emotional closeness leads to increased anxiety.
7. All behavior is purposeful and meaningful.
8. Behavior includes the individual's total response to stimuli.
9. What an individual perceives as happening to him is more influential in determining his behavior than what is actually happening to him.
10. The individual in the American culture satisfies most of his needs through relationships with others or groups of individuals.
11. Feelings of being accepted lead to increased trust and to increased self-esteem.
12. Consistency of nursing actions leads to increased trust.
13. Increased expression of anger leads to decreased anger and anxiety.
14. The need to defend implies perception of threat or attack.
15. Information essential to understanding a person and his problems can be obtained by the process of interviewing.
16. Successful interviewing depends upon attitudes of acceptance, objectivity, kindness and warmth.
17. A comfortable environment is conducive to successful interviewing.
18. Interviewing is more effective when geared to the interviewee's age and mental and physical capabilities.

SUMMARY

The nurse-patient relationship refers to the sequential phases of orientation, working and termination. A conceptual basis provides the foundation for implementing the nurse-patient relationship in the facilitation of the nursing process. Concepts such as confidentiality, involvement, empathy, acceptance, anxiety, trust, responsibility, and humor are integral components of the nurse-patient relationship.

The nurse-patient relationship is differentiated from a social relationship in that the focus is centered on the patient and upon meeting his needs. In the nurse-patient relationship, the nurse is responsible for her behavior. She continually examines her actions to determine her effect on patients.

BIBLIOGRAPHY

Brooks, Beatrice. "Aggression," *American Journal of Nursing*, LXVII, No. 12 (December, 1967), 2519-2524.

Burd, Shirley, and Marshall, Margaret. *Some Clinical Approaches to Psychiatric Nursing*. New York: The Macmillan Co., 1963.

Carter, Francis M. *Psychosocial Nursing*, 2d ed. New York: The Macmillan Co., 1976.

Congress for Nursing Practice. *Standards of Psychiatric-Mental Health Nursing Practice*. Kansas City, Mo.: American Nurses' Association, 1973.

Ehmann, Virginia. "Empathy, Its Origin, Characteristics and Process," *Perspectives in Psychiatric Care*, IX, No. 2 (March-April, 1971), 72-80.

Erikson, Eric. *Childhood and Society*. New York. W.W. Norton & Co., 1950.

Glasser, William, and Zunin, Leonard. "Reality therapy" in *Current Psychotherapies*. Edited by R. Corsini. Itasca, Ill.: F.E. Peacock Publishers, Inc., 1973, pp. 287-315.

Goldsborough, Judith. "Involvement," *American Journal of Nursing*, LXIX, No. 1 (January, 1969), 66-69.

Kalish, Beatrice. "What is Empathy?" *American Journal of Nursing*, LXXIII, No. 9 (September, 1973), 1548-1552.

Kelly, Holly S. "The Sense of an Ending," *American Journal of Nursing*, LXIX, No. 11 (November, 1969), 2378-2382.

May, Rollo. *The Meaning of Anxiety*. New York: Ronald Press Company, 1950.

Penningroth, Philip. "Control of Violence in a Mental Hospital Setting," *American Journal of Nursing*, LXXV, No. 4 (April, 1975), 606-609.

Phillips, Bonnie. "Terminating a Nurse-Patient Relationship," *American Journal of Nursing*, LXVIII, No. 9 (September, 1968), 1941-1943.

Rogers, Carl. "Characteristics of a Helping Relationship," *Personnel Guidance Journal*, XXXVII, No. 1 (September, 1958), 6-16.

Sullivan, Harry S. *The Psychiatric Interview*. New York: W.W. Norton & Co., 1954.

Ujhely, Gertrud. *The Nurse and Her Problem Patients*. New York: Springer Publishing Co., Inc., 1967.

CHAPTER 6

The Nursing Process as a Framework for Psychiatric Nursing

Jeanette Lancaster, R.N., Ph.D.

INTRODUCTION

How one views the nature of man largely determines the substance of nursing actions. Each individual brings to the nursing situation preconceived notions of man. These ideas have a direct bearing on the conceptual approach utilized as the basis for practice. By definition, a conceptual approach refers to the unified body of beliefs and theories comprising the framework in which actions take place. Nursing has borrowed heavily from other disciplines attempting to design a conceptual basis for practice. The integration of biological, psychological, sociological and philosophical concepts and principles has enabled nurses to establish a holistic view of man.

Man, viewed from a holistic perspective, is considered part of, not apart from, the environment in which he exists. In order to meet his daily subsistence needs, man interacts with both his internal and external environments. Man is viewed as an open-ended system constantly interacting with his environment, so as to maintain life and function as a member of his species. Each of man's responses to environmental insults represents his attempt to maintain homeostasis. The complexity of these adaptive efforts can be best appreciated upon realizing that one cannot select certain environmental components toward which a response is directed, but rather each person faces the total environmental impact.

An individual's behavior in coping with both his internal and external environment provides clues to his needs. A framework is essential in order systematically to assess an individual's needs at any given time. Psychologist Abraham Maslow postulates a theory of human behavior based on need-fulfillment. Although Maslow's theoretical formulations were discussed in Chapter 3, they are summarized here to guide the reader's thinking.

Maslow describes a progressive hierarchy of needs which must be gratified in sequential order, if the individual is to attain higher level needs. Baseline physical needs are met first, including physiological requirements for air, water and food. The second level of needs refers to safety needs such as an environment free from noxious input or abuse.

Once physiological requirements and safety needs are met, the need for love and belonging seeks fulfillment. This refers to each person's need to experience closeness with at least one other person. The fourth step in the needs hierarchy, esteem needs, refers to an individual's requirement for respect and acknowledgment of worth and value as a unique being. Self-actualization needs comprise the last stage in Maslow's hierarchy. These needs, only met after all others are attained, refer to man's ability to develop his own potential as fully and productively as possible.

Maslow (1954) states that higher order needs are fulfilled only after completion of lower order needs. Thus, an individual may be unconcerned about his need for esteem, if he is struggling to find money to pay his rent and utility bills. The threat of being without a place to live or without heat and lights takes precedence over higher order needs. Similarly, a hungry person has tunnel vision when it comes to need-fulfillment: all of his energy is mobilized in an attempt to obtain food.

While a hierarchy such as Maslow's provides a valuable assessment tool, a word of caution is urged. Not all human situations are as simple as they appear on first glance. Thus, a nurse who completes a sketchy patient assessment may choose to focus on needs not representative of the actual problem. A behavior, such as losing weight, has varied causes and likely arises from more than one of the needs defined in the hierarchy.

Not all physical problems relate to physical needs; instead, some physical problems have origins in a higher level need. Consider the example of a 36-year-old female admitted to the hospital with a recent history of rapid loss of weight. Diagnostic testing reveals no physiological process to be causing the weight loss. After careful interviewing, the patient is ready to tell the nurse that she has recently obtained a divorce after sixteen years of a stormy marriage. Since her husband left the house, she cannot tolerate the sight of food. For her, mealtime is the loneliest time of the day. Prior to her divorce, it was only at meals that she and her husband could talk without arguing. Thus, her weight loss reflects an inability to meet love and belonging needs. For this patient, a stormy marriage was less frightening than the loneliness of divorce. The most beneficial nursing approach at this point is to plan with the patient ways she can begin to meet her love and belonging needs. What resources are possible options for her? What help does she need? What action is she willing to take to meet her needs? It is only through nurse-patient interaction, that the true needs behind a person's behavior can be uncovered.

Maslow's theory of personality refers to moving beyond equilibrium and homeostasis to new growth levels. It is not sufficient to avoid disease and dysfunction: complete need fulfillment strives for emotional growth in the face of new challenges and environmental inputs.

If the nurse is to assist patients in attaining a more productive interface with the environment, it is important to apply the nursing process. By definition, the nursing process is "an orderly, systematic manner of determining the client's problems, making plans to solve them, initiating the plan or assigning others to implement it, and evaluating the extent to which the plan was effective in resolving the problems identified" (Yura and Walsh, 1973, p. 23). The nursing process is based upon the problem-solving approach, with the decision-making process as a central feature.

Implicit in the nursing process is the belief that both patient and nurse determine goals and plan interventions. The principles of the problem-solving approach, a scientific way of organizing information, are included in the nursing process. The steps in the problem-solving approach include:

1. Observation and recognition of the problem
2. Definition of the problem
3. Formulation of hypotheses
4. Implementation of hypotheses
5. Formulation of conclusions

Similarly, the stages of the nursing process include:
1. Assessment
2. Planning
3. Implementation
4. Evaluation

Although the steps in the problem-solving approach and nursing process overlap, the purpose of each is different. The problem-solving approach holds as its purpose the development of new information and theories. In contrast, the nursing process seeks to maximize an individual's interaction with either internal or external environmental forces. The methods differ in that the problem-solving approach can be completed in isolation, while the nursing process is an interactive process with both client and nurse seeking to enhance the client's coping abilities.

The problem-oriented record serves as a framework for documenting the nursing process. Indeed, it is the written communication component of the action-oriented process. The problem-oriented record facilitates communication by its concise, straightforward listing of the data base, problem list, plan and follow-up. Its structure "encourages logic, clear thinking and the assessment of data in that for each problem the supporting data for its existence is formulated (Ryback, 1974). The subjective and objective portions of the problem-oriented record differentiate between fact and inference by separating what is directly observed from that reported by the patient, family or other staff members.

The steps of the nursing process are often labelled assessing, planning, implementing and evaluating, while the problem-oriented record is divided into the sections of data base, problem list, plan and follow-up. In this text, nursing assessment is the step in which the data base is obtained; the problem list and plans are made during the planning stage, with action occurring in the implementation phase and follow-up being synonymous with evaluation.

The nursing process focuses upon the client or patient and the family constellation in which he exists. It is initiated through a comprehensive and systematic assessment designed to identify needs, order the needs according to priority and decide which are nursing needs. Assessment is begun during the first nursing interview.

Although for convenience sake, the nursing process is divided into four sequential stages, in actuality, there is wide overlap of stages with two or more occurring simultaneously. Frequently during the evaluation stage, new nursing problems are identified, and the process begins anew. In order to study the process, the steps are described as sequential with the reminder that the nursing process is a complex, interactive approach for providing responsible care to clients.

The initial nursing interview, generally conducted within the first 48 hours of hospitalization, has as its purpose assessment of the patient's immediate needs. Comprehensive assessment and formulation of a problem list and plan are ideally carried out at a planning conference attended by the entire treatment team. Collaboration is essential, if the treatment plan is to be consistent among members of varied disciplines and is to provide continuity.

The primary purpose of assessment is to collect data related to the patient's mental health in order to formulate a list of nursing care problems. Standard I of the ANA Standards of Psychiatric-Mental Health Nursing Practice describes assessment factors (Congress for Nursing Practice, 1973).

STANDARD I

Data are collected through pertinent clinical observations based on knowledge of the arts and sciences, with particular emphasis upon psychosocial and biophysical sciences.

Rationale

Clinical observation is a prerequisite to realistic assessment of a client's needs and for the formulation of appropriate intervention. Observations can be facilitated through knowledge derived from a broad general education. In addition, scholarship acquired in the study of psychosocial and biophysical sciences fosters acuity of perception and alerts the nurse to psychological, cultural, social and other relevant clinical data.

Assessment Factors

1. Data collecting activities involve observation, analysis and interpretation of behavior patterns of clients which indicate a need for growth promoting relationships.

2. Data collecting activities involve identification of significant areas in which clinical data are needed.
3. Data collecting activities involve utilization of knowledge derived from appropriate sources to gain a comprehensive grasp of the client's experience.
4. Data collecting activities involve inferences drawn from observations which contribute to a formulation of therapeutic intervention.
5. Data collecting activities involve inferences and treatment observations which are shared and validated with appropriate others.

Assessment continues throughout the nurse-patient relationship, with each contact providing additional data, validating information or necessitating revision of previous conceptions. Nursing assessment is a complex perceptual and interpretive function utilizing all available data regarding behavior and mechanisms of functioning for detecting deviations from the norm. It is accomplished through skillful observation, competent interviewing and purposeful listening. Assessing to obtain a data base is a screening tool often necessitating further data collection.

Decision-making and judgment, inherent in all phases of the nursing process, are essential assessment components. The nurse decides what to ask, in what manner and of whom—the patient and/or his family. Using judgment, she differentiates between focal areas for cursory or intensive attention.

Although the patient is the primary source of data, the nurse obtains information from family, friends, medical records and test results. Information received from other sources is validated for accuracy with the patient. Standard II notes client involvement in each stage of the nursing process (Congress for Nursing Practice, 1973).

STANDARD II

Clients are involved in the assessment, planning, implementation and evaluation of their nursing care program to the fullest extent of their capabilities.

Rationale

To a very large degree, the therapeutic process is a learning process. The same principle that applies to learning also applies to therapy; that is, the learner or client must be an active participant in the process. The ability to participate in such a process will vary from person to person and, at times, even within the same person. The word "therapy" is used here in its broadest sense; that is, any behavior or planned activity that promotes growth and well-being. Thus, "nursing care program" and "nursing therapy" are interchangeably used, although it is recognized that many other forms of therapy exist.

Assessment Factors

1. Client's capabilities to participate at any given time are assessed, always keeping in mind the ultimate goals mutually determined by the client and nurse.
2. Plans for achieving and reexamining the goals are developed with the client, making whatever readjustments are necessary to progress toward them.
3. Problems are identified in collaboration with the client to determine needs and to set goals.
4. Progress of clients toward mutual goal achievement is assessed.

On occasion, clients admitted to an inpatient psychiatric facility are unable to provide accurate information. Some are not oriented to time, place or person, whereas others, while fully oriented, are agitated and unable coherently to describe the events precipitating the hospitalization. If the client is unable to participate fully in the assessment, information is obtained from the individuals bringing him to the hospital or clinic. The nurse later confirms the information with the client. Since the client or family member may have a biased perception of the situation, the nurse is objective in her assessment and takes neither side in the conflicting information.

Data from the patient, family, members of the health team, as well as other significant people, are collected through observing, interviewing, collaborating and from reading the records. The nursing assessment is accomplished by comprehensive visual, auditory or tactile observations and examination of the patient. Observation is purposeful rather than haphazard with guidelines specifying what to observe. For example, during the initial interview, the nurse allows considerable time to observe characteristics such as emotional tone, rate of speech and nonverbal behavior. Observation is also objective in that impressions and opinions are validated with other staff, records, family members or the patient.

Ideally, data are collected in a setting free from distractions. Clients, often upset over the impending hospitalization, are provided with privacy as they attempt to adjust to an unfamiliar setting. It is embarrassing for a client to participate in an initial assessment in an area open to the curiosity of onlookers. Questions are paced to the respondent's ability to handle in-coming information. Open-ended questions seem less threatening, in that they allow the individual some flexibility in his choice of response. Sample assessment questions include asking for the client's perception of the problem necessitating hospitalization; or discussing whether it was his idea to come to the hospital. An individual's response to the question, "Why did you come to the hospital today?" is generally laden with information. He may respond that he came because, "My father, that no-good bum, called the police who jerked me out of bed to bring me here." Such a response would indicate a feeling of powerlessness by being "jerked out of bed," as well as anger toward the father, "that no-good bum."

Another client, recognizing his need for help, might respond to the question of why he came to the hospital by saying that he is afraid, lonely, depressed or anxious and hopes to find help in dealing with these painful feelings. The client may demonstrate overt psychiatric symptoms of which he is aware, such as hallucinations, or he may evidence behavior which appears symptomatic to others but not to him. For example, the client experiencing delusions of persecution may say, "They are out to get me, and I want protection." Consciously, he may deny having a psychiatric problem, yet by coming to the hospital voluntarily, he acknowledges his feeling of helplessness.

How the family views the problem may closely resemble or dramatically contrast with the client's perception. Much can be learned about the functioning of a family by asking the client first how he perceives the problem and then individually asking each other family member. One 16-year-old girl said that her problem was, "My folks just don't understand what life is all about. They freak out when I smoke dope or miss a day or two of school." In contrast, the father defined the problem as his daughter just "being no-good; just a tramp who takes drugs, skips school and will never make anything of herself. She's just like her mother, always taking a tranquilizer or sleeping pill." In marked contrast, the mother said that the only problem was, "My daughter hangs around with drug types who influence her to do things like skip school. She will outgrow this wild behavior. All kids have to act up a little."

In this family, the perception of the problem differs appreciably from one member to another. Since the daughter was brought to the hospital against her wishes, her desire to participate in the treatment program is likely to be minimal. Moreover, the family response to the interviewer's questions uncovered conflict unrelated to the daughter. In this situation, the family conflict seems the underlying problem, with the daughter's behavior being a symptom of the stress.

Comprehensive and systematic nursing assessment is obtained by utilizing a standardized tool. Data collection is seldom completed during the initial assessment, although the nurse obtains considerable objective information by sensitivity, perception and astute observation. It may be beneficial to interview the client separately from his family, so that the nurse can direct complete attention to the one being interviewed.

The following assessment tool can be utilized in the psychiatric setting.

ASSESSMENT INTERVIEW TOOL

I. **OBJECTIVE DATA**

   A. Thought Process and Verbal Ability
   An individual's thought processes, either clear and reality-based or disordered, are reflected in his language. The manner in which a client responds to assessment questions indicates whether his thinking is organized or characterized by loose and fragmented association between thoughts. It is important to recall that high levels of anxiety interfere with thought processes.

   Areas to Assess
   1. Communication Patterns
      a) Is the client spontaneous or hesitant when he speaks?
      b) Is blocking of thoughts noted? Does he stop in the middle of a sentence?

c) Does his communication make sense? Is it necessary to ask the client, "What did you mean by that?"
2. Sensorium and Intelligence
   a) Is the client oriented to time, place and person?
   b) Is his memory accurate for recent and remote events? Does he know what he did yesterday, as well as where he was born or grew up?
   c) Is he attentive to the questions or does he look around and ask, "What did you say?"
   d) Can the client think abstractly, or is his thinking concrete? How does he respond to proverbs such as "a rolling stone gathers no moss" or "people who live in glass houses should not throw stones"?
3. Thought Processes
   a) Is the client coherent? Does he seem to complete a thought, or jump from topic to topic in mid-sentence?
   b) Are his comments clearly or loosely associated?
   c) Are any of the following types of disordered thinking noted?
      (1) Blocking—a sudden interruption of thought or speech.
      (2) Mutism—refusal to speak
      (3) Echolalia—meaningless repetition of the nurse's words
      (4) Neologisms—new words formed to express an idea
      (5) Flight of ideas—skipping from one topic to another in a fragmented often rapid fashion
      (6) Perseveration—involuntary repetition of the answer to a previous question in response to a new question
      (7) Word salad—a mixture of words and phrases lacking comprehensive meaning or coherence
4. Thought Content—Are thoughts consistent with reality?
   a) Obsessions—unwanted, recurring thoughts
   b) Delusions—persistent, false beliefs not in keeping with the person's culture or education

c) Hallucinations—false sensory perceptions without external stimuli
d) Ideas of reference—incorrect interpretation of causal incidents and external events, as though they are personally directed toward the self

5. Contact with the Environment
    a) Is the person oriented to time, place and person? Does he know where he is, who he is and the date?
    b) Is he easily distracted by sounds and sights nearby?

6. Sample Questions
    a) Do you know the name of the hospital? (Client may not have been told).
    b) Were you born in this area of the state?
    c) What brought you to the hospital? A concrete response would be "an ambulance," whereas an abstract response would in some way relate to the patient's problem.
    d) Do you have thoughts that worry you?
    e) Do you sometimes think people are talking about you?

B. Nonverbal Behavior
It is easier to control what is said than to control nonverbal actions such as gestures, movements, tone of voice, posture and facial expression. A client may provide more information by his actions than his words.

Areas to Assess

1. General Appearance, Attitude and Activity
    a) Appearance—Is the client clean and well-shaven? Is his posture erect or slumped? Are his clothes appropriate to the season, setting and occasion?
    b) Attitude—How does he react to you? Does he appear angry, cooperative, sullen, overly compliant, evasive or cheerful?
    c) Activity—Are signs of anxiety noted such as moist hands, restlessness, swinging leg or foot, cracking

knuckles? Is there evidence of a tic, hyperactivity, retarded movement, posturing or grimacing?
2. Sample Questions
    a) Will you tell me a little about yourself?
    b) Have things been going badly?

C. Social Assessment
This information may be obtained from the client, his family, records or observation.
1. Socioeconomic, educational and religious background
2. Family structure
3. Family understanding of client's illness
4. Work habits
5. Who visits the client? How often do visitors come? How do the visits seem to go—is warmth, aloofness or anger evident? Where do visitors sit in relation to the client? Is the client included in the conversation?
6. Sample Questions
    a) Who lives in your home?
    b) What is wrong with _____? (Ask the family this question)
    c) Does the client smoke, drink or consume drugs? (Ask both client and family)

D. Medical Assessment
The nurse must remain continuously aware that medical imbalances can cause symptoms resembling emotional dysfunction. System irregularities are noted both in the initial exam and on a daily basis by astute observation.
1. Circulatory—skin color and texture distribution of body hair, edema, condition of nails, palpitations and chest pain
2. Respiratory—breathing rate, presence of abnormal or labored breath sounds, chest pain, chest movement and diameter
3. Gastrointestinal—appetite, elimination pattern, discomfort
4. Genitourinary—frequency, pain on urination, pain in genitalia, discharge

5. Neurological—vision, hearing, speech, tactile, level of consciousness, reflexes, muscle tone and coordination, gait
6. Extremities—pulses, edema, varicosities, range of motion

II. **SUBJECTIVE DATA**
This category refers to an assessment of the client's perception of his present situation, including his thoughts, feelings and behaviors.

   A. Present Illness and Current Coping Patterns
   A client's description of his current situation provides data about his contact with reality, ability to tolerate and handle stress, and the defense mechanisms he currently utilizes.

   Areas to Assess

   1. Client's reasons for coming to the hospital are discussed.
   2. What does the precipitating event mean to the client?
   3. How does the client handle stress?
   4. Sample Questions
      a) What was going on with you before you came to the hospital?
      b) Has anything like this happened to you before?
      c) What happened to upset you?
      d) What was your reaction when _____ occurred?

   B. Support Systems
   Each client constantly interacts with his environment in an attempt to attain homeostasis. Viewed from a systems theory framework, a client is one component (subsystem) of a larger system (family, group, community). The resources available to a client in his system provide support or intensify stress. Mental illness is seen as a system breakdown, in that the homeostatic state is upset with one person seeming more "out of phase" or in disequilibrium within the total system. Careful assess-

ment reveals system supports as well as factors mitigating against homeostasis. Frequently, family therapy is included in a program for reinstituting equilibrium in the system.

Areas to Assess

1. Whom does the client trust?
2. Whom does he believe cares about him?
3. How do the patient and family members act toward one another?
4. Who seems to be concerned about the client?
5. Sample Questions
    a) Whom do you talk with when you are upset?
    b) How would you describe your family?

C. Self-Assessment

How a person views himself affects all aspects of his life. One's self-view is learned through interactions with significant others throughout life. What a person believes about himself is largely a reflection of what others have said about him, and how they have responded to him. The way in which a client views himself determines his behavior. A person with feelings of inadequacy and worthlessness approaches situations differently than one whose self-view is characterized by security and assurance. The goals a person strives for are influenced by his self-concept. A person who feels worthless is unlikely to be motivated toward greater achievements. His orientation to life is colored with hopelessness and apathy.

Areas to Assess

1. How does the client view himself?
2. Is his self-view consistent with how others (including the staff) view him?
3. Does he appear motivated to change?

4. Sample Questions
   a) What do you like about yourself?
   b) What would you like to change about yourself?
   c) Do any changes in your ability to get along with others seem possible?

D. Awareness
   It is often easier to use defense mechanisms to handle stressful situations than to deal with reality. Clients may deny their true feelings, so as to insulate themselves from further pain. A client may also project his feelings onto others. The degree to which an individual is aware of his feelings and experiences in the "here and now" influences his ability to cope. It is easier to focus on events (actions) and thoughts than on feelings. Before a client can problem-solve and move forward, he must be aware of his feelings. In the assessment stage, the nurse collects data about ways in which a patient expresses and deals with his feelings. When he is angry, does he deal with the anger directly or handle it indirectly by withdrawing or turning the anger into somatic pain?

Areas to Assess

1. How does he handle feelings such as anger, sadness, joy?
2. Is he aware of his behavior patterns?
3. Sample Questions
   a) What do you do (say), when someone hurts your feelings?
   b) What was your reaction the last time something pleasant happened? Once essential data are collected, the next step is to formulate a nursing diagnosis or statement of the patient's psychiatric problem. This is completed through the development of the problem list in the planning phase. Standard III of the ANA Standards of Psychiatric-Mental Health Nursing Practice, defines this step in the nursing process (Congress for Nursing Practice, 1973).

STANDARD III

The problem-solving approach is utilized in developing nursing care plans.

Rationale

A nursing diagnosis is based on pertinent theories of human behavior. It is used to plan therapeutic intervention, taking into consideration the characteristics and capacities of the individual and his environment in order to maximize the treatment program for the client.

Assessment Factors

1. The individual's reaction to the environment is observed and assessed.
2. Themes and patterns of behavior are observed and assessed.
3. Nursing care plans are used as a guide to nursing intervention.
4. Nursing care plans are interpreted to professional and non-professional persons giving care.
5. Observations and reports of others are incorporated in the nursing care plans.
6. Nursing care plans are designed, implemented and reviewed systematically by the nursing staff

The data gathered are written in SOAP format. That is, the data are written as subjective, objective, assessment and plans in the progress notes. (Figure 6-1 indicates the data flow used in the problem-oriented record.)

The nursing process and problem-oriented record are completely merged in the acronym SOAPIER with the letters representing:

S — Subjective data (symptoms as identified by the patient or client)
O — Objective data (signs or nursing observations)
A — Assessment (nursing conclusion based on the subjective and objective data; nursing diagnosis)
P — Plans or nursing interventions which, in the nursing diagnosis, are related to the assessed patient problem

```
┌─────────────────────┐
│ DATA BASE           │
│ (Assessment)        │
│ Subjective data     │
│ Objective data      │
│ Nursing Diagnosis   │
└─────────────────────┘
          ↓
    ┌─────────────────────────┐
    │ Complete Problem List   │
    │ (Based on assessment    │
    │      above)             │
    └─────────────────────────┘
                ↓
        ┌──────────────┐
        │    PLAN      │
        └──────────────┘
                    ↓
            ┌──────────────────┐
            │ IMPLEMENTA-      │
            │    TION          │
            └──────────────────┘
                        ↓
                ┌──────────────┐
                │ EVALUATION   │
                └──────────────┘
```

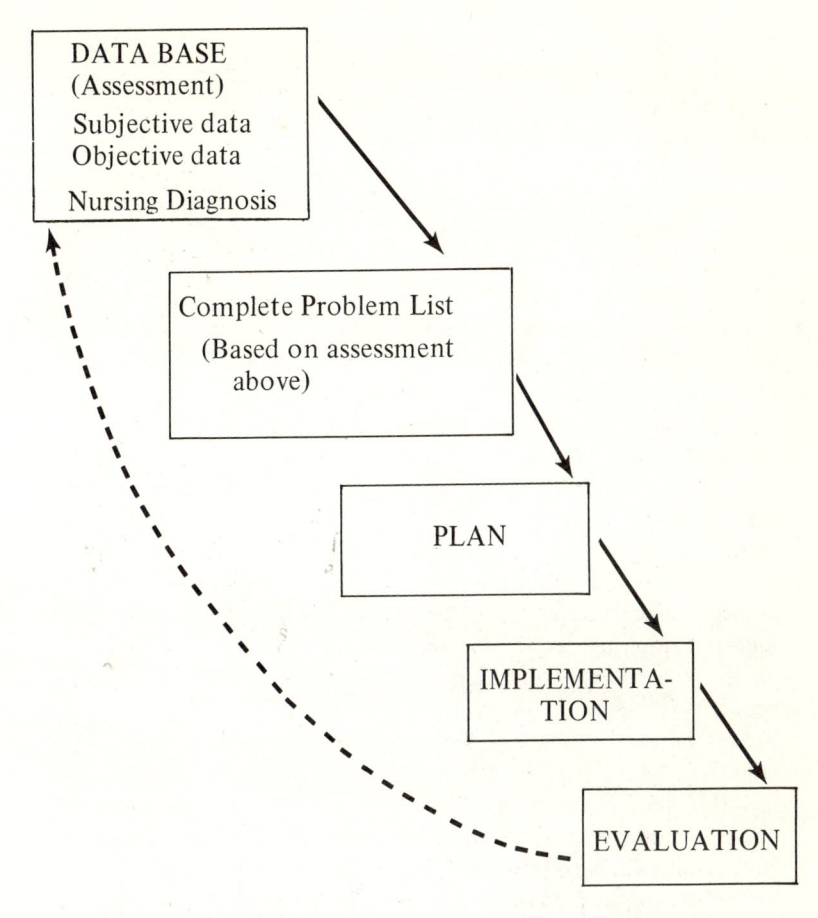

Figure 6-1: Data flow used in the problem-oriented record.

I — Implementation or nursing actions done for, with or to the patient or client

E — Evaluation, which is an appraisal of the outcome of the nursing process.

R — Revision based on the steps identified above (SOAPIE).

The problem list or nursing diagnosis is made jointly with the client. The goals must be attainable, with progress toward meeting them measurable. From an operational framework, "a problem may be defined as anything important enough to do something about or for which something has been done" (Ryback, 1974).

A nursing diagnosis is defined as the "judgment or conclusion which occurs as a result of nursing assessment." The nursing diagnosis is a statement of the nursing care goal derived directly from the identified patient problem. Nursing in the past has hesitated to use the term "diagnose" to refer to an identification of patient needs. Diagnose has long been associated with medical care and, until recently, seemed to have little relevance to other areas of health care. By definition, diagnose means "to recognize or identify by examination and observation" (Webster, 1961). Using the above definition, diagnosis has long been an integral component of nursing practice.

According to Mayers (1972) nursing diagnosis includes actual, potential or possible problems. Thus, the nursing diagnosis is essential to all three stages of preventive care: primary, secondary and tertiary.

In defining the problem, first consider the immediate circumstances. What is causing the current difficulty? Focus on the here and now, looking carefully at the presenting problem or chief complaint. The precipitating event leading to a client's contact with a health care agency is generally recent. What was the "straw that broke the camel's back?" What is the client's perception of the situation; what does the problem mean to him? In what way does he feel threatened? Once the immediate situation is presented, the nurse can move to the underlying problem. For example, if an adolescent comes to the hospital because the police picked him up for possession and consumption of drugs, the immediate situation may be to provide supportive care directed toward his physical needs, while he recovers from the drug abuse syndrome. Nursing care may later be directed toward the underlying problems of anxiety and loneliness.

Problems necessitating nursing actions arise when a person cannot meet his own needs and requires assistance in coping with current life situations and need attainment. Difficulties in coping also occur when a client attempts to meet his needs in an inappropriate fashion or in ways conflicting with societal norms and expectations.

Prior to planning nursing interventions, patient problems must be clearly and specifically listed. A well-stated problem must be both specific and patient-centered.

Following an enumeration of the problems, the next step is to assign priorities to the list. The most pressing problems are dealt with first.

As problems are clarified and refined, the original list is modified accordingly, with a notation made beside each problem which has been resolved or cancelled. To be functional, the problem list must be accurate, comprehensive and current. Not all complaints are noted on the list. Those seen as momentary, such as gastric distress relieved by an antacid, are not included. Each problem has its own correspondingly numbered plan, so that an observer can correlate problem and nursing plan.

A nursing plan organizes and provides direction and structure to what is done for and with a client. Based on the application of theory from nursing, as well as from related content areas such as the physical and social sciences, the plan strives to meet the identified needs of the client. Each plan is individualized, just as each client is unique.

The first step in planning nursing intervention is to develop clearly described objectives or goals for nursing action.

Nursing goals or objectives may be defined as the "expected physical or behavioral outcomes to be achieved through the nursing process" (Monken, 1975 p. 110). Goal statements, like the problem list, must be specific and patient centered. The desired outcome of the action must be clearly evident in the goal statement. Nursing goals should include the following:

1. Who — the person performing the activity
2. What — the specific action
3. Where — the location of the action or intervention
4. When — the time frame in which the action is to occur
5. For, with or to whom — the recipient of the action

A prerequisite in writing objectives is that the outcome or result be measurable. Thus, objectives are written in behavioral terms, with the verb in each objective being measurable. For example, behaviors such as to identify, to list or to describe are measurable in contrast to verbs such as to know, to think or to feel. The more specifically an objective can be stated, the more beneficial it is in planning nursing care. Writing objectives and making plans is no easy task; the task is simplified by using concise, descriptive language rather than opinionated or generalized terms. Examples of measurable objectives include:

1. Assist the client to identify three positive self-attributes
2. Describe two ways to express anger
3. List the last two times joy was experienced
4. Plan three actions for obtaining a job.

The nursing plan involves mutual decision-making with the client to establish priorities, as well as to determine short- and long-term goals. The client must have input into the plan or it is doomed to failure, due to his lack of motivation or his efforts to sabotage the plan. Moreover, since each client retains responsibility for his actions, he must have input into any plan developed for his treatment. The purposes of the planning phase are:

1. to assign priorities to the identified problems
2. to differentiate problems handled by nursing intervention, those handled by the client and family and those requiring referral to other members of the health team
3. to designate specific actions for meeting long- and short-term goals
4. to write the problems and describe the actions and expected outcomes on the record.

Nursing orders, or prescriptions, must be both specific and clearly related to the client problem. Nursing orders include what is to be done (action), when it is to be done, where and how (by what means).

Implementation is the deliberate action to meet the planning goals. Prior to implementation, alternatives are delineated and possible consequences described. An action is taken with the expectation that if _____ is taken, the _____
              planned action   expected result
will occur. In examining alternatives to plan implementations, all possible approaches of tackling the problem are considered, choosing the action having the most desirable consequences. The client's perception of the consequences of proposed actions and their meaning to him are of importance in selecting alternatives. The nurse may perceive the consequences of an action as of no importance, whereas the client, functioning from a different frame of reference with a unique set of needs, may perceive the consequences in an entirely different way.

During the implementation phase, the nurse uses her interpersonal, technical and intellectual skills to observe, communicate and make decisions. Using the problem list and plan as a blueprint, the nurse puts the plan into practice. Additional information is collected during this phase, as the nurse responds to verbal and nonverbal input from the client. Priorities are reevaluated, considering the client's response to the implementation of the planned actions. While the implementation phase has an action focus, it continues the process of assessment, planning and evaluation. This phase ends when the nursing actions are completed and have been recorded.

Accurate record-keeping is essential in implementing the nursing process. The problem-oriented record is utilized to provide a concise, non-repetitive format. In the problem-oriented record, duplication of content is decreased, as progress notes from all members of the health care team are written in chronological order in the same section of the record, rather than having a space designated for physicians, nurses and each speciality group on the health care team.

Each entry in the problem-oriented record is organized according to a specified format denoted by the acronym SOAP. This designation refers to the subjective, objective, assessment and planning information.

Subjective information includes all data reported by the client. The client's view of his present situation and his description of the problem are included as subjective data. Data to confirm or disagree with the client's subjective account are included in the objective component. This information is obtained from records, other health team members or by direct observation of the client. Standard VIII of the ANA Standards of Psychiatric-Mental Health Nursing Practice (Congress for Nursing Practice, 1973) describes the collaborative aspect of obtaining a data base.

STANDARD VIII

Nursing participates with interdisciplinary teams in assessing, planning, implementing and evaluating programs and other mental health activities.

Rationale

In addition to the nurse, the number and variety of people working with clients in the mental health field today make it imperative that efforts be coordinated to provide the best total program. Communication, planning, problem-solving and evaluation are required of all those who work with a particular client or program.

Assessment Factors

1. Specific knowledge, skills and activities are identified and articulated, so that these may be coordinated with the contributions of others working with a client or a program.
2. The value of nursing and team member contributions is recognized and respected.
3. Consultation with other team members is utilized as needed.
4. Nursing participates in the formulating of overall goals, plans and decisions.
5. Skills are developed in small group process for maximum team effectiveness.

Each identified problem has a specific number, which remains constant as long as the problem is a part of the record. All subsequent SOAP notes correspond with the number attached to the problem.

The assessment section is initially derived from analysis of subjective and objective sections. As the nurse becomes acquainted with the client, her assessment includes an expanded data base. Also, with each interaction, data are added, elaborated on or changed. Such on-going evaluation elicits additional assessment areas.

In the planning section, action is described in relation to each identified problem. Weed (1970) describes three content areas of the planning component:

1. Additional collection of data is required
2. Treatment plan
3. Plans for client education

Teaching is accomplished by one health care team member or as a result of collaborative efforts. The client is the core of the teaching effort, with his comprehension of the problem essential. Standard IV of the ANA Standards of Psychiatric-Mental Health Nursing Practice (Congress for Nursing Practice, 1973) describes collaborative efforts for health teaching.

STANDARD IV

Individuals, families and community groups are assisted in achieving satisfying and productive patterns of living through health teaching.

Rationale

Health teaching is an essential part of a nurse's role in work with those who have mental health problems. Every interaction can be utilized as a teaching-learning situation. Formal and informal teaching methods can be used in working with individuals, families, the community and other personnel. Emphasis is on understanding mental health problems, as well as on developing ways of coping with them.

Assessment Factors

1. The needs of individual, family and community groups for health teaching are identified, and appropriate techniques are used in meeting these needs.
2. The principles of learning and teaching are employed.
3. The basic principles of physical and mental health and interpersonal and social skills are taught.
4. Experiential learning opportunities are made available.
5. Opportunities with community groups to further their knowledge and understanding of mental health problems are identified.

Evaluation is the specific measurement of the effectiveness of the actions taken to intervene in the patient's problems. The evaluation phase is a time for reappraisal of the decisions made in earlier stages, as well as an evaluation of the actions taken. In initiating the evaluation phase, the nurse reviews the goals set by the original assessment, ascertaining whether the goals have been met, whether they were realistic in the light of additional information or whether omissions occurred.

As in all other phases, the client is involved in evaluation. Standard II of the ANA Standards of Psychiatric-Mental Health Nursing Practice (Congress for Nursing Practice, 1973) describes the evaluation phase as including the client.

Selected useful questions to ask during evaluation include:

1. What was the expected client behavior?
2. Was the expected behavior realistic, accurate?
3. What behavior was observed?
4. What goals have been met?
    a) What factors influenced goal attainment?
    b) What factors inhibited or limited goal attainment?
5. What additional data are indicated and from whom should they be obtained?
6. Are some problems partially resolved?
7. If the patient's behavior indicates that problems were not resolved, what were the reasons?
8. Do the nursing and medical care conflict or complement each other?
9. Are new problems evident?
10. Were the nursing actions based on principles from the physical, biological or behavioral sciences?

Evaluation is often a neglected phase of the nursing process, possibly because tools for evaluation are not readily available and, to date, evaluation has not been a widely acknowledged component of the nursing process. While evaluation is stressed on paper, few verbal comments are directed toward this aspect in many clinical agencies. Too often, one evaluates only when an inspection is imminent. Moreover, if the patient gets better and leaves the hospital, staff may decide that intervention worked and fail to take time to assess what contributed to the effectiveness of the implementation. If the patient fails to get better, nursing staff decides he has limited resources and motivation, that is, he "is choosing not to get well—to keep his old coping mechanisms."

At times, the nurse's perception of the situation is inaccurate and hinders evaluation. Supervision and guidance by peers and administrative personnel prove valuable when the situation seems unclear. In the planning stage, a variety of alternative approaches is identified. In evaluating the approach used, if the outcome is nonproductive, additional alternatives are examined. The nurse, at times, is involved in the situation to the extent that neither she nor the client can perceive alternatives. Outside resource persons can help consider options and approaches. Both peer evaluation and supervisory sessions provide valuable information and feedback in the nurse-patient relationship.

Nursing education seeks to stimulate peer and supervisor evaluation by the use of written nursing process records and process recordings. The written work is shared with an instructor and, on occasion, with peers in an attempt to validate the accuracy and comprehensiveness of the written work.

SUMMARY

In applying the nursing process, it is essential to be aware of the order most individuals utilize in need-fulfillment. Physiological needs take precedence over higher level needs such as love, belonging and esteem.

The stages of the nursing process include: assessment, planning, implementation and evaluation. Each step has implications for the other steps with an implicit feedback system in the process. For example, on occasion, the outcome of the evaluation stage of a nursing action sheds light on additional problems and indicates the need for further assessment.

The problem-oriented record serves as a framework for documenting the nursing process. It provides a logical, concise medium for recording the steps of the nursing process. An accurate and complete assessment is essential to the implementation of the nursing process, as all other stages are built on the assessment. The assessment provides the data base, which includes the subjective and objective data in the problem-oriented data base component of the record. Following an assessment, the nursing diagnoses are identified and an action-oriented plan is described and implemented. Evaluation of the plan is essential to determine if the actions were adequate to meet the patient's needs.

PRINCIPLES

1. All behavior includes the individual's total response to stimuli.
2. The response of an individual is the best that he is capable of making at the given moment.
3. Inherent in every individual is a potential for striving forward.
4. Increased consistency of the nurse leads to an increased ability of the patient to trust the nurse.
5. Information essential to understanding a person and his problems can be obtained by the process of interviewing.
6. Interviewing is more effective when geared to the interviewee's

age, as well as to his mental and physical capabilities.
7. Successful interviewing depends upon attitudes of acceptance, objectivity, kindness and warmth.
8. Each individual seeks to meet physiological needs, before he turns his attention to meeting higher level needs.

Nursing Diagnoses Commonly Seen in Psychiatric Settings*

1. *Anxiety, Mild*
   Increased questioning
   Restlessness
   Increased awareness
   Increased attending

2. *Anxiety, Moderate*
   Voice tremors
   Voice pitch changes
   Rate of verbalization
   Shakiness
   Pacing
   Increased muscle tension
   Narrowing focus of attention
   Diaphoresis
   Increased heart rate
   Increased respiratory rate
   Increase in verbalization

3. *Anxiety, Severe*
   Inappropriate verbalization
   Purposelessness
   Perceptual focus scattered
   Perceptual focus fixed
   Tachycardia
   Hyperventilation

4. *Anxiety, Panic*
   Difficulty in verbalization

---
*Kristine Gebbie (ed.), *Summary of the First National Conference/Classification of Nursing Diagnoses*, St. Louis: C.V. Mosby Co., 1975.

Immobilization
Inability to focus on reality
Dilated pupils
Pallor

5. *Confusion*
   Disoriented to person (and/or time, place, object, purpose)
   Inappropriate verbal and/or nonverbal behavior
   Statements reflecting recognition of confusion
   Other possible defining characteristics:
   Impaired attention span
   Restlessness
   Purposeless responses (activity)
   Inappropriate activity (responses or affect)
   Anxiety
   Agitation
   Apprehension
   Fright
   Verbosity
   Confabulation
   Rambling speech
   Dependent and demanding attention-getting behavior
   Withdrawal
   Belligerence
   Combativeness
   Facial expression specific to confusion
   Hyperactive

6. *Grieving, Acute*
   Loss of significant object
   Expression of distress at loss
   Denial of loss
   Guilt
   Anger
   Sorrow
   Choked feelings
   Changes in eating habits
   Alterations in sleep patterns
   Alterations in activity level
   Altered libido
   Altered communication patterns

7. *Grieving, Anticipatory*
   Potential loss of significant object
   Expression of distress at potential loss
   Denial of potential loss
   Guilt
   Anger
   Sorrow
   Choked feelings
   Changes in eating habits
   Alterations in sleep patterns
   Alterations in activity level
   Altered libido
   Altered communication patterns

8. *Grieving, Delayed*
   Loss of significant object at least one year in past
   Expression of distress at loss
   Denial of loss
   Guilt
   Anger
   Sorrow
   Choked feelings
   Changes in eating habits
   Alterations in sleep patterns
   Alteration in activity level
   Altered libido
   Altered communication patterns

9. *Manipulation*
   Lack of empathy
   Self-centered
   Covert use of others to meet own goals
   Overt use of others to meet own goals
   Avoidance of open communication
   Conscious attempt to influence others
   Unconscious attempt to influence others
   Attempt to play people against each other

10. *Self Concept: Alterations in Body Image*
    Alterations in verbalization regarding body

Alterations in response to body change
Self-motivation and self-destruction
Denial of altered body state
Alteration in perceived focus of control
Expressed feelings of hopelessness
Expressed feelings of helplessness
Expressed feelings of powerlessness
Other possible defining characteristics:
    Alteration in ability to accept positive reinforcement
    Alteration in ability to make change, grow, adapt
    Alteration in ability to adapt redependency and independence

11. *Sensory/Perceptual Alterations*
Disoriention in time
Disoriention to place
Disoriention to persons
Altered abstraction
Altered conceptualization
Change in problem-solving abilities
Report of change in sensory acuity
Measured change in sensory acuity
Change in behavior pattern
Anxiety
Apathy
Change in usual response to stimuli
Indication of body image alteration

12. *Sleep-Rest Activity, Dysrhythm of*
Restless when asleep
Restless when awake
Change in activity level
Dozing
Insomnia
Difficulty in arousing
Delayed response to stimuli
Increased response to stimuli
Irritability
Verbalization of sleep disturbances
Verbalization of fatigue
Lethargy

13. *Thought Processes Impaired*
    Impaired attention span
    Discrepancy between chronological age and development level
    Inappropriate behavior
    Impaired recall ability
    Decreased ability to grasp ideas
    Decreased ability to order ideas
    Impaired ability to reason
    Impaired ability to conceptualize
    Impaired judgment
    Impaired perception
    Impaired decision-making

BIBLIOGRAPHY

Black, Kathleen. "Appraising the Psychiatric Patient's Nursing Needs," *American Journal of Nursing*, LII, No. 6 (June, 1952), 718-720.

Congress for Nursing Practice. *Standards of Psychiatric-Mental Health Nursing Practice*. Kansas City, Mo.: American Nurses' Association, 1973.

Maslow, Abraham. *Motivation and Personality*. New York: Harper & Row, Publishers, 1954.

Mayers, M.G. *A Systematic Approach to the Nursing Care Plan*. New York: Appleton-Century-Crofts, 1972.

Monken, S.S. "After Assessment—What Then?" *Nursing Clinics of North America*. Vol. 10, No. 2 (March, 1975), 107-120.

Ryback, Ralph. *The Problem-Oriented Record in Psychiatry and Mental Health Care*. New York: Grune & Stratton, Inc., 1974.

Webster. *Webster's New Collegiate Dictionary*. Springfield, Mass.: G. & C. Merriam Co., 1961.

Weed, Lawrence. *Medical Records, Medical Education, and Patient Care*. Cleveland, Oh.: Case Western Reserve University Press, 1970.

Yura, Helen, and Walsh, Mary. *The Nursing Process: Assessing, Planning, Implementing, Evaluating*. 2d ed. New York: Appleton-Century-Crofts, 1973.

PART III: Clinical Entities In Psychiatric Nursing

CHAPTER 7

Depression and Suicidal Behavior

Linda Colvin, R.N., M.S.

"Sadness, hopelessness, dejection, emptiness, a feeling of low self-esteem—these are the affective content of depression" (Swanson, 1975). Almost everyone has known transient depression, usually precipitated by a loss. The loss may be real, such as the death of a loved one or loss of job or status, or it may be a feared or imagined loss. Regardless of the nature of the loss, dejection and lowered self-esteem result.

Depression as a mood or affect is universal and normal. Most people at some point experience a depressed feeling resulting from a blow to self-esteem or the actual or threatened loss of something of value.

This chapter focuses on depressive neuroses, psychotic depressive reactions and suicidal behavior. The "blues" and grief are briefly discussed to distinguish them from the diagnostic categories of depression.

After a disappointment or loss, one may feel sad or "blue." This is a transient period of lowered spirits, in which the person is aware of the event causing the depressed mood. Sadness and a dejected feeling often accompany physical illness, and end when a person resumes normal activities.

During the "blues" episode, one may suffer crying spells, irritability, decreased ambition and difficulty in concentrating. As confidence in one's ability to function returns, and routines resume, the sadness lifts.

Grief

Following the death of a loved one, a person goes through a period of grief; thinking centers around the lost person. During grief, symptoms of depression such as crying, restlessness, numbness, guilt, sadness, inability to sleep or diminished appetite emerge in realistic balance with the loss suffered.

Within four to eight weeks, normal acute grief, an adaptive process, nears completion. The symptoms decrease as the person "works through" feelings about the loss. Although one suffers during the grieving process, one rarely sees oneself as a "bad" or worthless person.

Depressive Neurosis

This disorder is manifested by an excessive reaction of depression due to an internal conflict or to an identifiable event such as the loss of a love object or cherished possession. (Committee on Nomenclature and Statistics of the APA, 1968).

Psychotic Depressive Reaction

This psychosis is distinguished by a depressive mood attributable to some experience. Ordinarily, the individual has no history of repeated depressions or cyclothymic mood swings. The differentiation between this condition and depressive neurosis depends on whether the reaction impairs reality testing or functional adequacy enough to be considered a psychosis. (Committee on Nomenclature and Statistics of the APA, 1968).

From these definitions, depressive neurosis and psychotic depressive reaction can be considered together, the major difference being a matter of degree. "Studies using multivariate statistical techniques have consistently failed to separate a neurotic group from a psychotic group. The neurotic-psychotic distinction appears to form a continuum of grades of severity" (Klermangl, Gerald L. "Overview of Depression," from Freedman, Alfred M., Kaplan, Harold I., and Sadock, Benjamin (eds.). *Comprehensive Textbook of Psychiatry*. Vol. II. 2d ed. Baltimore: Williams & Wilkins, 1975, p. 1010).

Through the years, writers have discussed depressed people. Hippocrates, in the fourth century B.C., regarded melancholia as the result of black bile. Aristotle suggested the use of wine, music, aphrodisiacs and catharsis as the treatment for melancholia. The poet, Edna St. Vincent Millay (1969, p. 188), presents a striking picture of the depressed person:

> I know a hundred ways to die
> I've often thought I'd try one;
> Lie down beneath a motor truck
> Some day when standing by one.
>
> Or throw myself from off a bridge—
> Except such things must be
> So hard upon the scavengers
> And men that clean the sea.
>
> I know some poison I could drink.
> I've often thought I'd taste it
> But mother bought it for the sink,
> And drinking it would waste it.

Dynamics of Depression

Before discussing application of the nursing process to the depressed individual, it is important to set forth the theoretical framework in which depression is considered to develop. Various theories are available regarding the etiology of depression. The theoretical position taken in this chapter is that depression occurs in response to a loss in which the individual, suffering from low self-esteem, cannot deal constructively with the ramifications of the loss and functions with considerable unresolved anger.

A closer look at what leads to inability to deal constructively is necessary. The development of low self-esteem is central to the etiology of depression. Self-esteem is affected by self-image, superego, ego ideal and ego functions. According to psychoanalytic theory, a healthy development includes learning to differentiate self from others, relating effectively with others and developing a consistently high and lifelong level of self-esteem. For these developments to take place, the child needs loving parents who help him face frustrations in amounts he can handle. The environment of parental affection and acceptance allows him to develop a high self-esteem and enter into interpersonal and educational activities independent of his parents. As he succeeds in these activities, his high level of self-esteem is strengthened.

If, during development, a child undergoes extreme emotional traumas, the child may develop low self-esteem and be predisposed to depression in later years. Such childhood traumas include death or loss of a parent; lack of parental acceptance, love or affection; rejection from one or both parents; parental devaluation; frustrations experienced too early and before adaptive mechanisms are available; and failure in early social activities or in early educational activities.

A closer look at the loss of a parent in childhood is indicated, for it is recognized as a potential predisposing factor in depression. The theory holds that a child having ambivalent feelings about the lost parent fears that dislike or anger toward the parent caused the death (magical thinking). Feelings of guilt over the death, buried (repressed) as the person develops, become a source of intrapsychic conflict which are ignited by a loss in adult life.

Low self-esteem may develop due to the lack of love and acceptance necessary for sound personality development and a generalized sense of worthiness. Other factors influencing self-esteem are disfigurement, unattractiveness, guilt feelings or failure in performance. Accordingly, the combined forces of low self-esteem and a stress in adult life leave the person in a state diagnosed as a depression.

A look at adult stresses provides clues the nurse picks up from the patient's history, which lead to the final diagnosis. These include college failure, emotional rejections, marital crises, conflicts at work, job failures, loss of status, major financial setbacks, loss of money or material possessions, death of a family member or friend, or loss of a close friend, as through moving.

The unresolved childhood problems and the adult trauma combine to leave one overwhelmed with feelings of worthlessness, guilt and extreme sadness.

Other factors possibly leading to vulnerability to depression include genetic traits, hereditary predisposition and biochemical make-up.

Depressed persons may be angry persons who have learned faulty or nonfacilitative ways of dissipating the anger. Rather than deal directly and consciously with the angry feelings, these persons summon tremendous psychic energy to keep the feelings below the level of awareness. Freud refers to the anger turned inward as retroflexed rage; anger misdirected toward oneself, rather than handled in a direct fashion, is common with depressed persons.

An example of the dynamics of depression can be operationally summarized as follows:

1. Development of low self-esteem in childhood
2. Loss of a valued object (either a real or imagined loss)
3. Ambivalent feelings toward the valued object (a mixture of simultaneously held positive and negative feelings)
4. Guilt over the negative or hate part of the ambivalence
5. Burying or hiding this guilt from awareness (the belief is held by the person, "I shouldn't feel this way")
6. Anger and aggression turned inward toward the self, since the person cannot tolerate conscious negative feelings toward the valued object.

DEPRESSION AND PHYSIOLOGICAL DISEASES

Since the same behavior or symptoms are observed with psychological stress as with physiological stress, the nurse needs to be aware of the medical conditions which (1) may lead to depression and (2) may present as depression. Behavior changes and symptoms may be diagnosed as the results of a psychogenic disorder, when, in reality, they are the results of an unrecognized systemic disease. On the other hand, symptoms may be diagnosed as a systemic disease, when they actually reveal a psychogenic disorder. Symptom description, history and a complete physical examination lead to the correct diagnosis and treatment.

Illnesses such as malignant, metabolic and degenerative diseases seem to be depression-producing. Specifically, cancer, heart disease, cerebrovascular accidents, multiple sclerosis and Parkinson's disease frequently lead to depression.

Medical diseases including infectious hepatitis, carcinoma of the head of the pancreas, malnutrition, frontal lobe tumors and some anemias present depressive sequelae. Drugs, such as reserpine, steroids, Rauwolfia derivatives and phenothiazines can produce depression. Also, the period when a patient is being taken off steroids may induce depression (Wintrobe, 1974, p. 1889).

SYMPTOMS OF DEPRESSION

Emotional and Psychological Symptoms

The depressed person reports that he feels blue, sad, unhappy, depressed, bored, indifferent to surroundings, empty, lonely or gloomy. He may plead guilty of a variety of transgressions against others, feel hopeless in the face of an overwhelming atmosphere of gloom and be totally inadequate to deal with the onslaught of events. Life often seems meaningless, and one approaches each new activity with a feeling of numbness and emotional insulation. Regardless of what one attempts, the end result is the same—an oppressive feeling of despair and concern that one may have acted in an unacceptable fashion. Many comments indicate self-reproach about past as well as present activities. Being exceedingly self-critical and derogatory, such a person acknowledges few accomplishments.

Statements reflecting decreased self-esteem include, "My family would be better off without me," "I'm so useless now" or "I don't deserve to live."

Due to ruminations of an obsessive nature, the depressed person is not sought out by others, who soon tire of hearing repetitious discussion and complaints.

Physical Symptoms

The depressed person presents as an unhappy, dejected-appearing individual. The typically depressed facies is characterized by strained, drawn features with a pervading mood of discouragement, apathy and fatigue. At times, such a person may alternate between crying and attempting to force a bleak, unsuccessful smile. Discussion reveals that it takes considerable effort to get through activities of daily living; washing his face and combing his hair may seem difficult tasks. Actions are characterized by psychomotor slowdown of speech, walking and gestures. Lassitude or lack of energy may be the first indication of the onset of a depression. The physical lassitude precedes feelings of despair and hopelessness.

The depressed person reporting an increased sensitivity to cold wears sweaters and covers himself at night with several blankets, when others in the same environment appear comfortable in short-sleeve clothing. It seems as though the depressed person is *trans-*

posing internal feelings of coldness and barrenness to the environment and then experiencing the coldness, as though it were present all around.

An intellectual slowdown is typically noted in the depressed person. Thinking may be exceedingly difficult, with ideational content limited to a few topics. These topics may revolve around somatic ailments seeming hypochondriacal in nature. It is as if one cannot direct attention outside one's own physical being. Spontaneous speech is limited, with the person responding to questions as briefly as possible, providing little indication of private thoughts.

Social withdrawal is noted in the depressed person. One may present an obstinate unwillingness to meet people, avoiding new social contacts. One further finds it difficult to be in the presence of people who once were friends, even intimates. At times, the depressed person may walk the long way around to avoid speaking to a friend.

These behavioral changes—unkempt appearance, dark clothing, loss of interest in hobbies, avoidance of friends—are important in the diagnosis of depression, because they are often the first indication of the onset of depression noticeable by friends and relatives.

The depressed person reports sleep disturbances—one of the earliest and most consistent signs of depression—including fitful dozing, unpleasant and terrifying dreams, difficulty falling asleep (usually indicating depressive neurosis), early morning awakening (usually indicating psychotic depressive reaction) with difficulty returning to sleep or constant escape into sleep. The depressed person is not refreshed by the sleep. One may report constipation or a fear of cancer of the bowel.

Appetite may be decreased or absent. Frequently nauseated at the thought of food, such a person does not eat adequate amounts, thereby losing weight and becoming dehydrated. It is not uncommon for the depressed person to present an unkempt appearance, neglecting to comb or wash the hair. Diminished sexual activity and/or menstrual irregularity or amenorrhea may occur.

Nursing Management

As set forth in Chapter 6, nursing management in the hospital setting includes gathering a data base, identifying the patient's problems and making plans for care.

The problem list for a person diagnosed as depressed includes some or all of the following:

1. Feelings of sadness, despair, emptiness
2. Feelings of failure
3. Feelings of worthlessness
4. Feelings that one is unloved, uncared for and guilty
5. Retarded physical activity and/or withdrawal
6. Difficulty in dealing with angry feelings
7. Inability to make decisions
8. Slowed thought processes
9. Nausea or refusal to eat
10. Constipation
11. Sleep disturbances
12. Suicidal ideas

Following the development of a problem list, nursing actions are planned.

1. Feelings of sadness, despair, emptiness
Plan: Some time during each nursing shift must be spent with the depressed patient. By providing quiet, non-threatening companionship, the nurse communicates acceptance of the patient.

Although the nurse may think she is having little impact on the patient, she must recognize that environmental inputs have an effect. The patient is influenced by the nurse's attitudes, verbalizations and actions. Patients are acutely sensitive to all that goes on around them, while appearing isolated, as though in a world of their own.

The nurse's positive regard supplies encouragement and helps increase the level of self-esteem.

When the patient speaks, it is important to listen carefully. Listening so as to understand the patient's message serves to lessen painful feelings of sadness by conveying the feeling that someone does care and recognizes the patient's distress. Listening also communicates that one is understood and, thus, decreases some of the loneliness of depression.

2. Feelings of failure
Plan: Enlist the patient in unit activities in which success is possible. This may be a slow process, since it is necessary to move at the

patient's own pace. It is important not to push the patient into activities until readiness to participate is evident. Care is taken not to suggest activities in which the patient may do poorly and, thereby, reinforce feelings of inadequacy. Often, it is helpful to introduce the patient into activities by working cooperatively first on a one-to-one level. As the patient becomes increasingly comfortable in the one-to-one relationship, a move is indicated into a one-to-two relationship by introducing another patient or staff person into the nurse-patient interaction. Last, the nurse may help the patient move into a one-to-group situation, with support provided in a group situation, until the patient is able to tolerate the presence of others without direct nursing presence.

3. Feelings of worthlessness
Plan: Once the nurse becomes aware of the patient's withdrawal, possibly due to overwhelming feelings of worthlessness, it is important to persist in forming a relationship with the patient. Due to depressive symptoms of sadness, fear, anticipation of failure and worthlessness, the patient discourages overtures from the nurse, who would like to spend time with him. At first, the nurse may sit with the patient with little or no interaction. By sitting and accepting quiet behavior, the nurse may help the patient recognize that he is deemed worthwhile by at least one person.

Since the patient has a self-view of worthlessness, comments to the contrary are assessed as fake; words of encouragement are seen as phony and are not incorporated by the patient into a self-system. Thus, words of encouragement and support are kept brief while the patient is severely depressed.

An aggressively cheerful attitude on the part of the nurse seems alien to the patient, who cannot respond to this cheerfulness and, thus, feels more worthless.

By her verbal and non-verbal behavior, the nurse conveys to the patient that the view of self as worthless and unlikeable is not shared by her. This attitude of acceptance eventually has an impact.

With the patient who feels worthless, consistency and dependability in nursing actions are stressed. If the nurse says she will return at a certain time, she must do so or send word to the patient that she has been detained. The patient personalizes lack of consistency on the part of the nurse by thinking, "I can see why she wouldn't come back; there are a lot of other patients who need her care now. Who really wants to come in and see me anyway?"

4. Feelings that one is unlovable and guilty

Plan: The basic interpersonal task of the nurse is gradually to lessen the patient's feelings of rejection, guilt and worthlessness.

Caring and involvement with patients occur in the minute-to-minute relationships nurses maintain. The term "here and now" has tremendous impact on the nurse-patient relationship. Each time a patient feels secure and recognizes support from a significant person, feelings of being unlovable are shaken.

Brief, non-essential encounters with a patient serve to intervene in a negative, unlovable self-view. Walking by the room of Mr. M., a 55-year-old depressed patient, the nurse entered, calling him by name and fluffing his pillow. Mr. M., barely looking at her, mumbled, "Why do you bother with me?" The nurse's reply, "Because I care about you," communicated human compassion and concern.

As the patient begins to improve, the ways he emotionally pushes away people who could care and love can be cooperatively examined.

By initiating a teaching program with emphasis on ways to interact with others, the nurse offers the patient new ways to solve problems. Frequently, it is helpful to use role playing and chair reversal for the patient to learn what he is doing and how to change. The following is an example of the use of role playing.

Mrs. B., a 45-year-old depressed female, states, "My daughter and I used to be so close and got along so well until she turned 13. Then she didn't like the things we did together, and she quit loving me. Now we argue about everything, and she not only doesn't love me, she hates me just like everyone else."

The nurse suggested that they role play an interaction between Mrs. B. and her daughter. The nurse played the 13-year-old daughter, and Mrs. B. played herself, the mother. During the role play, it became clear that Mrs. B. was placing unrealistic demands on her daughter, thus leaving her daughter feeling trapped and ready to fight. Mrs. B. was afraid her daughter was growing up, and that she would lose her and her love. Feeling that she was unlovable, Mrs. B. was actually placing her daughter in a position that could cause her to reject her mother. The nurse explained her insight concerning the problem, and by using role reversal and letting the mother play the 13-year-old daughter and the nurse play Mrs. B., Mrs. B. became aware of what she was doing. She was then ready to learn new ways to deal with her daughter and others, thus improving relationships and allowing others to love her again.

5. Retarded physical activity and/or withdrawal

Plan: It is impossible to force another into activities or relationships. The depressed person, often slow to move, shuns contact with others. It is essential that the nurse move in the relationship at the patient's pace. She must be constantly alert for cues that the patient can tolerate interaction. By avoiding others, the withdrawn patient shuns the opportunity to experience satisfying interpersonal relationships, simultaneously raising barriers against rejection by others.

The person who chooses withdrawal as a way of coping with internal stress is often frightened of others: such a person may fear that rage will surface and cause loss of control of the situation. Although avoiding the nurse, the patient may desperately desire some contact with another. Thus, as mentioned, the nurse is constantly alert for signs on the patient's part of a desire for contact. Moreover, the withdrawn patient may feel hopeless and anticipate rejection and failure in forming a relationship. Rather than be misunderstood, rejected or treated with contempt, the patient shuns contact with others.

If the patient continues to be withdrawn for a considerable length of time, it is possible that members of the nursing staff will likewise withdraw. If this mutual withdrawal occurs, the nurse-patient relationship reaches a stalemate, with the patient's withdrawal reinforced by the nursing actions.

The anxiety and discomfort due to the nurse's inability to tolerate silence, hostile remarks or lack of control with a withdrawn patient can be instrumental in preventing the nurse from seeking contact with the patient.

The nurse might experience feelings of rejection, failure, hurt, disappointment or hopelessness. She may then avoid the patient to prevent future feelings that are uncomfortable. The following interaction between Mrs. A., the staff nurse and a withdrawn patient, Mr. S., may help to clarify how mutual withdrawal can come about:

Mrs. A. approached Mr. S., who had been lying on his bed all morning.

Mrs. A.: "Mr. S., I would like to talk with you for a little while."

Mr. S.: "Leave me alone."

Mrs. A.: "You've been in your room several hours, and I thought that we might spend some time together."

Mr. S.: "I don't want to talk...." (silence)

Mrs. A.: "I'll leave, if you want to be alone."

Mrs. A. did not approach Mr. S. again during his hospital stay, except to administer his medications.

The nurse can prevent this mutual withdrawal from occurring. This next interaction is very similar to the one just presented; however, the nurse had a plan to show Mr. S. that she cared about him. She realized that the relationship might take a long time to develop, and that she must start by using nonverbal communication and by helping him with his most basic needs. She also realized that brief contacts at frequent intervals might be easier for Mr. S. to tolerate. Ready to tolerate silence, she was aware that she might experience feelings of failure, disappointment or hurt at some point in the relationship.

Mrs. C.: "Mr. S., I would like to sit here with you for a few minutes."

Mr. S.: "Leave me alone."

Mrs. C.: "I've noticed that you have been alone for quite awhile, and I would like to spend a few minutes with you."

Mr. S.: "I don't like to talk to anyone anymore—just leave."

Mrs. C. sat in silence approximately one minute. "I respect your statement that you don't want to talk. I will be back after lunch to spend some more time with you." She then straightened his bedside table and placed the water and a magazine within easy reach. She noticed a large crease in the sheet and as she said, "I know that this must be uncomfortable," she pulled the sheet smooth and left.

Later, Mrs. C. returned with his favorite hot drink and spent about five minutes with him. In this slow way, the relationship developed. The importance of this relationship to Mr. S. justified the time Mrs. C. gave him.

6. *Difficulty in dealing with angry feelings*

Plan: Talking with a depressed patient is certainly important, and the value of listening cannot be overestimated. Also, diversional activities can be provided, so that the patient can have at least a brief respite from suffering. Activities such as pounding metal into a useful tray or art piece, sanding a piece of furniture or playing an active vigorous sport help the person channel anger in a less destructive manner onto the exterior rather than internal environment. One can rid oneself of hostility without feeling guilty. Expressing hostility with words may spur a flood of guilt feelings. One may fear that an expression of anger will open a flood gate of pent-up emotions and devastate the person toward whom the wrath is directed. Patients often need to learn to handle angry feelings in small doses. No one learns overnight how to hold in a multitude of feelings; hence, expression of feelings is learned slowly.

When a depressed person shows signs of anger or makes statements that indicate anger, it is important that the nurse accept the feelings. A patient can slowly begin to verbalize feelings as well as release them by activities, once aware that it is all right to have and express these feelings.

7. Inability to make decisions

Plan: Often the patient feels an inability to answer questions correctly, to decide what to say. Thus, no matter how a question is answered, concern over having said the wrong thing flares. Therefore, if the nurse finds it necessary to ask the patient questions, she should keep them simple.

At this point, the nurse should not ask the patient to make decisions. The patient feels unworthy to make decisions, unable to decide on even minor things. For example, while selecting the foods from the menu, the nurse might say, "I suggest that you have roast beef, corn, green beans, a hot roll and ice cream for dinner tonight." To ask the patient to decide between roast beef and chicken, corn and carrots, roll and corn bread, green beans and peas, ice cream and pudding is forcing decisions the patient is not ready to make. Forced to make decisions, he may become agitated and worry about whether the choice was the right one. During this period, the nurse presents the patient with suggestions rather than choices.

A frequently used aid for the patient is a schedule, to be on hand at all times. This schedule will include everything from getting up and brushing teeth in the morning to taking rest periods, watching television and eating. By using this schedule, the patient can stay busy and involved without making any decisions.

The nurse uses her assessment skills to determine if the depression has subsided. As the patient seems less depressed, the nurse provides reassurance and encouragement toward making choices again. She watches for feelings of worthlessness or fear of having made the wrong decision. A great deal of nursing judgment is necessary to decide when the patient is ready to make decisions. For example, an acutely anxious patient may be unable to decide what foods to eat. As the depression lessens and the person is less anxious, the nurse, noticing the patient looking over the menu, encourages decision-making.

8. *Slowed thought processes*
Plan: Frequently, the patient finds long explanations upsetting; therefore, it is necessary to give brief explanations about the care administered. Because the patient's thinking is slowed, it is essential that the nurse take time to perform procedures for the patient, remain calm and pleasant and demonstrate competence.

9. *Nausea or refusal to eat*
Plan: The patient who is depressed often feels too unworthy to eat (problem #3). The nurse makes careful observations of when, where and how much the patient eats. Following an assessment, the nurse can set aside time for eating when she can stay with the patient during the meal. By staying, the nurse encourages the patient to eat and also helps bring about a more worthwhile self-view.

She may find it helpful to collaborate with the dietician, in order to plan meals which the patient likes or at least finds less nauseating. For example, fried foods may be less tolerable than fresh fruit.

As the depression subsides and the nausea ceases, the nurse reevaluates the necessity of staying with the patient during each meal time.

10. *Constipation*
Plan: Since the nurse realizes that constipation may be the result of a number of conditions, she collaborates with the physician concerning necessary medications or treatments.

As with the previous problems, keeping accurate records concerning elimination will indicate the severity of the problem and the success of the treatment.

11. *Sleep disturbances*
Plan: Once again, observation is a key nursing function. Observing the person and keeping accurate records helps to ascertain the type

of sleep disturbances the patient is having and allows for collaboration with the physician concerning the need for medication.

After the nurse has assessed the situation, she can use basic nursing measures such as back rubs, warm milk, hot showers and sitting at the patient's bedside to help him relax and rest.

Checking frequently during the night allows the nurse to assess how much sleep the patient is getting and provides a source of comfort to the patient to know about the checking. If a nurse finds a patient awake, she should stay until sleep returns. This action often provides the security, acceptance and caring needed.

12. Suicidal ideas

This is a major problem and is therefore dealt with in greater detail than the previous problems.

SUICIDE

Etiology

An understanding of the reasons for self-destructive action is basic for planning competent nursing actions. Although it is true that some depressed patients are suicidal, not all suicidal persons are depressed.

Freud identified man's two significant instincts as Eros and Thanatos. Eros, the instinct for life, is shown through the sexual urge. Thanatos, the death wish, is shown through anger and aggression toward others. Freud explained that man represses his anger toward others and turns it inward upon himself. The death wish, followed by an ego which is split between the demands of the id and the demands of society, leads to feelings of guilt and shame. This battle between the id and society's demands results in an internal weakness. This person is then predisposed to suicide. A stress such as the loss of a loved one, failure or a powerful surge of emotion, may precipitate a self-destructive attempt. Basically, Freud saw suicide as an aggressive act toward others that was turned inward. He indicated that the stressful event brings out confusion, guilt and shame which activate the death wish, and the person kills himself instead of the stressor or object that he wants to destroy (Freud, 1957, p. 1243-1258).

At the end of the ninteenth century, Emile Durkheim (1951) conducted a study of suicide which has become a classic. In this study, three kinds of suicide were identified: Egoistic, Altruistic and Anomic. Basically, Egoistic suicide results when a person is not integrated into a group. This person might say, "I'm just another number." There is a lack of social cohesion, and the person is forced to rely on his own resources. Altruistic suicide, on the other hand, results when the individual is closely bound to his society and/or family; he destroys himself in order to help the group. The third type of suicide, Anomic suicide, results when a person with a clearly defined set of roles and basic need fulfillment experiences a change in his life. Divorce or loss of wealth occurs, and the person loses his clear set of roles. Not knowing how to act, he feels overwhelmed and tends toward self destruction (Warga, 1974).

While these ideas on suicide are helpful, the exact reason that a person turns to suicide is unclear. Other ideas view suicide as a bid for attention, as acting out behavior or as punishment of others.

Based on Freud's ideas and Durkheim's studies, the potential for suicide is determined to a large extent by the interaction of the basic instincts (Eros and Thanatos), personality development (which leads to low self-esteem), the society in which the person developed (social cohesion or lack of cohesion) and the person's current environmental stresses (feelings of loss or desertion).

There is general agreement that the suicidal act follows a precipitating event. This precipitating event varies greatly from person to person. The event or problem may be the loss of a loved one, ill health, change in social status (up or down) or any number of other things. Feeling isolated and rejected, the individual may try to work out his problems, but when it seems to him that everything has failed and nothing has brought him relief, he loses hope and turns to thoughts of suicide. At this point, suicide may seem the only solution to an overwhelming problem.

Nursing Management

First, it must be determined that the person is suicidal. This is assessed early by the nurse, who obtains a data base on each new patient. When the nurse detects signals given out by the person that he is considering suicide, a plan is initiated. Nurses must be aware of their feelings concerning suicide. Anxiety toward suicide can lead to denial by the nurse and, thus, signals are missed.

A closer look at the signals, or clues, indicating suicidal potential are divided into the following categories:

I. Clues obtained from the history—Greater potential for suicide if:
   1. male over 50
   2. no family ties
   3. absence of close emotional bonds to people
   4. history of previous suicide attempt
   5. recently received bad news
   6. recent loss or death of a loved one
   7. progressive degenerative disease
   8. auditory hallucinations commanding him to kill himself
   9. bizarre delusion that by destroying himself, he is making a religious sacrifice (usually the patient is diagnosed as schizophrenic or having organic brain syndrome).
   having organic brain syndrome)

II. Physical and emotional clues:
   1. feelings of hopelessness and overwhelming guilt
   2. decreased interest in everything
   3. loss of sex drive
   4. carelessness about personal appearance
   5. constant brooding
   6. irritability
   7. poor appetite
   8. insomnia

III. Actions as clues:
   1. giving away prized possessions or getting financial affairs in order prematurely
   2. buying a casket
   3. playing with ropes, razors or other items which might be used in a suicide

IV. Statements as clues:
   1. coded communication—"I won't be around much longer for the doctor to worry with."
   2. non-direct communication—"Farewell." "I just can't take it any more."
   3. direct communication—"I'm going to kill myself."
   4. written communication—a suicidal note

V. Diagnosis as clues:

1. severe depression
2. schizophrenic syndromes
3. organic brain syndrome
4. personality disorders

A person considering suicide does not generally demonstrate all of these signals. The more of the characteristics the person has, the greater the potential for self-destruction.

Plan: Once the nursing judgment is made that the person is considered to be suicidal, a plan is initiated immediately. The traditional approach includes removing all potentially dangerous items from the person's environment. This is almost impossible to accomplish, unless the patient is placed nude in a totally empty room. This isolation and removal of possessions may be conceived by the patient as proof that he is worthless. His feelings of loss and rejection are personified. It does seem sensible to remove razor blades, ropes and medications from the environment, but the most important aspect of care is the provision of a caring, therapeutic environment. The nurse provides this environment in the following eight ways:

1. *Therapeutic relationship*

A therapeutic relationship begins when the nurse conveys interest and an unshakable attitude of acceptance toward the patient. Knowing that even one person accepts him and is interested in him might be enough to influence him to abandon his suicidal plans. If even one person is able to establish rapport with the patient, this may well be the best protection against suicide.

2. *Communicate the potential for suicide to team members*

Protecting the person from self-destruction is a team effort. In the case of suicide, not to communicate to others on the team is doing the patient a disservice. The nurse often relates to the patient on a significant level, and she may be the first team member to pick up the clues of a potential suicide. Even if the clues seem insignificant, it is important to have a team meeting including the physician. The only time that one can be totally sure that a person is seriously self-destructive is after he has succeeded; then it is too late to help him.

3. Stay with the person

By staying with the person who is suicidal, the nurse can provide constant watchful care, be available to listen and give him a sense of assurance that until he is able to control his self-destructive impulses, control will be provided. The patient is under constant observation, with the focus on supporting him throughout his current crisis.

4. Accept the person

The nurse demonstrates an unshakable attitude of acceptance toward the person. A person who sees suicide as his only choice may change his plans if he feels accepted by even one person. Acceptance helps reassure the person that he is a worthwhile human being.

5. Listen to the person

After the patient knows that the nurse is interested in him and accepts him, he may ventilate his hostility, pain or disgust for life. He may need to be encouraged to express himself by such statements as, "What has been happening to you lately?" This can help him identify, examine and share the source of his pain. Listen calmly as he tells what has happened to him. Listen with the sharp sense known as the third ear for any hidden messages. Check with him to see if there are people that he feels do not listen to him. If he answers "Yes," give him guidance in finding constructive and appropriate ways to get them to listen. Family therapy is an excellent approach for families to learn to communicate with one another. Check with him to be sure he knows that the nurse is listening to him. If the person feels that someone knows, hears and understands the intense pain he feels, then the suicide act is less likely.

6. Secure a promise that he will make no suicide attempt

Get the suicide idea out into the open. The person has a certain amount of relief when he has told a significant other person of his suicidal ideas. Present the fact that if he destroys himself, he cannot get better. Secure a promise or contract from him that he will make no suicidal attempt.

7. Give the person a message of hope

The nurse can talk with the person, without being overly cheerful, concerning ways in which life can be better. The person under intense mental strain feels pain and despair; he sees no hope that life can be better. He may not be sure that he wants to die, but he does not want to live life as it is. After letting him express how painful his life has been, offer a message of optimism that life can be better, that his seemingly insolvable problem can somehow be worked out, although the process may be difficult.

8. Give the person something to do

Provide a meaningful activity to let out tension and hostility, such as sanding furniture, pounding clay or playing an active sport. By helping him participate in these activities, the nurse provides opportunities for him to see that he is a worthwhile person, and she also allows him a medium for expressing his feeling of aggression and hostility constructively. By encouraging him to eat, bathe and meet his other basic needs, the nurse is helping him to be involved once again in the interactions of living. The nurse can help guide his activities by providing times for eating snacks of fresh fruits and by providing times for rest and sleep.

Long-term goals for a suicidal person are individually determined. Psychotherapy is often indicated to help the person develop a more realistic and positive self-concept. He needs to learn ways to express his feelings to others. He needs to learn ways to have successful interpersonal relationships, to feel acceptance by others and have a feeling of belonging.

CASE STUDY: DEPRESSIVE BEHAVIOR

Mrs. A. was admitted to the unit by her older brother, who summarized Mrs. A's life for the nurse. Although born at a time of parental financial difficulty, life was uneventful until Mrs. A. was 6 years old, when her mother died and Mrs. A. assumed many household chores. While her father cared about her, he had to work hard and spent little time with her. Assuming the responsibility of cooking for her father and older brother and making household decisions, she finished high school and business college. Although social activities were limited, she met a young man who worked in the same office. Once they married, Mrs. A. experienced happiness for the first time since early childhood. She was a good mother to her two children and enjoyed her home and family. When her oldest child, a son, married and left home, she felt a great sense of sadness and loss. However, she continued to care for her daughter and husband and, at times, enjoyed activities and the home.

Two years after the son was married, Mrs. A.'s husband died. This was six months before her admittance to the hospital. At first, Mrs. A. had shown very little grief and did not cry.

On admission, Mrs. A. cried frequently and reported feelings of guilt and worthlessness. She lost interest in her friends and social events. Her older brother brought her to the physician with complaints of constipation, anorexia and difficulty falling asleep. Mrs. A.'s history, general appearance and crying spells led the physician to believe that hospitalization was warranted.

After talking with Mrs. A. in the quietness of her room, much of the following data base was obtained.

I. OBJECTIVE DATA
  A. General appearance, attitude, and activity
    1. Appearance: wearing a wrinkled house dress, hair uncombed, no makeup
    2. Attitude: she appears sad, gloomy, answers the nurse's questions slowly
    3. Activity: looks at the floor, sits for long periods without looking up or moving, moves slowly when encouraged
  B. Communication patterns
    1. When encouraged to talk, she dwells on how guilty and worthless she is
    2. Her communication is understandable
  C. Contact with the environment
    1. She is oriented to time, place and person
    2. She is not distracted by sights or sounds in the room
  D. Sensorium and intelligence
    1. She is oriented
    2. Her memory is accurate for recent and remote events
    3. She is not as attentive as expected, and she states that she would like to rest
  E. Thought processes
    1. She is coherent

F. Thought content
   1. She continually dwells on her own self-worthlessness
   2. No delusions
   3. No hallucinations reported
G. Social Assessment
   1. Mrs. A. is in the upper-middle-class socioeconomic group; she is a high school graduate, with business school training
   2. Her parents are deceased: mother died when Mrs. A. was 6 years old
   Her husband died 6 months ago
   Living relatives: married son, older brother and a 16-year-old daughter who lives at home
   3. The children do not seem surprised by their mother's condition; however, they do seem concerned. Her older brother, who brought her in, reports that she has been sad off and on throughout the years, but not this bad.
   4. She does not smoke. She states that she drinks alcohol approximately twice a year.
   5. The family visits daily and state they are very anxious for Mrs. A. to be discharged.
   6. The family is very friendly toward the staff, and they have agreed to family conferences and/or therapy.
H. Medical Assessment
   1. She reports that she is constipated
   2. She is nauseated at the sight of food; weight loss of 8 pounds
   3. She has a lot of trouble getting to sleep

II. SUBJECTIVE DATA
   A. Present Illness
      1. Mrs. A.'s reason for coming to the hospital is: "My brother was worried about me not eating, sleeping, and my lack of energy. I cry most of the time, and I would like some medicine to get rid of this constipation."
      2. Precipitating event: Mrs. A. tells of her husband's

death six months prior. This may be the precipitating event, as she states that he was her hope in life, her love and her security. She, however, does not relate this loss to her present crying, nausea, insomnia or constipation.
3. She states that she has had "sad spells off and on for as long as she can remember." (Objective data: no previous hospital admittance to a psychiatric unit.)

III. STATEMENT OF THE PSYCHIATRIC PROBLEM
  A. Neurotic Depression
  B. Problem List:
    1. Feelings of sadness
    2. Feelings of worthlessness
    3. Inability to make decisions
    4. Slowed thought processes
    5. Lack of appetite
    6. Constipation
    7. Insomnia

IV. PLANNING PHASE
A nursing conference was indicated to begin planning the nursing actions and overall treatment plan. Because of problem #3, inability to make decisions, the patient was not initially involved in the planning.

In the conference, the problems were discussed and priorities were set. Problem #1, feelings of sadness, and problem #2, feelings of worthlessness, were considered to be the primary nursing problems. Problems #3, inability to make decisions, #4, slowed thought processes and #5, lack of appetite, were also discussed and nursing actions planned. Due to the fact that problem #5 necessitated collaboration with the dietician and the fact that problems #6 and #7 required collaboration with the physician, a team conference was initiated by the nursing staff. (Later, long-term planning involved the social worker, recreational therapist, occupational therapist, art therapist, her minister, her family and, of course, Mrs. A.)

The team came up with the overall plan to begin Mrs. A. in psychotherapy with the clinical specialist in psychiatric-mental health nursing and the admitting psychiatrist. They initiated ego-supportive measures and, later in the course of treatment, they used insight therapy. Electroshock treatment was ruled out. An antidepressant, in adjunct to psychotherapy, was indicated. Medications for constipation and insomnia were also a part of the overall treatment plan. The problems and plan were placed on the record.

A. Feelings of sadness
   1. *Plan:* The primary nurse assigned to Mrs. A. (this was a consistent person on each shift) will spend at least one hour with Mrs. A. two times during the shift.
   2. *Expected outcome:* By using quiet companionship, the nurse allows Mrs. A. time to express her feelings of sadness. She will feel accepted, cared about and encouraged. She can share her sadness with another person. This sharing and being heard will help to lessen her painful feelings of sadness.
B. Feelings of worthlessness and guiltiness
   1. *Plan:* Initially, do not act overly cheerful with Mrs. A. Keep words of encouragement brief. Use nonverbal behavior to indicate that she is not seen as worthless or unlikeable. Examples: a smile, a touch, a gift of a magazine, a fresh flower from the garden, staying with her when not required or expected to do so. These caring actions, compliments or strokes are to be continued throughout Mrs. A.'s stay.
   2. *Expected outcome:* Mrs. A. will feel less worthless. She will begin to feel more worthwhile, as the nurse's attitude of acceptance begins to have an impact on her. Her feelings of rejection, guilt and worthlessness will gradually lessen. She will learn to give and receive positive remarks and gestures from significant others in her environment.
C. Inability to make decisions
   1. *Plan:* Ask only simple questions. Present her with a suggestion rather than a choice. Make a schedule for her which includes everything for her to do during the day. As her depression subsides, slowly add

choices for her to make. Allow her to make choices. Provide encouragement after each choice.
   2. *Expected outcome:* Mrs. A. will not become anxious about her decisions or worry about decisions in the initial stages of therapy, because she will not have any decisions to make. In the later stages, she will be able to make decisions without fear of making the wrong choice.
D. Slowed thought processes
   1. *Plan:* Remain pleasant, calm and competent when with the patient. Give her brief explanations about medications or care that she receives. Avoid long explanations.
   2. *Expected outcome:* She will find being with the nurse comforting rather than confusing. Eventually as the depression subsides, her thought processes will clear.
E. Lack of appetite
   1. *Plan:* When and how much Mrs. A. is actually eating must be assessed. The dietician has planned a nutritious menu including foods Mrs. A. indicated she preferred. On Mrs. A.'s schedule, make it clear as to when she is to eat each meal. Stay with her during the entire meal, conversing with her and, when necessary, encouraging her to eat.
   2. *Expected outcome:* Mrs. A. will begin to eat. Her nutritional needs will be met. She will cease losing weight. As feelings of worthlessness decrease, she will regain her appetite.
F. Constipation
   1. *Plan:* Keep accurate records as to frequency and consistency of elimination. Give appropriate medication as ordered.
   2. *Expected outcome:* Constipation will cease.
G. Insomnia
   1. *Plan:* Give the appropriate medication as prescribed. Spend time with Mrs. A. just before she goes to sleep. Use any nursing measures, such as a back rub or warm milk, to help her relax. Tell her each night to call if she cannot get to sleep. Tell her that she

will be checked out frequently throughout the night. Check on her frequently and record her sleep patterns.
2. *Expected outcome:* Mrs. A. will feel secure and safe. She will be able to sleep without the previous difficulty.

The problem list changed for Mrs. A. as the problems, one by one, became inactive. Due to the treatment regimen, which included these nursing actions, Mrs. A. returned to her home where she became a competent mother for her teenage daughter and an active community worker.

Evaluation of the plan was a necessary part of the nursing process. Success was determined by how near the patient came to the identified expected outcomes.

PRINCIPLES

1. Repression of angry feelings leads to symptom formation.
2. Unsatisfied need for love leads to disappointment and alienation from others.
3. Childhood traumas often lead to low self-esteem.
4. Low self-esteem combined with adult loss or stress leads to depression.
5. Nurse's positive regard for patient supplies encouragement and leads to increased self-esteem.
6. Self-esteem is enhanced by acceptance.
7. Quiet, non-threatening companionship communicates acceptance.
8. Perception of acceptance by significant others leads to increased self-acceptance.
9. Nurse's "thereness" leads to decreased feelings of aloneness.
10. Listening serves to lessen painful feelings of sadness and decreases loneliness.
11. Suicidal acts follow a precipitating event and may seem the only solution to an overwhelming problem.
12. Suicidal threat may be lessened when one has rapport with even one person.
13. A person unable to control his self destructive impulses needs someone else to provide control for him.

SUMMARY

In summary, the focus is on depressive neuroses, psychotic depressive reactions and suicidal behavior. Depressive neuroses and psychotic depressive reaction are examined together, since the major difference between the two categories is a matter of degree.

A theoretical framework in which depression develops, symptoms of depression, nursing management including a problem list and plan of action, a theoretical framework in which suicidal behavior develops, characteristics of a suicidal person, and the nursing management for the suicidal person are included.

A case study of a depressed person is presented so that the student can see the actual gathering of a data base and the development of a plan of care. Overall, this chapter is a basic look at depression and suicide with some simple, concrete actions for the nurse to use in caring for the patient.

BIBLIOGRAPHY

Bahra, Robert J. "The Potential for Suicide," *American Journal of Nursing*, LXXV, No. 10 (October, 1975), 1782-1788.

Burgess, Ann W., and Lazare, Aaron. *Psychiatric Nursing in the Hospital and the Community*. 2d ed. Englewood Cliffs, N.J.: Prentice-Hall, Inc., 1976.

Committee on Nomenclature and Statistics of the American Psychiatric Association. *Diagnostic and Statistical Manual of Mental Disorders*. 2d ed. Washington, D.C.: American Psychiatric Association, 1968.

Durkheim, Emile. *Suicide*. New York: Free Press of Glencoe, 1951.

Freud, Sigmond. "Mourning and Melancholia," in the *Standard Edition of the Complete Psychological Works of Sigmund Freud*. Vol. 14. London: Hogarth Press, 1957, pp. 1243-1258.

Huston, Paul. "Psychotic Depressive Reaction," in the *Comprehensive Textbook of Psychiatry*. Vol. II. 2d ed. Edited by Alfred Freedman, Harold Kaplan and Benjamin Sadock. Baltimore: Williams & Wilkins Co., 1975.

Millay, Edna St. Vincent. "From a Very Young Sphinx," in *Edna St. Vincent Millay: Collected Lyrics*. New York: Harper Torchbook, 1969, p. 188.

Swanson, Ardis. "Communicating with Depressed Persons," *Perspectives in Psychiatric Care*, XIII, No. 2 (March-April, 1975), 63-67.

Warga, Richard. *Personal Awareness: A Psychology of Adjustment*. Boston: Houghton Mifflin Co., 1974.

Wintrobe, Maxwell, et al. *Harrison's Principles of Internal Medicine*. 7th ed. New York: McGraw-Hill Book Co., 1974.

CHAPTER 8

Psychophysiological Disorders

Joan Goe, R.N., M.N.

INTRODUCTION

From the time of the rise of the Descartian philosophy of the dual nature of mind and matter in the seventeenth century (Rogers, 1970, p. 19) to the mid-twentieth century, medicine and other disciplines which focused on the care and study of man held a concept of man which separated him into the segments of mind and body. During the following World War II, a trend away from the segmentalized conception of man was noted. Again, scientists began to reaffirm the ancient principle that the mind and body are interdependent and interactive, that they are, in fact, a single organ (Weiss and English, 1957). Bertalanffy (1967), a biologist of the twentieth century, expressed a belief in the indivisability of man as follows: "There is no sharp distinction between bodily functions, unconscious and conscious mind . . . In the last resort, they may be the very same thing" (p. 100).

OVERVIEW OF SYSTEMS THEORY

What is a system? Undoubtedly, this question could be answered in several different ways, each equally valid. For present purposes the most appropriate answer is "a system is a way of looking at the world" (Weinberg, 1975, p. 52). It may be conceptualized as a collection of components or phenomena that have an interactive effect upon one another. One basic premise of systems theory is that it is impossible to understand a phenomenon independent of the systems of which it is a part. Another basic premise of systems theory holds that an impact made on one component or portion of a system affects the functioning of the total system. Contrasting the systems theory with a linear model, it is noted that in the linear model, A leads to B, which in turns leads to C and finally to D and the outcome. In the linear concept of causality, A is not affected by B, nor B by C, and the outcome does not have an impact on A, B or C. That is, the linear model is a unidirectional rather than an interactive model. The difference between a linear concept of causality and a systems concept of outcome is illustrated in the following diagram.

Linear Model

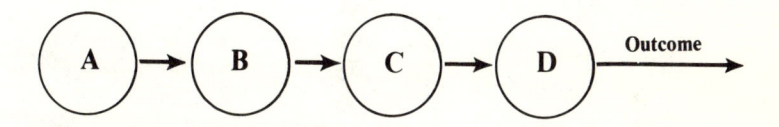

A → B → C → D —Outcome→

Systems Model

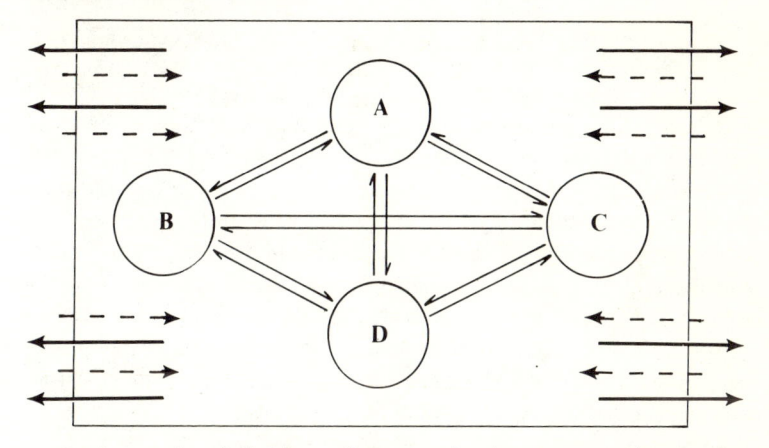

Basic to the definition of system is the constant interaction among the components of the system. In addition to the intrasystem exchange, there is the constant interaction between the system and its environment. Resources in terms of energy, information and materials are taken in from the environment. The system, in turn, discharges by-products of system activity into the evironment. These by-products are information, energy and material.

In addition, any unit or component of a system may also be a portion of one or more additional systems. That is, Component A of System One may also be a component of System Two and System Three. Component A may be the vehicle of exchange between Systems One, Two and Three. This concept is illustrated below.

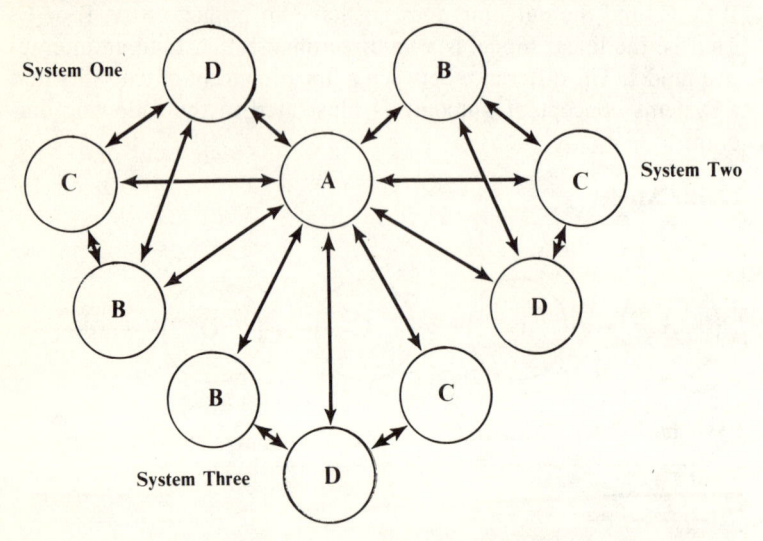

Each system, in turn, fits into the matrix of life in terms of suprasystems and subsystems. Generally speaking, two or more systems are linked together in some manner to form the suprasystem. One may accurately view the world as a suprasystem and the various nations, such as the United States, the Soviet Union, France and the United Kingdom, as subsystems. Likewise, if one views the United States as the suprasystem, then the various states become subsystems. This concept of expanding and contracting systems can be applied to biological states, psychological states, social situations and environmental systems.

Man as an Open System

Each individual is a special situation of an open system in a state of constant interaction with his environment. Martha Rogers (1970,

p. 49) succinctly states this as follows: "People are inseparable from the natural world." These suprasystems, of which each human is a part, are not only of a physical nature but include social systems as well. Activity of man is dependent upon the exchange between the individual and his environment. Visible or outer-directed activities involve an interchange between an individual and his suprasystems. That is, these interchanges are based on the exchange of information between the individual and those around him. Energy and materials in the form of food, water, oxygen, carbon dioxide and excretions are exchanged with the physical environment.

Not only is an individual a component of several interactive suprasystems, he also is a system which encompasses a multitude of interdependent, interactive subsystems. With even a cursory overview of a basic anatomy and physiology textbook, this concept of bodily subsystems is impossible to escape. What may escape the novice is the complex interaction among these various subsystems. Metabolic and other internal activities are dependent upon a constant exchange among the various bodily subsystems, as well as the exchange with the outer environment.

As a result, the subsystems of man are not purely of a biological nature but are composed of psychological and emotional facets as well. Internal man is of both a biological and non-biological nature. As has been pointed out, there is little purpose in attempting to demonstrate where biology ends and psychology begins. In the last analysis, they may be the very same.

THE NATURE OF HEALTH AND ILLNESS

Attempts to understand man by the process of reducing him to his subsystems and studying these is doomed to be inadequate. Any real understanding of the person is based on the conceptualization of the individual in terms of his totality: his subsystems and suprasystems, the systems which he encompasses and systems of which he is a part. Thus, health must be viewed as an integration of the whole being, an integration of the dimensions of mind, spirit and body. Loss of integration results in some manifestation of disequilibrium or illness (Dunn, 1973). Smooth functioning or a state of dynamic equilibrium in the subsystems of the individual and within the environmental suprasystems of which an individual is a part predisposes him to health. Loss of equilibrium either in the internal or the external systems causes the individual a loss of well-being and may result in disease.

Health or disease is not an all-or-none situation. Well-being or lack of well-being is on a continuum, not fixed in nature. Each individual's relative state of well-being fluctuates along the continuum on a daily basis, so that his health is in a state of constant flux. Contributing to this flux are various personal and environmental factors which affect the relative well-being of the individual. Such factors as a fortunate heredity, optimal nutrition, avoidance of pathogens and trauma, adequate sleep and exercise and supportive individuals are widely recognized as contributing to integration of the individual. Conversely, such factors as a less fortunate heredity, exposure to environmental hazards, poor nutrition, metabolic and emotional imbalances and destructive social constellations are stressful situations which contribute to disruption of the individual's integrity.

Factors external to the individual are only a portion of the mosaic of health. Internal factors, unique to the individual, are equally important. These unique internal factors determine how the person in question interacts with external forces. No two people interact with a given external situation in an identical manner. Hence, the outcome is never duplicated in totality.

The inseparability of body and mind is additionally reinforced by the body or somatic therapies currently used in some psychological and psychiatric circles. Wilhelm Reich, one of the earlier psychiatrists of this century, advocated a theory that fused the concepts of mind and body into a unitary phenomenon. Initially, Reich's theories were largely ridiculed or ignored. In the last decade, however, these theories have been adapted for, added to and incorporated into such therapies as Rolfing and Gestalt psychotherapy. A basic tenet of the Gestalt school is that a person does not possess a body—a person is his body. Personhood and the body are inseparable, for they are a unified phenomenon.

Hans Selye (1956) in his classic volume, *The Stress of Life*, speaks of the interactive nature and inseparability of mind and body when he discusses psychosomatic and somatopsychic disorders. Psychosomatic disorders are those disabilities that result in organic pathology due to psychological stress. Somatopsychic disorders are those psychological dysfunctions that are the result of organic pathology, brain damage excluded.

Hence, from both the perspectives of the natural scientists, von

Bertlanffy and Hans Selye, and from the behavioral scientists, Reich and the Gestaltists, the inseparability of mind and body, psyche and soma, are reiterated. Health and illness, like mind and body, are not mutually exclusive, but a unitary process. There is no sharp demarcation between illness and health. Health is a continuum along which each individual is in a never-ending flux, sometimes moving toward greater degrees of health, sometimes moving towards disequilibrium and disease.

PSYCHOPHYSIOLOGICAL DISORDERS

Psychophysiological disorders are a collection of disorders in which emotional factors play a major but not necessarily the only causative role. These disorders are associated with disturbances in the functioning of the sympathetic or the parasympathetic components of the autonomic nervous system (Eaton and Peterson, 1969, p. 143). Psychophysiological disorders range in seriousness from minor inconveniences to life-threatening emergencies. Most students are familiar with the nuisance of pre-examination nausea and vomiting or diarrhea. Generally speaking, they are aware that the basis of their discomfort is the threat of the impending examination. It is more difficult, however, to realize that a perforated peptic ulcer is also a psychophysiological disorder resulting from a disequilibrium of the autonomic nervous system.

Before proceeding with the discussion of psychophysiological disorders, the term "psychophysiological" needs to be discriminated from three other terms: psychosomatic, malingering and conversion reaction. Earlier in the chapter, the term psychosomatic was used in a historical perspective in discussing some of the earlier theorists. This term has been dropped, for the most part, from scientific literature because the term itself implies a dual nature of man, a division between mind or psyche and body or soma. Thus, to avoid reinforcement of conceptually splitting an individual into the components of mind and body, the term "psychophysiological" is frequently used and is currently standard nomenclature. In the most basic sense, malingering is present when an individual deliberately fakes an illness or disability for primary or secondary gains. This may be the primary gain of avoidance of some unpleasant task or a secondary gain to attempt to receive compensation for injury. Conversion reactions are unconscious processes of an hysterical nature, in which the individual displays or subjectively reports certain and often bizarre symptoms for which there is no organic basis or correlate. In summarizing the differences between malingering or conversion reactions and psychophysiological disorders, it is important to remember that the person with a psychophysiological disorder is neither pretending to be ill nor is his disability all "in his head." He has a very real disorder which, in fact, may take his life, unless he receives the appropriate nursing and medical therapies. Lachman (1972, p. 5) makes this point clear when he states, "Conversion reactions . . . are neurotic disorders characterized by development of an illness symptom" in which "there is no physical damage; in fact there is no detectable tissue change." He contrasts this with psychophysiological disorders in the following manner: "Neither is . . . the patient producing his symptoms deliberately nor malingering; but the psychosomatic patient does directly suffer real tissue damage . . ." (Lachman, 1972, p. 5).

Causes of Psychophysiological Disorders

The tendency to look for a singular cause for a disease or a disorder was perpetuated by the dramatic outcomes of the work of Koch and Pasteur. The concept of specific cause, while producing a dramatic ability to control massive epidemic diseases, is inadequate to explain the occurrence of many diseases and disorders—some infectious diseases included. As a result, looking for the "cause" of diseases or disorders in terms of systems or multicausality rather than for the cause in terms of linear causality holds more possibility for current problems. Although a single factor does not result in disease or disability, one of the variables which has been suggested as a major contributing factor in the development of pathology is the emotional state of the affected individual. The emotional state of the individual has a profound and dramatic impact on his lower brain and ultimately his autonomic nervous system.

The work of Kiritz and Moos (1974) suggests a complex interaction between environmental dimensions, personality characteristics and physiological indices. These researchers found that the social milieu may either moderate or mediate the physiological aspect of a disease process. Those social factors found to have positive outcomes in terms of the recovery from illness were identified as "support," "cohesion" and "affiliation."

Psychological factors, in addition to cultural variables, compound and have an impact upon the physiological manifestations of the individual. Identification of psychological variables which are indicative of the development of physiological symptoms has been attempted by various researchers. In a study of individuals affected by inflammatory bowel disease, McMahon, *et. al.* (1973) found these patients to score significantly higher on measures of hypochondriasis and hysteria as determined by the Minnesota Multiphasic Personality Inventory. In a separate study, a relationship between abasement—as measured by the Edwards Personal Preference Scale—and resting temperature, pulse, and respiration and changes in these vital signs was found (Pilowsky, 1973). Conclusions, based upon the results obtained by these and other researchers, in addition to the theoretical concepts of von Bertalanffy, support the interactive and interdependent nature of the spheres of man labeled "mind" and "body" and their conceptualization as a "unitary event."

In addition to looking for multiple causes of disease, there is a multiplicity of theories advanced to explain the occurrence of psychophysiological disorders. Yet, no one theory of psychophysiological disorders seems to be adequate to explain all instances. Differing theories are useful in different circumstances to various categories of health care practitioners. The more common theories to explain psychophysiological disorders include the psychoanalytic model and explanations based on learning theories and stress theories.

Before proceeding with discussions based on these theories, it is well to review some of the basic premises presented earlier in this chapter. The first significant point is that psychophysiological disorders are based upon the conceptualization of man as a unitary phenomenon, as a holistic entity, rather than as a collection of unrelated or loosely related systems. Psychology and physiology are manifestations of the same phenomenon, rather than expressions of a person who possesses a mind and possesses a body. The second crucial premise is that whatever affects one suprasystem of which the individual is a component, or subsystem which he encompasses, affects the entire system of the individual. That is, if a person experiences an insult in his cardiovascular subsystem, all of his other subsystems are affected. The subsystems of man are not exclusively biological in nature, hence, he is affected in his cognitive functions, his emotional and psychological states. The individual affected with a cardiovascular disorder, in turn, has an impact on all of the social suprasystems of which he is a part. His family is affected, as well as his friendship and employment groups. The response of his suprasystems to his altered health status is fed back to the afflicted person, influencing his adaptation and adjustment to his altered state of being. These interactions among components and systems, subsystems and suprasystems, continue until the system disintegrates.

Psychoanalytic Explanations of Psychophysiological Disorders

In outlining the psychoanalytic explanation of psychophysiological disorders, Eaton and Peterson (1969) list six relevant factors. These factors, as pointed out by these writers, are often interrelated and are not to be thought of as mutually exclusive categories. The categories described include somatization, organ language, stress, emotional specificity, undischarged emotion and personality type (Eaton and Peterson, 1969, pp. 146-147).

The first category, somatization, is defined as an "ego defense mechanism in which conflicts are represented by physical symptoms involving parts of the body innervated by the autonomic nervous system." Somatization, which involves the autonomic nervous system, is to be discriminated from the conversion reactions that involve the sensory or the motor nervous system (Eaton and Peterson, 1969, p. 146).

In the second category, organ language, symptoms are the vehicles of symbolic communication. These communications may be quite specific or of a rather general nature. Symptoms typical of organ language include nausea and vomiting, flatulence or cardiac symptoms. These symptoms have been quite specifically interpreted as, "I find this a nauseating experience," anger and disgust and as "a broken heart." In a more general nature, the experienced need to be taken care of may be expressed in the form of symptoms which lead to a pervasive helplessness and dependency (Eaton and Peterson, 1969, p. 146).

Stress, as the third category, has been implicated in a higher incidence of psychophysiological disorders than has any other single factor. It has been suggested that stress, interacting with some other variable or variables, determines the site of organ involvement. These other relevant variables quite possibly include the most genetically susceptible organ (Eaton and Peterson, 1969, p. 147).

The fourth category identified by Eaton and Peterson is that of emotional specificity, which involves physical manifestations produced by a prolonged emotional state such as anger, fear, sadness or helplessness. The physiological correlates of the various emotional states are not the same; hence, one would expect differing outcomes following a prolonged experience of these various states (Eaton and Peterson, 1969, p. 147).

Undischarged emotion, the fifth category, is a prolonged state in which the individual is prepared for some sort of action or expression of feelings. Once these actions have been taken, the emotional state abates. If action is not taken, the prolonged state of tension is capable of producing damage to some organ or system (Eaton and Peterson, 1969, p. 147).

The final category identified is that of personality type. This, as a variable to explain the occurrence of psychophysiological disorders, is based on a theory that holds that typical personality types can be identified for each of the major categories of psychophysiological disorders. "Personality profiles" have been developed for certain diseases and disorders. However, notable exceptions have occurred, and high percentages of individuals with a given disorder do not have the typical personality profile (Eaton and Peterson, 1969, p. 147).

Stress as a Factor in Psychophysiological Disorders—Stress may be conceptualized as a syndrome or a mosaic of interactive bodily responses to perceived threats, either real or fancied, to the well-being of the individual. Bodily responses typically associated with the stress syndrome include hormonal changes, alterations in kidney functioning and in the functioning of the autonomic nervous system, as well as elevations in blood pressure, pulse and respiratory rates.

Stressors are of a widely varied nature including threats of physical injury or deprivation, loss of a meaningful individual, changes in status and adaptations of a physical, social or psychological nature. Not all that is stressful is of a negative nature. Certain situations, widely accepted as stressful, are deliberately sought out by a great many people. Common examples of "positive stressors" are contests—political, athletic, business or academic. Courtship and marriage are so much a part of the social aspects of life, in general, and so widely pursued by so many people that their potent stressor capabilities are frequently forgotten.

What is perceived of as stressful, or is a stressor to one individual, is not necessarily perceived in a similar manner by another person. For instance, a snowstorm is probably perceived as a minor inconvenience to the general population in Montana. The driver from a southern state perceives (probably a realistic perception) the same snow as a threat to his physical well-being. The crowding and confusion of a major city is accepted by the native as a normal state of life, while to the rural visitor the same situation is probably acutely stressful, making a heavy demand on his powers of adaptation.

Temporary states of physiological response to stressful situations seem to produce no structural changes or permanent alterations in physical functioning. However, prolonged stress response may lead to permanent pathology. For example, during the height of an athletic contest, one expects to see the blood pressure, pulse and respiratory rates of the participants increase. Shortly after the contest is over, the vital signs return to the normal resting rates. Contrarily, the competition associated with business, politics or interpersonal conflicts is not so circumscribed in nature. These stressful situations are of a more prolonged nature and, indeed, frequently become a way of life. It is in these situations that one expects to see permanent elevations in blood pressure and pulse rate. Typically, during the early phases of essential hypertension, the episodic elevations in blood pressure are associated with emotionally stressful periods. As the disease progresses, the elevation in blood pressure becomes a consistent rather than an episodic finding. Over a prolonged period of time, these physiological alterations often lead to arterial damage as well as ventricular hypertrophy.

Psychological stressors may have a profound affect on vagal nerve activity resulting in an increased secretion of hydrochloric acid. Temporary stimulation of the vagus nerve with a short-term increase in hydrochloric acid production does not generally cause structural changes in the gastric or duodenal mucosa. However, prolonged vagal stimulation with associated gastric hyperacidity is commonly accepted as an important factor in the formation of peptic ulcers.

Elimination of all stress from living is neither possible nor desirable. Stress is associated with positive change and growth as well as with the inevitable tragedies and losses in life. However, in as much as prolonged or unremitting stress is associated with the occurrence of disease and disability, the individual needs to learn how to alleviate unnecessary stress and to manage inevitable stress in a positive manner.

Learning as a Factor in Psychophysiological Disorders—A strong point supporting learning as a theoretical explanation for psychophysiological disorders is made by Lachman (1972, p. 34) when he states "... that with few exceptions psychosomatic disorders are learned." Two of the basic principles of learning theory hold that 1) an individual learns behavior that he is motivated to acquire relatively quickly, and 2) the individual repeats behavior which is reinforced by the environment. The relevancy of these two principles is described in the following illustration:

> Tommy, as a child, needs the attention of his mother on a relatively continuous basis. Tommy's mother is an active, intelligent woman with many interests, Tommy being only one of these. Tommy discovers he can capture his mother's attention when he is ill. By the time he is in his teens Tommy learns, at the unconscious level, to control his bodily processes in such a way as to produce the symptoms associated with a typical classical migraine headache.

The paradigm of the psychophysiological sequence may be illustrated as follows:

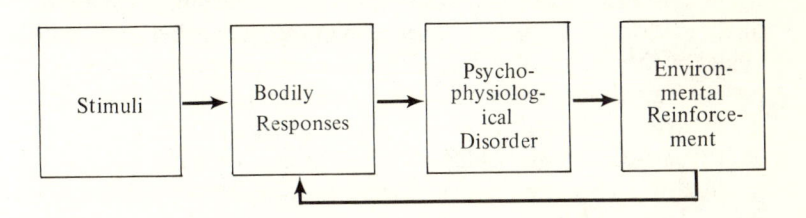

Stimuli → Bodily Responses → Psychophysiological Disorder → Environmental Reinforcement

In this situation, the stimuli are Tommy's experienced needs for his mother's attention. Fluid retention and localized transient ischemia of the central nervous system comprise a portion of the bodily responses associated with the psychophysiological disorder of the migraine headache. Environmental reinforcement is provided in terms of his mother's concern and attention.

Central to understanding psychophysiological disorders as a learned response are the following points:

1. The individual does not deliberately control his physiological processes to produce the bodily responses associated with the disorder.
2. This type of learning is of an unconscious rather than of a conscious nature.
3. At some time in the past, the symptoms or the disorder itself resulted in the individual's receiving some type of gratification or reinforcement. In other words, there was a payoff.
4. Not all rewards or reinforcements are positive. Negative reinforcement or acknowledgment is generally preferable to no acknowledgment.
5. The individual cannot "will away" the disability.
6. The individual can learn alternate patterns of behavior, if he is motivated to do so.

Summary of Theoretical Explanations

Regardless of the theoretical explanations of the causes of psychophysiological disorders that one is considering, there are several underlying principles applicable to all theories discussed earlier. None of the preceding theories negates the concept of multicausality in the disease process or the total system involvement in threats to the organism. Hereditary and environmental factors are considered relevant forces in determining what bodily structures are vulnerable to the development of pathology. The smoker is more likely to develop respiratory disease than the nonsmoker. The individual with a familial history of cardiovascular disease is more prone to the development of hypertension and, ultimately, coronary artery disease than is the person with a different heredity.

Psychoanalytic, stress and learning theories need not be used in a mutually exclusive manner in attempting to understand the occurrence of a psychophysiological disorder in a given individual. Stress is undoubtedly an important factor in the disease process. This does not rule out the role of learning. An individual experiences stressors either from internally or externally imposed factors. How he deals with these stressors and his bodily stress responses can be a learned process.

Classifications of Psychophysiological Disorders

According to Lachman, psychophysiological disorders may be

classified into eight broad categories according to the bodily subsystem primarily involved. These broad categories are (1) cardiovascular disorders, (2) respiratory disorders, (3) gastrointestinal disorders, (4) genitourinary disorders, (5) musculoskeletal disorders, (6) endocrine disorders, (7) skin disorders and (8) sensory disorders (Lachman, 1972). Other theorists may use a somewhat different classification system.

Cardiovascular Disorders

Typical changes noted within the cardiovascular system following episodes of heightened emotional states include: alterations in heart rate and rhythm, elevations in blood pressure, constriction or dilatation of the diameter of the blood vessels, changes in corpuscle counts and chemical composition of the blood. Specific cardiovascular disorders identified by Lachman as being of a psychophysiological nature include coronary occlusions (heart attack), tachycardia, bradycardia and arrhythmias. Other disorders included in this classification are migraine headaches, essential hypertension and anginal syndrome (Lachman, 1972, p. 75).

Respiratory Disorders

Hyperventilation syndrome, vasomotor rhinitis, sinusitis, laryngitis, bronchial asthma and chronic bronchitis are respiratory disorders considered to be of a psychophysiological nature (Lachman, 1972, p. 106). Underlying these disorders are such varied physiological changes as muscle spasm, alterations in the lumen of the respiratory passages, allergic responses including inflammation and edema, and changes in the pattern of breathing.

Gastrointestinal Disorders

Gastrointestinal disorders considered to be of a psychophysiological origin are ulcers, gastritis, colitis, chronic constipation and chronic diarrhea. Physiological changes associated with these disorders involve those processes which are controlled by the autonomic nervous system. These changes include alterations in the rate, quantity and quality of gastrointestinal secretions and alterations in peristalsis, either an increase, a decrease or reverse peristaltic activity (Lachman, 1972, p. 91).

Genitourinary Disorders

Disorders of the genitourinary system are grouped into three major categories by Lachman. These categories are (1) disorders of sexual functioning, (2) disorders of reproductive functioning and (3) disorders of urinary functioning. Disorders of sexual functioning in the male include impotence, premature ejaculation and retarded ejaculation. In the female, frigidity and vaginismus are disturbances of sexual functioning. Disturbances in the reproductive functioning of the female include menstrual difficulties and spontaneous abortions. Inability of the male to produce sperm may be a disturbance in reproductive functioning of a psychophysiological nature. This type of disturbance is referred to as psychosomatic infertility (Lachman, 1972, pp. 132-138).

Sexual and reproductive functioning in both the male and the female are activities mediated by the autonomic nervous system. This control may be in the form of direct innervation or via the endocrine system. Penile erections and ejaculation in the male and vaginal lubrication in the female are functions of the autonomic nervous system. Hormonal alterations associated with the menstrual cycle and fertility, as well as the hormonal components necessary to maintenance of pregnancy, are largely under autonomic control. Testicular activity including hormone production and spermatogenesis in the male are also controlled by the autonomic system.

Genitourinary disorders associated with disturbances of urinary functioning, in both males and females, are reflected in difficulty in urination, frequent urination, involuntary urination and nocturnal enuresis persisting into the adult years (Lachman, 1972, p. 138). Passage of urine includes voluntary activity and an involuntary component. The autonomic nervous system controls the involuntary component.

Musculoskeletal Disorders

Rheumatoid arthritis, rheumatism and bone degeneration, according to Lachman (1972, pp. 142-143), are musculoskeletal disorders which may have a psychogenic base. Rheumatoid arthritis is an inflammatory process of the joints. It tends to be progressive, causing profound changes in the structures of the involved joints and often leads to their destruction. Rheumatism is also an inflammatory disorder, but primarily it involves the muscles rather than the joint structures. Bone degeneration of a psychogenic origin is probably associated with errors in calcium metabolism. Calcium metabolism is primarily controlled by the endocrine system which, in turn, is under the influence of the autonomic nervous system. Another psychogenic explanation for bone degeneration involves the circulatory system. This explanation holds that there is an inadequate supply of blood to provide for the cell's needs for oxygen and removal of waste products. Lachman (1972, p. 143) also suggests that tooth decay may be a psychophysiological disorder, in that some disturbances in calcium metabolism can be attributed to the autonomic nervous system.

Endocrine Disorders

The endocrine system includes the following structures: the pituitary and thyroid gland, the adrenals, the parathyroids, the pancreas and the gonads. The activity of these glands is under the direction of the autonomic nervous system and is extremely sensitive to emotional stimulation. The various endocrine glands are interdependent, exerting a continuous reciprocal effect upon each other. Hormones secreted by the endocrine glands directly control many bodily processes and affect all other aspects of bodily functioning. Lachman (1972, pp. 149-153) has noted the onset of hyperfunction of the thyroid gland, hypofunction of the adrenal cortex and the pancreas to be associated with emotionally stressful situations. Keeping in mind the concept of multicausality in the occurrence of disease conditions allows for both the influence of heredity and the presence of emotionally stressful situations in the onset of diabetes and other endocrine disturbances. Additional disturbances in physiology associated with the endocrine system include menstrual irregularities, fluid retention and hirsutism. The intimate relationship between the endocrine system and the autonomic nervous system underlies the sensitivity of endocrine functioning to emotionally-laden situations.

Skin Disorders

Structures considered to comprise the skin in addition to the dermal and epidermal cells are the hair, glands, blood vessels and muscles of the skin. Activity of these cells—including glandular activity, vasodilation, vasoconstriction, tissue perfusion, capillary permeability and muscle tone—is directly or indirectly mediated by the autonomic nervous system. Disorders of the skin are characterized by such varied manifestations as excessive sweating (triggered by emotional factors rather than by heat or physical activity), hives, rashes, lesions or unusual texture of the skin and hair loss. An allergic type skin disorder such as hives, rashes or eczema may or may not have a psychogenic base. Lachman (1972, pp. 122-123) indicates that stressful situations and learning play a role in some cases of this nature. It has also been suggested such varied skin disorders as acne, Raynaud's disease and rapid hair loss have a psychogenic base.

Sensory Disorders

The sensory subsystems of the body include the visual, auditory, olfactory and gustatory apparatuses in addition to the labyrinthine mechanism and the kinesthetic sense organs. Psychophysiological disorders of the sensory subsystems are those disorders induced, at least to some degree, by activity of the autonomic nervous system. Psychogenic disorders involving activities of the motor or sensory nervous systems are considered to be conversion reactions. Lachman (1972, p. 159) points out that research into psychosomatic disorders involving the sensory apparatuses has not been undertaken on a widespread basis. He does however indicate that, theoretically at least, such visual disturbances as myopia, hyperopia and other refractive errors could have a psychogenic base. Studies do support that Meniere's disease and the visual disturbances of glaucoma and angiospastic retinopathy do have a psychogenic component in their etiology (Lachman, 1972, pp. 157-159). Physiological changes associated with psychophysiological disorders of the visual apparatus probably include excessive autonomic activity of the fibers of the eye associated with lacrimal, pupillary and vasomotor responses. An additional effect of autonomic activity is spasms of the retinal vessels induced by emotional factors. Swelling and excessive vasomotor activity of the nasal mucosa is characteristic of excessive autonomic stimulation.

SUMMARY

The classification of psychophysiological disorders presented here is only one possible system. Moreover, one must understand that several premises underlie the meaningful usage of this or any other classification system. First, to begin to understand psychophysiological disorders, one must keep in mind that only in unusual circumstances is there a single cause of a disease or disorder. In most cases, there are several contributing factors such as heredity, toxic environmental substances and stressful situations arising from either internal or external forces. Second, if the individual suffers with a psychophysiological disorder of any one of the eight subsystems presented in this classification system, all other bodily subsystems will ultimately be affected. In addition, there is a continuous interactive exchange between the individual and the larger environment. The environment contributes to or interferes with the individual's recovery. Third, psychophysiological disorders have as one contributing etiological factor the influence of the autonomic nervous system.

NURSING MANAGEMENT OF PSYCHOPHYSIOLOGICAL DISORDERS

Optimal treatment of the individual with a psychophysiological disorder requires a multifaceted approach. It is imperative that this individual receives the traditional medical therapies. However, this is but one facet in a holistic or comprehensive treatment program. Since traditional therapies are adequately dealt with elsewhere (in texts of Medical-Surgical Nursing or Medicine), the discussion in this text addresses the nontraditional nonmedical management of psychophysiological disorders.

For current purposes, psychoanalytic theories of psychophysiological disorders are not utilized in discussing nursing management. Discussion of nursing management addresses those interventions based on a systems theory of disease. The systems theory of disease and disability, when contrasted with the psychoanalytic model, negates the concept that a given emotional response or "personality type" leads, in a linear fashion, to the occurrence of a specific pathological condition. The occurrence of pathology in a given individual is the result of complex interactions among multiple variables. These variables are unique for each individual in his given situation. Linear theories of cause and effect are simplistic in contrast to systems conceptualizations.

With regard to the multicausal concept of disease, as opposed to the linear concept, it is apparent that the nurse cannot do something "to" or "for" the patient which will result in cure or alleviation of his physical or emotional distress. The systems approach implies that the patient is responsible for his own well-being: he alone can alter the ways in which he responds to his internal and external environment. The patient must be willing to assume some accountability for both the occurrence of the disorder and for active participation in his treatment and recovery. The treatment process is further expedited if significant individuals, such as family members or friends, are incorporated into the treatment plans.

The nursing process for the patient with a psychophysiological disorder includes the usual components of assessment, planning, implementation of the plan and evaluation. It is crucial that the patient be included, in a meaningful way, in each stage of this process.

Assessment of the patient with a psychophysiological disorder is a complex and continuous process. Accurate assessment depends, in large measure, on the ability of the nurse as an interviewer and the adequacy of the history taken. A comprehensive history identifies such contributing factors as heredity, personal living habits, work, recreational and social habits. In addition, the community and larger environment play a role in the occurrence of the disability. Identification of significant contributing factors necessitates a thorough understanding of the etiology of the disorder. That is, if an individual has a duodenal ulcer, a thorough nursing assessment requires the nurse to have a comprehensive understanding of the multitude of factors favoring the development of the ulcer. This understanding enables the nurse to identify those personal, social, and environmental factors contributing to the development of ulcers in a particular patient.

The assessment portion of the process also includes a determination of which contributing factors can be eliminated or modified. For example, certain pulmonary disorders, of a psychophysiological nature, are exacerbated by stressors such as air pollution. Sources of air pollution include cigaratte smoking, being in the company of smokers, auto exhaust and industrial air wastes. Pollens and dust from the natural environment may also be contributing factors. Each individual has limited control of stressors such as auto exhaust, pollens or dust in the air. However, he may be able to avoid or limit his exposure to these pollutants.

In addition to environmental and physiological factors contributing to a psychophysiological disorder, a thorough nursing assessment attempts to uncover relevant psychosocial factors such as a highly competitive profession, a rigid and excessive time structure with multiple deadlines, or a tense living situation with strained interpersonal relationships. Factors the patient is willing or able to modify or eliminate are individually determined.

After identification of factors contributing to the psychophysiological disorder, a list is made of those factors the patient is willing to modify. If a patient is unwilling to change his patterns of living, it is extremely difficult to intervene in the system. While the nurse or physician cannot make changes for the patient, they can provide medications, treatments and instructions aimed at alleviating symptoms.

After alterable stressors have been identified, the nurse and patient jointly develop a plan for implementation. The plan includes the behavioral changes the patient is willing to make. Such plans are stated in terms of patient behavior. Thus, if the plan calls for increased social interaction, it must include specifically what the patient will do, when he will do it and with whom. A behaviorally stated plan would be, "I will call Sarah tonight and make arrangements to go to dinner this weekend." The plan "to socialize more," is vague, and, generally, no real change in behavior will occur.

Behavioral changes having an impact on the total situation of the patient must be maintained over an indefinite period. Activity carried out on a one-time basis or for a short period of time is useless. Problems do not develop overnight; they develop over a period of years. Thus, they cannot be magically resolved in a short time. The patient must be willing to develop and maintain a less stressful life style.

As the plan is implemented, the nurse needs to monitor closely the progress of the patient in terms of what he successfully carries out, and what portions he fails to accomplish. Those portions not implemented need to be evaluated in terms of feasibility and patient acceptability. The plan needs to be revised, so the goal of the intervention can be achieved in an alternate manner. This is illustrated in the following example:

> A.T. is a nurse working in the Student Health Center of the local university. One of the patients she is working with is R.Z., a 24-year-old male with a medical diagnosis of psychogenic hives. During

the assessment process, it is determined that R.Z. has the most problems when he presents orally in his Sociology Seminar. R.Z. reports he has always been self-conscious, socializes rarely and has few dates. His grades are excellent. Assessment implies that R.Z. needs to learn ways to be more comfortable with peers. Without consulting the nurse, R.Z. makes arrangements to take an attractive undergraduate to a dance. The night of the dance, he not only develops hives but has an acute asthmatic attack requiring admission to the infirmary. After the acute phase, the nurse works with R.Z. to plan for increasing his social sphere in manageable ways. R.Z. decides to take a gourmet cooking class in which both sexes participate.

Evaluation of the effectiveness of the implemented plan is an ongoing process and not a terminal activity. Evaluation, concurrent with the intervention, is aimed at determining if a goal is attained. Evaluation is not the process of ascertaining whether specific plans were implemented or not. Rather, it is a method by which the effectiveness of these plans can be compared to some criteria. Generally speaking, evaluating the effectiveness of the intervention for the patient with a psychophysiological disorder is gauged by the alleviation or control of the disorder or its symptoms. Such changes as the amount of skin areas involved in the lesions of the disease, changes in vital signs or a reduction in the amount of medication needed may all be legitimate evaluative criteria.

In the preceding example, actual involvement in and completion of the gourmet cooking class is one small segment of the total intervention. Successful completion is not an evaluative criterion. At this point, we do not know whether this plan was effective in alleviating R.Z.'s psychogenic hives. The real goal is for R.Z. to be able to speak before a group of his peers without developing hives. When this occurs, one can say the basic problem has been alleviated.

CASE STUDY

Ms. L. was referred by an internist to the nurse clinical specialist at H____Medical Clinic, with a diagnosis of essential hypertension. The nurse obtained the following information from the physician's notes. Ms. L. is 35 years old, white, divorced and self-employed. She was first seen two months previously for a routine physical examination. The listed address was that of an upper-middle-class neighborhood. At the time of the first visit, the following data were obtained: temperature 98.4, pulse 108, respiration 16, blood pressure 158/110, height 5'6", weight 120 pounds. The physical examination found no abnormalities of any body systems. The E.C.G. and chest x-ray were normal. All laboratory examinations of blood and urine were within normal limits. All other data were normal.

Ms. L. has been seen on a bi-weekly basis since the initial visit for monitoring of blood pressure and pulse. The systolic reading fluctuated between 150 and 160. The diastolic pressure varied between 96 and 116. The pulse ranged between 90 and 114. At the time of the last visit, the physician informed Ms. L. of her diagnosis of essential hypertension and suggested a regime of dietary salt reduction and medications of a mild diuretic and tranquilizers. Ms. L. was unwilling to begin medications, until other forms of therapy were explored. The physician agreed that Ms. L. could explore alternate therapy, with the condition she return to his office in two months for an evaluation. He suggested that Ms. L. talk with the nurse clinical specialist about her health problems. Ms. L. agreed, and the referral was made.

Ms. L. was initially scheduled for a one-hour interview with the nurse for the purpose of data collection and identification of personal and environmental factors contributing to the elevated blood pressure. Ms. L., on time for the appointment, was attractive, well groomed and expensively attired.

During the interview, Ms. L. stated that she had grown up in a financially comfortable home where she was the middle child, having an older and a younger brother. Her father was a successful professional man, who had died unexpectedly of a heart attack when Ms. L. was 23 years of age. Her mother had remarried three years after his death and currently lived in a distant city.

Ms. L., having completed a masters degree in business, owned and operated a successful travel agency. Both of her brothers were established professional men, married and had children. The older brother lived about 75 miles from Ms. L.'s home. Her younger brother lived in the same city. Ms. L. had married at the conclusion of her undergraduate work and completed graduate study during the first years of the marriage. With the financial support of her husband, a lawyer, she started the travel agency. Both Ms. L. and her husband were extremely involved in career advancement and their professional lives. Their marriage had "just seemed to die due to neglect." They were divorced after five years of marriage with no children. Mrs. L. was not remarried, but Mr. L. had remarried and had two children.

Ms. L. described her work as being busy and full of pressure, even with six employees. The volume of business required that she work ten to twelve hours for five or six days each week, rarely taking a real vacation—only "a few days off now and then." Her social life was active, with frequent entertaining at home or dining out with friends. She admitted that she "rarely really eats a meal at home" but snacked when she did not eat out. Free time on weekends was usually spent in activities with her brother's children.

Her personal habits included smoking one and one-half to two packages of cigarettes daily. Her daily alcohol consumption, limited to two drinks, was not seen by Ms. L. as a problem. Her sleeping patterns usually included five to six hours in bed each night. Although Ms. L. experienced episodic insomnia, she did not use sleeping medications.

Ms. L. described herself as "an impatient person" who has difficulty dealing with delays or frustrations and who frequently becomes angry with the incompetencies of others. She is even more critical of herself when she makes a minor error.

At the conclusion of the first meeting, the following factors were mutually identified by Ms. L. and the nurse as potentially contributing to the hypertension:

1. cigarette smoking
2. excessive caffeine consumption
3. lack of adequate sleeping time
4. excessive work demands and over-scheduling of available time
5. inadequate provision for real recreation and diversion
6. lack of regular exercise
7. inconsistent eating habits
8. personal responses to frustration.

The second session was scheduled for the following week with the objective of planning for change. Ms. L. was asked to identify, prior to the session, factors she would be willing to change and how she would be willing to alter her patterns of living.

The following week when Ms. L. met with the nurse, she had already initiated an important change. She had not smoked a cigarette since the preceding week's appointment. She identified the following changes she would "like" to make: "get more exercise" and "learn how to relax" rather than be "so up-tight and high-strung all of the time."

In the planning phase, the nurse understood how crucial it was to help the patient translate her goals into concrete behavioral terms. After talking with Ms. L. about the "how" and "what" of meeting the goals, the following plans were made:

1. Ms. L. would begin jogging at the Y.W.C.A. on Sunday, Monday, Thursday and Friday. She would follow Dr. Cooper's aerobic guide* (Cooper, 1968).
2. Ms. L. would use "imagery" and "progressive relaxation techniques" twice daily. She would return for instructions the following day.**
3. To provide time for this regime in her daily schedule, Ms. L. would hire part-time clerical help to enable her personal secretary to relieve her of some of her administrative responsibilities.

Ms. L. returned the following day for instruction in "imagery" and "progressive" relaxation. After the period of initial instruction, Ms. L. was provided with a cassette tape of the instructional dialogue and was requested to carry out the exercise twice daily using this tape. The exercises were to be done once in the morning before work and again in the evening.

The nurse met with Ms. L. on a weekly basis for the next seven weeks. At these weekly meetings, Ms. L. and the nurse discussed her progress, further refined the problem list, and identified ways to modify her response to frustration in order for her to spend less time "being angry." During the discussions, Ms. L. discovered that some of the problems she had identified earlier were also resolving. Her

---

*Dr. Kenneth Cooper, in his book, *Aerobics,* outlines a graduated program of exercise for individuals of varying ages. His wife, Mildred Cooper, adapts this program to an exercise regime for women. The program of Dr. Cooper's is based on aerobics, or the body's utilization of oxygen, as opposed to anaerobics. Aerobic exercises include running, walking, bicycling and swimming. Isometrics, push-ups, and weight lifting are anaerobic exercises.

**Imagery and progressive relaxation techniques are accomplished by asking the client to be situated in a comfortable position. At the request of the therapist, he is asked to image a peaceful and pleasant scene. While holding this scene in mind, he is instructed to relax the major muscle groups in turn. This procedure is continued until all parts of the body are relaxed.

episodes of insomnia were lessening. With less anxiety about sleeplessness, Ms. L. found herself retiring at an earlier hour. She also felt better in the morning and was eating a light breakfast. Her coffee consumption also decreased markedly. At the conclusion of each discussion, Ms. L. practiced imagery and the progressive relaxation techniques, with the nurse providing the dialogue rather than using the cassette recorder.

At the end of the two-month trial period, Ms. L.'s blood pressure was 144/92, her pulse 86. With this progress, the physician encouraged Ms. L. to continue working with the nurse and return to see him in six months.

The nurse met with Ms. L. bi-weekly for two months. The meetings were then scheduled for once a month to measure the blood pressure and pulse and to provide a structure in which the instituted changes in Ms. L.'s life style could be reinforced.

At the end of the six months, Ms. L.'s blood pressure was 134/78 and her resting pulse was 70. She had not resumed smoking and was continuing to use imagery and the progressive relaxation techniques twice daily. Ms. L. was instructed to see the physician at six-month intervals. Ms. L. and the nurse determined that meeting together every other month was adequate for Ms. L. in order to maintain her motivation and not slip back into her old habits.

SUMMARY

The successful outcome of this form of treatment of a psychophysiological disorder requires a high degree of commitment on the part of the patient. The patient must be willing to examine his life style critically to determine how he is contributing to his own problems. He must also be willing to change himself and his environment, in order to remove or alleviate stressors contributing to his problem. Altering the stressors cannot be done *for* the patient but is done *by* the patient.

The role of the professional nurse is to share knowledge about the etiology of the disorder, assess the patient's situation with him, and assist him in formulating realistic and helpful plans for change. Following the planning stage, the nurse is responsible for providing positive reinforcement as the patient successfully implements the plan. If the patient fails in the implementation of his plan, the nurse examines with the patient what frustrated implementation and assists in the development of a revised plan. It is also the responsibility of the professional nurse to evaluate the success of the interventions in terms of whether they were adequate to accomplish the needed changes in the patient's situation. That is, did the interventions alleviate the patient's problem?

PRINCIPLES

1. Each individual is enmeshed in a matrix of psychological, social and physiological systems.
2. Each individual is a component of a multitude of interdependent and interactive suprasystems.
3. Each individual encompasses a complex network of interactive subsystems of both a psychological and physiological nature.
4. Each individual is an integrated whole. Mind and body are inseparable.
5. Force applied against any component or portion of the subsystems or suprasystems of an individual affects the whole individual.
6. Illness is the composite outcome of stressors applied to the individual's physiological, psychological or social subsystems or suprasystems.
7. Effective nursing care is care of the whole individual, rather than activity directed at a specific subsystem.

BIBLIOGRAPHY

Benson, Herbert, Beary, John, and Carol, Mark. "The Relaxation Response," in *Biofeedback and Self-Control*. Chicago: Aldine Publishing Co., 1975, pp. 467-475.

Bertalanffy, Ludwig von. *Robots, Men and Minds*. New York: George Braziller, Inc., 1967.

Cooper, Kenneth H. *Aerobics*. Philadelphia: J.B. Lippincott, Co., 1968.

Dunn, Halbert. *High-Level Wellness*. Arlington, Va.: R.W. Beatty Co., 1973.

Eaton, Merrill, Peterson, Margaret, and Davis, James. *Psychiatry*. 2d ed. Garden City, N.Y.: Medical Examination Publishing Co., Inc., 1969.

Kiritz, Stewart, and Moos, R.H. "Physiological Effects of Social Environments," *Psychosomatic Medicine*, 36 (January, 1974), 96-114.

Lachman, Sheldon J. *Psychosomatic Disorders*. New York, John Wiley & Sons, Inc., 1972.

McMahon, A.W., et al. "Personality Differences Between Inflammatory Bowel Disease Patients and Their Healthy Siblings," *Psychosomatic Medicine*, 35 (January, 1973), 91-103.

Pilowsky, I., et al. "Hypertension and Personality," *Psychosomatic Medicine*, 35 (January, 1973), 50-55.

Rogers, Martha. *Introduction to the Theoretical Basis of Nursing*. Philadelphia: F.A. Davis Co., 1970.

Selye, Hans. *The Stress of Life*. New York: McGraw-Hill Book Co., 1956.

Weinberg, Gerald M. *An Introduction to General Systems Thinking*. New York: John Wiley & Sons, Inc., 1975.

Weiss, Edward, and English, O. Spurgeon. *Psychosomatic Medicine*. Philadelphia: W.B. Saunders Co., 1957.

CHAPTER 9

Neuroses

Ann K. Kirkham, R.N., M.S.

INTRODUCTION

Neuroses are relatively mild psychiatric disturbances, characterized by excessive anxiety and depression, disrupted bodily functions, unsatisfying interpersonal relationships or obsessions and compulsions. Eight types of neuroses are defined by the American Psychiatric Association in the *Diagnostic and Statistical Manual of Mental Disorders* (Committee on Nomenclature and Statistics of the APA, 1968). This chapter will examine the general characteristics of these neuroses; the anxiety common to all types of neuroses; the theories of etiology; and the specific behavior patterns and nursing interventions appropriate to each of the eight neuroses. Finally, a case study will illustrate the development of the nursing process with the neurotic patient.

Generally, neuroses manifest themselves in the following ways:

1. Onset is acute. Unlike personality disorders, neuroses are not lifelong disturbances, although prodromal symptoms of a more persistent nature may be manifested.
2. Debilitation is mild. Frequently, neurotic individuals can function adequately in their occupations, since behavior and social interaction are not always affected by their symptomatology.
3. Symptoms of anxiety are displayed.
4. Contact with reality is not lost, although the view of reality may be distorted.

Because of rigid conscience development, neurotics tend to have many socially acceptable traits. Often they are reliable, responsible, honest and moral, and they are willing to conform to society's norms. However, rigid superego development often causes neurotics to become inhibited, especially when dealing with hostile or sexual thoughts, feelings or impulses. They may become overly sensitive to criticism by others, and feelings of inadequacy may thwart their high ideals and aspirations. Since neurotics are usually aware of their suffering and mental anguish, they frequently seek help from professionals such as family physicians, ministers or marriage counselors.

Neuroses can be readily distinguished from psychoses. Unlike the psychotic, the neurotic

1. is aware of the existence of a psychological problem
2. is able to adapt to the psychological problem
3. maintains a sense of reality
4. functions socially and remains in touch with the outside world
5. frequently exploits symptoms for secondary gain.

Since anxiety is the common denominator of all neuroses, much of the individual's psychic energy is spent on worry, doubt and fear. Thus, the primary gain derived from the neuroses is relief from anxiety. Sometimes the patient derives secondary gain, an incidental result of the symptoms, in which the individual discovers other advantages to being neurotic than anxiety reduction. For example, the neurotic may find that people pay more attention to him, demand less of him or allow him to be more dependent. Or perhaps his symptoms give him an acceptable reason for changing an unwanted role or job. When he learns how his symptoms can make life easier, the neurotic process, with its primary and secondary gains, is self-perpetuating, because it decreases anxiety and is self-defeating, and because it decreases the person's effectiveness.

Although the neurotic may at first appear to be within normal limits in attitude and behavior, several symptoms typically depict a maladaptive defense against overwhelming anxiety. For example, conversion is an unconscious process by which the neurotic exemplifies his conflict as a physical symptom. A phobia is a persistent and unrealistic fear of an object or person; an obsession is a persistent uncontrolled thought. Dissociation is the mental defense of separating emotion from a situation or one item from another. By recognizing conversion, phobias, obsessions and dissociation as symptoms of a neurotic process, the nurse can more readily understand the source of the patient's anxiety.

ANXIETY: THE COMMON DENOMINATOR

Anxiety, as opposed to fear, is the common manifestation of the neurotic. Unlike fear, which is the tangible reaction to specific known danger, anxiety is the reaction to a vague, often objectless danger. While fear warns people of impending threat from without, anxiety warns of impending threat from within, such as an impulse that is repulsive and unacceptable to the ego or a repressed thought or desire that is struggling to consciousness.

Anxiety may be classified as normal or pathological. Both types of anxiety are characterized by feelings of uncertainty, helplessness and an intense sense of personal discomfort. Normal anxiety is a warning and serves to prepare the person for defense or change in regard to the danger. This type of anxiety can be motivating and useful, for example, when it motivates a student to study diligently for an exam. Pathological or neurotic anxiety, however, continues after the need for warning has passed.

Normal anxiety is often distinguished from neurotic anxiety by assessing the individual's awareness of a disagreeable emotional state. With normal anxiety, the person consciously experiences anxiety and, thus, keeps it proportionate to the threat. If, for example, the anxiety surrounding a new experience is felt and acknowledged at a conscious level, and possibly even discussed with others, this anxiety is normal as long as it remains proportionate to the threat. Normal anxiety, then, does not involve repression. Neurotic anxiety, however, results from repressed conflicts. The anxiety serves as a warning that the unresolved conflict is surfacing once again. Thus, the person displays a stereotyped reaction to problems repressed and unresolved in the past. Often, the person is uneasy, apprehensive and tense and expresses a feeling of impending doom. For example, one patient described her neurotic anxiety this way: "I was just standing in the kitchen rolling out cookie dough and all of a sudden—for no reason—I felt this sudden letdown feeling, like the bottom had dropped out of the world. It was a feeling similar to what I felt when I was told my dad died . . . but I hadn't even been thinking of him."

Differentiation between neurotic and normal anxiety is also made by assessing the realism of the threat, since neurotic anxiety is provoked by an imaginary or unrealistic threat. For example, the patient who insists on being near the nurses's station, because of the unfounded conviction that the intercom will not work, is displaying neurotic anxiety. However, if the intercom has actually malfunctioned, the patient is displaying normal anxiety and coping skills.

Besides distinguishing between normal and neurotic anxiety, other classification systems identify anxiety in terms of degree. In one system:

Level + 1 = ability to comprehend is increased, powers of observation are sharpened.
Level + 2 = anxiety begins to affect the individual's comprehension.
Level + 3 = observational power is markedly decreased and hearing is diminished.
Level + 4 = the individual feels helpless, fearful, panicky, unable to do anything. This level of anxiety cannot be tolerated for long.

Another anxiety classification system divides anxiety into mild, moderate and severe degrees:

Mild: The person is able to comprehend most of what is happening in reality.
Moderate: The person has limited ability to comprehend what is happening in reality.
Severe: The person cannot focus on what is happening in reality.

In its mildest form, anxiety can be manifested subjectively by a vague sense of apprehensive expectation; in its most severe form, by an overwhelming feeling of panic. The degree of anxiety is not related to the distinction between normal or neurotic anxiety. Anxiety is increased by the severity of the threat (whether real or perceived) and by the success of anxiety-relieving behavior. Since anxiety tends to increase in severity if not dealt with adequately in the early phase, it is important for the nurse to be able to identify anxiety early.

Specific symptoms and behavior patterns are typically associated with anxiety. The physiological symptoms of anxiety include:

1. insomnia
2. increased perspiration (hyperhidrosis)
3. tachycardia (rapid pulse)
4. muscle tension
5. restlessness and irritability
6. tremor
7. gastrointestinal disturbances, such as vomiting, anorexia, and diarrhea
8. urinary frequency
9. increased B/P
10. hyperventilation
11. pupil dilatation (mydriosis).

Types of behavior commonly evoked by anxiety include:

sullenness	denial
quarreling	defensiveness
irritability	panic
crying	restlessness
anger	withdrawal
complaining	

For successful nursing intervention with neurotic patients, it is first necessary to deal with the symptoms and behavior related to anxiety. Four steps are useful in intervening with the anxious patient (see Table 9-1 on p. 254):

1. Recognize that the patient is anxious
2. Assist the patient into recognizing the anxiety
3. Encourage the patient to understand the anxiety
4. Help the patient cope with the threat he faces

Recognizing anxiety (step 1) requires both an understanding of the common symptoms of anxiety and an ongoing assessment of the patient's behavior. Once the nurse identifies anxiety, the primary intervention is the initiation of a trusting nurse-patient relationship. Sometimes the nurse's physical presence is sufficiently therapeutic to ease the patient's anxiety. Assisting the patient to recognize the anxiety (step 2) may be achieved by discussing with the patient his presenting behavior and underlying feelings. For example, the nurse notices that Mrs. C. is behaving anxiously:

Nurse: "I noticed you have been pacing up and down the hall for the past thirty minutes."
Mrs. C.: "I can't seem to get hold of myself."
Nurse: "You can't get hold of yourself?"
Mrs. C.: "Yes, I feel scared."
Nurse: "When did you begin to feel this way?"
Mrs. C.: "After I talked with my daughter on the phone. My husband is bringing her to the hospital to see me."

Once the patient realizes that anxiety exists, it is possible for the nurse to encourage the patient to understand the anxiety (step 3).

Nurse: "And that's when the scared feeling came over you?"
Mrs. C.: "Yes, I really don't want her to see me here. What will she think? She's only 7!"

The nurse, by reflecting and clarifying, helps Mrs. C. to see for herself the threat behind her anxiety.

Nurse: "What do you believe she will think?"
Mrs. C.: "I'm afraid she'll think I'm crazy and need to be locked up, because I'm dangerous!"

Helping the patient cope with the threat (step 4) now becomes the nursing objective. This can be accomplished through two courses of action: (1) by helping the patient learn new ways of coping with the threat and (2) by helping the patient reevaluate the threat (is the threat as bad as it may appear?).

If the nurse follows the first course of action, she might suggest alternatives to overcome the threat. For Mrs. C., some of these alternatives might be to:

1. call her husband and ask him not to bring her daughter
2. wait and see if she is correct in fearing that her daughter thinks she is dangerous
3. comb her hair, put on makeup and "rehearse" or role-play a warm greeting for her daughter
4. plan to visit with her husband and daughter in a homelike atmosphere like the visitors' lounge
5. purchase a toy for her daughter in order to "break the ice."

The possible choices and alternatives are only limited by the creativity of the nurse and patient. Alternatives should be based on the patient's needs and coping abilities rather than on the nurse's preference. The nurse defeats the purpose of the intervention by denying the patient an opportunity to decide which alternative is most appropriate. If the patient decides that none of the proposed alternatives is appropriate, the nurse accepts this as the patient's choice. Not to decide—is to decide. The patient must be made aware that an integral component of choice is the acceptance of the responsibility for the choice and for the consequences of whatever course of action is chosen. The nurse should not allow herself to be manipulated into deciding for the patient, for such intervention does not promote the patient's independence and insight.

If the nurse follows the second course of action and assists the patient in reevaluating the threat, the primary concern is to avoid discounting or minimizing the patient's perception of the threat. Whether the threat is unrealistic or imagined, the threat and associated anxiety are very real to the patient. When the nurse tries to argue the patient out of anxiety by discounting the fear as unfounded and unrealistic, the patient usually experiences further threat and increased anxiety due to the lack of understanding and subsequent isolation. Therefore, if the objective of the nursing intervention is to assist the patient to reevaluate the threat, the questioning must be carefully phrased so the patient, not the nurse, draws the conclusion that the threat is not really as bad as it appeared. In the example of Mrs. C. and her fear of rejection by her daughter, the nurse might ask questions such as:

"Is your daughter easily frightened?"
"What is your daughter's idea of 'crazy'?"
"Has your daughter ever been fearful of you or anyone else before?"

As the nurse explores the threat with Mrs. C., a more realistic view of the daughter's expected reaction might ensue.

Frequently, student nurses are not sure whether they should guide the conversation or allow the patient to verbalize freely on many topics. The conversation control depends on the nursing objective. In the preceding example, the nurse's objective is to assist Mrs. C. in reevaluating her neurotic fear of rejection by her daughter, who is coming to visit her. Therefore, the nurse guides the interview within the context of the patient's ideas about her daughter's fear of "crazy" people, as well as the patient's fear of rejection. Should Mrs. C. begin talking about unrelated matters such as the attire of another patient, the nurse carefully redirects Mrs. C.'s attention with a question such as: "Have you decided what you are going to wear when your family comes to visit?" The changing of the subject may be the patient's means of avoiding an uncomfortable topic.

TABLE 9-1

Nursing Process

ASSESSMENT →	PLANNING →	INTERVENTION →	EVALUATION
Patient displays anxious behavior	Nurse recognizes anxious behavior	Nurse enables patient to recognize anxiety	Patient displays decreased anxiety
		Nurse assists patient in gaining insight into anxiety	
		Nurse helps patient cope with threat behind the anxiety by learning new ways of coping with threat or reevaluating the threat	Nurse reinforces the decreased anxiety

In order to apply the above process skillfully, the nurse must:

1. be aware of her own feelings, for anxiety is contagious
2. find ways to control her anxiety, frustration or anger
3. maintain a genuine attitude of interest and concern
4. listen attentively and actively
5. promote autonomy by offering alternatives but *not by suggesting.*

THEORIES OF ETIOLOGY

Most of the etiological theories about neurosis share a common premise: that conflict plays an integral part in the development of the disorder. The conflict might be intrapsychic or socio-personal or inter-personal. The following are four principal theories of etiology:

Anxiety Theory

Freud proposes that neurotic disorders grow from attempts to resolve unconscious emotional conflicts. Conflicts arise from the individual's conscience and an unacceptable hostile or sexual desire. These conflicts arouse anxiety, which is then dealt with in a maladaptive manner. The maladaptive response is manifested by neurotic symptoms such as phobias, obsessions, conversion reactions or depression. Since these maladaptive behavior patterns reduce the anxiety, they are self-perpetuating.

Blocked Personal Growth Theory

Abraham Maslow (1970) theorizes that neurosis results from conflict regarding progressive growth versus maintenance of the growth level already achieved. In other words, the individual is preoccupied with meeting basic human needs and, therefore, is unable to move beyond the basic stages to self-actualization; he expends his energy in defense rather than advancement. Similarly, the pursuit of false or delusive values also creates a self-defeating situation, in which self-actualization is unattainable. In other descriptions of blocked personal growth, immature conscience development is emphasized as a primary cause. According to this theory, the individual experiences unresolved guilt, but the conscience is not functional enough to control instinctive ego-centered behavior. As a result, symptoms of neurosis are established to reduce anxiety, and attempts at further growth are blocked. An example of this might be the husband who, knowing that finances are tight, buys himself a luxurious cashmere topcoat and then feels guilty and self-rejecting, when he discovers the store won't refund his money.

Psychoanalytic Theory

Psychoanalyst Karen Horney proposes a theory that challenges

Freud's ideas about the dynamics of neurosis development. While Freud focuses on the conflict between desire and conscience, Horney defines the central conflict as one between child and parent: specifically, between the child's expression of hostility and the parents' inability to tolerate such expressions. The following is the process by which the neurosis is developed. Unable to tolerate even a minimal display of hostility, the parents respond to the child's behavior with rejection, irritation and coldness, so that loss of love and security become a danger in the child's mind. The child then correlates this danger with his own aggressive impulses and hostile behavior, and thus reasons that the expression of negative feelings threatens his survival in the family. As the neurosis develops, the child sees even his aggressive thoughts as threatening, and believes that the absolute abstinence of hostile expression is a life-saving measure. Although the perception of hostile expression as a threat to life is not experienced on a conscious level, the child learns to react to separation with extreme anxiety and to repress anger, hostility and aggression. When the child grows up, he represses even the association between hostility and parental rejection or loss of security. Unconsciously, the individual substitutes dependency on something (job, money) or someone (wife, husband) as a symbol of security and avoids situations that resemble desertion or increase anxiety. According to psychoanalytic theory, the neurotic process may originate at any stage of development when threat is great enough to cause repression. However, in the normal course of child development, several circumstances are especially threatening to the parent-child relationship. The birth of a sibling, separation from mother or major caretaker, and the Oedipal or Electra situation all demand parental sensitivity to the child's heightened need to express hostility.

Maladaptive Learning Theory

This theory proposes that neurosis develops when an individual uses trial and error to determine a defense that will decrease the anxiety. Once a defense is found, the individual automatically relies on the same mechanism in similar situations. While this learned behavior decreases anxiety, it also blocks the learning of new and more adaptive behavior.

CLASSIFICATIONS OF NEUROSIS

Anxiety Neurosis

The simplest of all the neuroses, this psychiatric disturbance is manifested purely by anxiety. Any or all of the signs and symptoms of anxiety presented earlier in this chapter may be experienced by the patient, either in attacks or as a continuous problem. An anxiety neurosis might have a spontaneous remission, become chronic or develop into a more complex disturbance. Since prolonged periods of anxiety are intolerable, defense mechanisms can transform an anxiety neurosis into another type of neurosis.

Hysterical Neurosis

This neurosis is associated with an involuntary loss or disorder of physical function, and the physical impairment is thought to be symbolic of an underlying intrapsychic conflict. The onset of symptoms occurs suddenly, usually during an emotionally charged interaction. The relationship between psychic conflict and physical disability that characterizes hysterical neurosis is clear in the case of Mrs. M. Following a fight with her husband, Mrs. M. loaded her three sleeping children into the family car and drove recklessly toward a friend's home. The car went out of control and crashed. Although Mrs. M. and the two older children were thrown to safety, the car door jammed while the mother watched the youngest child burn to death. When rescuers arrived, Mrs. M. was unable to see, although she had no physiological reason for the blindness. Later, when she talked about the incident during therapy, Mrs. M. suddenly regained her sight.

There are two basic types of hysterical neuroses. The first, called the *conversion* type, is a neurosis in which a physical symptom reflects an intrapsychic conflict and results in a repression of the conflict, thereby reducing anxiety. This physical expression of underlying anxiety is not the same as a psychosomatic disorder, such as a stomach ulcer, because there are usually no tissue changes that would be life-threatening.

Conversion symptoms include:

1. Anesthesia, especially "glove" or "stocking" numbness of limited areas of the hands or feet

2. Blindness
3. Deafness
4. Paralysis
    a. Aphonia—inability to speak
    b. Muscular twitches (tics)
    c. Peculiar movements
5. Convulsions, often during periods of complete awareness

A conversion reaction is characterized by an attitude of indifference in regard to the symptom. This attitude is sometimes called "la belle indifference."

A classic case of conversion neurosis concerns a spinster who began to experience paralysis of the right arm. During in-depth psychotherapy, the patient revealed extreme ambivalence toward her aging, demanding father, for whom she was responsible. Feeling both hostility toward her father and an intense subconscious desire to do away with him, she was torn between the need to be a dutiful daughter and the need to live a life of her own. To resolve this intrapsychic dilemma, the patient's "caring" arm became paralyzed, thus relieving her of her burden and rendering her incapable of murdering her father.

Another example of a case of conversion neurosis involved a young bride who disliked her job as a third-grade teacher. Torn between her desire to please her new husband by earning a paycheck and her desire to have time to be the "perfect housewife," Mrs. A. tried to excel in both roles. After many stressful months, Mrs. A. awoke one morning and found she couldn't move. Forced to give up her teaching position, she convinced herself that the paralysis was actually due to muscular dystrophy. Although the paralysis gradually subsided, Mrs. A. never taught school again, even though she and her husband had both worked so that she could get her college degree in elementary education.

The second classification of hysterical neurosis, the *dissociative* type, occurs when a person walls off parts of the consciousness in an attempt to deal with anxiety. This results in the following types of behavior:

1. amnesia—the temporary or permanent loss of memory
2. fugue states—fleeing from a situation without memory of the flight

3. somnambulism—sleep-walking, in which the somnambulist may not remember his actions
4. multiple personality—a pathological condition in which the personality is split into several distinct and unique portions.

An example of the fugue state in a dissociative type of hysterical neurotic is seen in Mrs. L., an outpatient being treated for neurosis. After a marital argument, her husband pushed her out of their car and tried several times to run over her. Following this experience, Mrs. L. did not remember borrowing a car from a friend and driving to another state. Even though the trip was 650 miles, the patient did not remember stopping to buy gas, to eat or to ask directions.

Since the symptoms express a message about the hysterical patient, the nurse should continually assess physical symptoms. It is important to chart any change in symptoms, as well as the events preceding the change and the patient's reaction to the change, so that the health team can identify the patient's progress in giving up the neurotic symptom. Also, continued assessment of the symptomatology enables the health team to differentiate between the malingerer and hysterical neurotic with a conversion reaction. Unlike the hysterical neurotic, who is motivated by an unconscious need, the malingerer consciously feigns symptoms in order to gain something desirable or to avoid something undesirable. Examples of malingering are pretending to have a whiplash injury in order to collect insurance or feigning visual problems to dodge the draft.

The nurse must guard against the temptation to promote the patient's symptom by inadvertently introducing secondary gains. By pampering a patient suffering hysterical blindness, the nurse rewards the patient for the blindness and makes it more difficult for the patient to give up the symptom. A good rule of thumb is to ignore the symptom but never the patient. For example, instead of trying to get a paralyzed patient to walk, the nurse should try to discover the psychological need for paralysis. By listening carefully, not only to what he says but to what he doesn't say, the nurse can obtain significant data regarding the symptoms.

Whether caring for a patient suffering from the hysterical neurosis, dissociation or conversion reaction, the nurse must remain non-judgmental. Frequently, there is a tendency to laugh off or ridicule people who have no physiological reason for their disabilities.

For the nurse who is accustomed to caring for patients with physiological problems such as sickle cell anemia, paralytic polio or nerve deafness, it is sometimes difficult to understand a patient whose behavior indicates a non-physiological etiology. This patient, however, needs understanding just as significantly.

Phobic Neurosis

In phobic neurosis, the neurotic reduces or alleviates anxiety through the defense mechanisms of projection and displacement. Through projection, the neurotic attributes his anxious thoughts and feelings to others, thus transforming his anxiety into fear. He then displaces this fear onto a neutral object, deed or situation. This defensive process changes internal anxiety into an irrational fear or phobia of external conditions. Now the neurotic need only avoid the phobic situation, object or deed to overcome fear; this is far more tolerable than facing inescapable anxiety within himself. The degree to which the phobias interrupt the patient's life depends upon the strength of the neurotic conflict, the frequency with which the patient must deal with this conflict, and the degree to which external conflicts are rekindled.

Nursing care of the phobic neurotic may include assisting the patient to understand that the phobia is the symbolic representation of a more basic anxiety. Studies have repeatedly shown, however, that insight into the origin, symbolism and function of the phobia has little effect on the patient's willingness to risk venturing into the phobic situation. Therefore, systematic desensitization has become a frequently utilized technique in the treatment of phobias. There are many variations of systematic desensitization, however the following are the basic steps in the process:

1. Train the patient in relaxation techniques
2. Establish an anxiety hierarchy (a list of anxiety-producing situations ranked in terms of intensity)
3. Repeatedly reinstate the feeblest item in the relaxed patient's list of anxiety-provoking situations, until no more anxiety is produced
4. Progressively work up the list of anxiety-producing situations

Regardless which variation of this technique is employed, the therapist encourages and supports the patient at each level of desensitization. For example, in treating a young woman who was so distressed by her phobia of snakes that she was unable to leave her home with confidence, levels of desensitization behavior ranged from looking at black-and-white illustrations of snakes to actually handling a harmless snake. The nurse encouraged the patient to use relaxation techniques while undertaking each step of the process. Further, the nurse provided support as the patient set her own pace and, within twelve weeks, the patient's mobility was no longer inhibited by the phobia.

Frequently, patients who overcome a phobia feel a greater sense of confidence in their ability to solve problems and control their lives. The nurse should make a conscious effort to reinforce these secondary gains.

Depressive Neurosis

The neurotic depressive reacts to loss with excessive sadness and lack of resiliency, whether the loss be of a love object, of status or of material possessions. Even after a reasonable period of time, the depressive mood does not return to normal. Typically, this type of neurotic demonstrates a lowered self-confidence, loss of initiative and enthusiasm and decreased activity but a high level of anxiety and apprehension. The depression is said to be mercurial: that is, at one point the person is in the depths of despair; yet with only a change of subject, he is animated and laughing. Frequently, the neurotic depressive has difficulty concentrating and complains of physical symptoms, such as trouble going to sleep. Together, these characteristics make the person with a depressive neurosis a potential suicide candidate.

Loss situations often trigger extreme depression because they reactivate repressed conflicts the patient experienced earlier in life, such as the loss of a significant person during childhood. Further, depression may occur following the loss of a loved one for whom the patient felt hostility, as well as love. Thus, grief may be intertwined with feelings of guilt and self-condemnation.

The nursing care of the depressed patient is covered in detail in Chapter 7. During any type of therapy, the nurse must constantly avoid reinforcing the patient's depression through secondary gains such as sympathy.

Neurasthenic Neurosis (Neurasthenia)

The neurasthenic neurotic is chronically tired and weak, has difficulty concentrating and spends an excessive amount of time sleeping, though the quality of sleep is poor. One of the most diagnostically significant things about the neurasthenic is that this fatigue is selective. During a golf or bridge game, for instance, the person's energy level is high, but in the face of family or occupational tasks, energy drops and the person becomes listless.

The classic case of neurasthenia is the "tired housewife syndrome." The housewife is "trapped" in an overly dependent role with a husband, who pays little attention to her. Prolonged frustration, discouragement and hopelessness reduce motivation and lead to listlessness and fatigue. These symptoms enable the housewife to avoid dealing with the true cause of anxiety, because she is too tired or too sick.

Nursing care of the neurasthenic is usually met with great resistance, because the patient continually searches for a physiological basis for the neurotic symptoms. The primary nursing intervention is aimed at helping the patient understand the nature of the problem. By encouraging independence and self-confidence and by discouraging self-pity, the nurse can build up the patient's ability to face unpleasant situations energetically.

Depersonalization Neurosis

The chief manifestation of this type of neurosis is a prolonged feeling of unreality either about oneself or one's external environment. Other manifestations include dizziness, distortions of time and space and, occasionally, the sensation that one is out of his body and is observing himself from a few feet overhead. Secondary anxiety often results when depersonalization experiences cause the patient to think he is going crazy.

The distinction between depersonalization and deja vu is important. While depersonalization is a sensation of strangeness, deja vu is a sensation of familiarity in which one feels that a situation or experience has happened before when, in actuality, it has not. Most people have deja vu experiences. Transient depersonalization is also a common experience, especially in children or in people who are suddenly submerged in a new culture. Depersonalization neurosis, however, appears to be a rarely observed syndrome.

Although prolonged stress and psychological fatigue are fairly common precipitating factors, the dynamics of this neurosis are not fully understood. Many theories of etiology are proposed, but no one theory is generally accepted. Since depersonalization is one of the first symptoms to appear in neoplasms of the brain, the patient should be assessed from a medical as well as a psychological standpoint. The course of depersonalization neurosis in approximately half of the cases is a long-lasting, chronic one. Sometimes the symptoms are sporadic, and the patient may be symptom-free part of the time.

Although the nursing care of the depersonalization neurotic has not been determined, it is possible to offer guidelines for intervention. First, the nurse should ease the patient's anxiety and fear by reassuring him of the availability of the staff. Even if the staff is scheduled for other non-delayable functions, the patient should know that help is available, and that he does not have to endure the fright alone. Second, the nurse should reassure the patient that he is not "going crazy." By having the patient define "going crazy," the nurse can then explain how his symptoms bear little or no resemblance to this description.

Hypochondriacal Neurosis

By demonstrating an exaggerated, morbid interest in the concern about bodily functions and health, the hypochrondriac avoids particular anxieties related to living and also achieves interpersonal gain. The patient is usually an avid reader of medical material and, therefore, frequently diagnoses and treats his symptoms. He is particularly suspicious of the excretory and digestive systems, although his preoccupation may be generalized to include any disease of which he learns.

The symptoms of the hypochondriacal patient are usually vague, alternating from one bodily function to another. An important phenomenon to note is that, although the patient may complain of serious disorders, he does not demonstrate the appropriate anxiety or fear that would be expected from a person suffering from disorders of such magnitude. The neurotic's sincere belief in his symptoms rules out malingering, even though the "illness" gives the patient an excuse for avoiding important life goals and, at the same time, provides a secondary gain through the sympathy and attention shown by significant others.

Sometimes this type of neurotic is programmed by a hypochondriacal parent to be overly concerned with his physical health. If a child is ill or injured early in life and experiences the secondary gains of exaggerated parental concern regarding his condition, he is likely to continue this pattern into adulthood. Other predisposed patients might display symptoms of hypochondriacal neurosis at mid-life, when they realize that their lives are more than half over, and they have failed to achieve their desired goals.

The hypochondriacal neurotic who is being treated as an outpatient is likely to undergo insight psychotherapy. However, the patient whose pathology is severe enough to cause hospitalization requires nursing care similar to that provided the schizophrenic (Kyes, 1974). Nursing care of the schizophrenic patient is covered in detail in Chapter 12.

Obsessive-compulsive Neurosis

This neurosis is manifested by the carrying out of compulsions and/or by the intrusion of obsessions upon the neurotic's consciousness. An obsession is an unwanted or recurring thought, urge or idea that may seem nonsensical or even morbid to the neurotic. A compulsion is a seemingly meaningless act that must be performed in order to relieve immense, unbearable anxiety. Performance of compulsions can become so frequent that the person's life is severely disrupted or debilitated. One of the most well-known examples of obsessive-compulsive behavior is Lady Macbeth's ritualistic handwashing, aimed at ridding herself of guilt for participation in the murder of King Duncan. Besides freeing the person of guilt, obsessive-compulsive behavior might also enable the frightened neurotic to control his world. Through a rigid and systematic life style, the patient becomes reassured that he can predict and prevent undesirable events, and only when this routine is disrupted does he feel threatened and anxious.

The obsessive-compulsive neurotic, then, is prone to feel guilty and inadequate and, thus, is vulnerable to threatening situations. The primary objective of nursing care is to help the patient understand why he perceives the compulsive behavior as necessary. The following nursing interventions have been found to be effective with the obsessive-compulsive:

1. Accept the ritualistic behavior without displaying shock, amusement or criticism.
2. Allow the patient to carry out the ritualistic behavior until he can be distracted into some other activity. To deny the patient this behavior is to increase his anxiety to an intolerable level.
3. Set limits on the patient's behavior only with the objective of preventing physical harm to himself or others.
4. Establish a routine for the hospitalized patient, and avoid anxiety-producing changes.
5. Notify the patient in advance if changes in routine must occur.
6. Assign a private living area for the patient, if possible.
7. Assess the patient's physical condition carefully. The compulsive hand-washer may have skin breakdown; his food and fluid intake might be inadequate, due to preoccupation with the ritual or due to the ritual itself.
8. Assign tasks that can be done to perfection, such as folding towels for one shelf of a small closet.
9. Provide opportunities for the patient to accomplish something positive, such as a creative project in occupational therapy.

When talking with the patient, the nurse should follow specific guidelines:

1. Encourage the patient to verbalize his feelings.
2. Gear conversation to accentuate the patient's value as a person.
3. Avoid discussion of the patient's illness, unless he initiates the subject.
4. Observe the patient carefully for symptoms of mounting anxiety and intervene before compulsive behavior begins, if possible.
5. Encourage a constructive one-to-one conversation, when the patient's anxiety has decreased following a compulsive ritual; remember, however, that the patient may be embarrassed about his behavior.

Some of the problems that interfere with reaching the goal of extinguishing the ritualistic behavior may be caused by other people. The nurse should be alert to the possibility that other patients and/or uninformed staff might ridicule the patient, thus increasing guilt feelings and compulsive behavior. Since compulsive behavior serves to decrease anxiety, the patient who continues this behavior will not actively seek help. Therefore, the nurse must plan time for intervention, lest the patient be forgotten.

SUMMARY

This chapter deals with the relatively mild psychiatric disturbance of neurosis. The neurotic, when compared to the psychotic, knows that a psychological problem exists, maintains contact with reality, can adapt to the psychological problem, and frequently exploits symptoms for secondary gain. The common denominator in all neuroses is anxiety, a feeling of fear or uneasiness as a reaction to a vague, often objectless danger. However, less severe forms of anxiety can serve as a warning and help to prepare the person to counter the danger through defense mechanisms or change.

Four steps are useful in intervening with the anxious patient:

1. Recognize that the patient is anxious.
2. Assist the patient to recognize the anxiety.
3. Encourage the patient to understand the anxiety.
4. Help the patient cope with the threat he faces, either by reassessing the threat or by proposing alternative ways of reacting to the threat.

In order to apply this process skillfully, the nurse must first be aware of her own feelings, for anxiety is contagious. She must find ways to control her own anxiety, frustration or anger. To intervene therapeutically, she must maintain a genuine attitude of interest and concern, and she must listen attentively and actively. When the nurse offers alternative ways of responding to anxiety, she promotes the patient's autonomy; conversely, if the nurse makes decisions for the patient, she thwarts the patient's ability to overcome his neurosis.

CASE STUDY

On admission to a minimum security unit, Mrs. C., a 30-year-old mother of two daughters, displayed extreme anxiety and fear. For several weeks prior to admission, she experienced the following difficulties: problems making decisions, sensitivity to opinions of others, persistent insomnia, inability to concentrate and emotional upset. Stating that she "cried at the drop of a hat," Mrs. C. said she wished she knew what she "was so worried about." Although she could not pinpoint any particular event that caused her difficulties, she said that her "nervous breakdown" started when she was unable to sleep for several nights; during that time, Mrs. C. drank coffee and smoked almost constantly. Her history revealed similar but less severe periods of anxiety. Although the patient's husband tried to understand her crying and nervousness, he frequently became exasperated.

Mrs. C. was one of six children. Since her father was frequently unemployed, the family was maintained primarily by the mother's frugality and hopefulness. The mother did ironing to earn money for basic needs, and the children were expected to work as soon as they were old enough to find jobs.

I. OBJECTIVE DATA
   A. General Appearance, Attitude and Activity
      1. Appearance: neatly dressed; hair straight, short and neat; fingernails bitten very short
      2. Attitude: tried to answer questions and carry on conversation; frequently apologized for not remembering the subject of the conversation; extremely polite
      3. Activity: smoked almost constantly; darted eyes from one object or person to the next; fidgeted with rings and ashtray; smiled infrequently
   B. Communication Patterns
      1. Content: focused on her inability to sleep and to make decisions; frequently commented on fear of what her children and neighbors are "going to think;" expressed concern regarding the staff's attitude toward her
      2. Pattern: talked rapidly, with many unfinished sentences; was easily distracted and had difficulty coming back to subject when interrupted
   C. Contact with Environment
      1. Oriented to time, place and person
      2. Easily distracted by others
      3. Easily startled

D. Sensorium and Intelligence
   1. Memory: appeared to remember accurately both recent and remote events with the exception of incidents immediately preceding hospitalization; did not remember anything about the day of hospitalization, such as how she arrived at the hospital or who was with her
   2. Concentration: had "difficulty concentrating on anything"
   3. Thinking: was able to think concretely and abstractly
   4. Intelligence: maintained a "B" average in high school and successfully completed two years of college

E. Thought Processes
   1. Thoughts in logical sequence
   2. Answered opinion questions after thinking about the question for some period of time; answered factual questions promptly

F. Thought Content
   1. Was concerned about the opinions of her children and others regarding her hospitalization
   2. No hallucinations reported

G. Social Assessment
   1. Education: high school graduate with two years of college
   2. Socioeconomic status: husband, a civil engineer of middle socioeconomic status
   3. Religion: Baptist
   4. Family: married eight years; two daughters, 7 and 5 years of age; patient's mother died of cancer two years ago, father lives thirty miles away
   5. Family's understanding of illness: on patient's admission husband stated, "She is so nervous I'm afraid she'll fall apart;" husband called patient every evening, was instructed by patient to tell no one except her father of her whereabouts; husband told children that Mrs. C. was "visiting grandfather"

6. Habits: "chain" smoked; drank alcoholic beverages when at parties or "when it is expected"
7. Visitors: husband visited patient once in one week; Mrs. C. instructed husband not to visit often, because she was afraid the neighbors would find out where she was; patient's father visited once and left phone number where he could be reached

H. Medical Assessment
1. Present complaints: frequent headaches, worsening in late afternoon; palpitations and increasing tremor of hands, which patient considered to be embarrassing; poor appetite; weight loss of 8 pounds in past month, for patient "was just not hungry;" stomach felt "knotted up;" insomnia, sometimes relieved by a glass of wine and warm bath
2. Date of last physical exam: three months prior to admission

II. SUBJECTIVE DATA

A. Present Illness
1. Reason for admission: voluntarily admitted self to hospital because the patient felt she "needed a rest"
2. Precipitating event: patient became more and more nervous after husband began traveling out of town for extended periods of time; insomnia became very severe two days prior to hospitalization; husband was to leave on a business trip the day of hospitalization
3. Previous treatment: patient was given a prescription for Valium, 10 mgm., t.i.d., p.r.n. for nervousness, one year ago

III. STATEMENT OF THE PSYCHIATRIC PROBLEM

A. Anxiety Neurosis

B. Problem List
1. Insomnia
2. Increased anxiety
   a) Headaches

            b) Palpitations
            c) Poor appetite
            d) Increased startle reflex
        3. Concern regarding hospitalization

IV. PLANNING PHASE

A nurse, whom the patient had approached on several occasions, initiated a conference with the patient to begin identifying problems, nursing actions and overall treatment goals. The patient identified three problems: insomnia, increased anxiety and concern regarding hospitalization. Each available treatment modality (one-to-one therapy, group therapy, occupational therapy and recreational therapy) was explained to Mrs. C. Exhibiting interest in recreational therapy but fear of group therapy, Mrs. C. then expressed a desire to see a psychiatrist once a week. The patient also requested that "when things got rough" she be able to talk with the nurse who accepted primary responsibility for the nursing care.

The nurse and patient presented the plan to the team and arranged a weekly appointment time with the psychiatrist. After the schedule for recreational therapy for the ensuing week was given to Mrs. C., the patient and the primary nurse presented the problem list. Mrs. C. and the team then agreed upon expected outcomes and a plan for reaching these outcomes. They scheduled a meeting in two weeks, at which time the team's (patient and personnel) progress toward the expected outcomes would be evaluated. New problems would be identified and plans would be modified as indicated. The problem list, including the expected outcome and the plan, was then recorded on Mrs. C.'s chart as follows:

A. Insomnia
   1. *Plan:* As soon as the patient identifies insomnia, she will notify the primary nurse or nurse on duty of her inability to sleep. The nurse will encourage Mrs. C. to verbalize the anxieties or concerns that keep her from falling asleep. Together, they will explore the problem to assess if the threat is real, imagined or exaggerated.

2. *Expected Outcome:* Mrs. C. will be able to fall asleep fifteen minutes after retiring. She will be able to sleep undisturbed for at least six hours.
B. Increased Anxiety (headaches, palpitations, poor appetite, increased startle reflex)
   1. *Plan:* The primary nurse will teach Mrs. C. the behaviors and physiological signs and symptoms of anxiety. The nurse will facilitate the patient's early recognition of anxiety and encourage her to understand what precipitated it, to learn new ways of coping with it, to reevaluate the threat and to assess the reality of the situation. They will explore the possibility of the patient's experiencing secondary gain from the anxiety.
   2. *Expected Outcome:* Mrs. C. will be able to recognize early signs and symptoms of anxiety in herself and will be able to cope satisfactorily with the threat related to the anxiety. She will experience an increased appetite, a decreased startle reflex, decreased palpitations and headaches and a progressively decreasing level of anxiety.
C. Concern Regarding Hospitalization
   1. *Plan:* Mrs. C. will explore this concern with the primary nurse. She will reevaluate the threat that she presently associates with telling friends, neighbors, and her daughters that she is in a "mental" hospital. The nurse may initiate insight-promoting methods such as psychodrama or role-playing, as appropriate, to help Mrs. C. understand the situation. The nurse will also offer alternative methods of dealing with the concern of others' responses to the patient's hospitalization.
   2. *Expected Outcome:* The patient will not be concerned about other peoples' opinions of her hospitalization.

Evaluation, an ongoing, continuous process, will take place between the patient and the primary nurse. If any problems remain unresolved, the nurse and patient will assess the validity of the expected outcome and the feasibility of the plan. If parts or all of the plans are not carried out, they will assess and correct the difficulty.

PRINCIPLES

1. Unresolved conflicts between members of the health team who care for the patient can have an adverse effect upon the patient's well-being.
2. Feelings of anxiety can have an adaptive or motivating value and thus can lead to constructive action.
3. High levels of anxiety decrease comprehension.
4. Anxiety is frequently associated with three underlying states of mind; helplessness, isolation and insecurity.
5. Every person needs to see himself as able to satisfy his wants.
6. Every person needs to see himself as able to control his own life and to contribute to the control of his environment.
7. Every person needs to see himself as useful and productive.
8. A threat to the self-image provokes anxiety.
9. Neurotic anxiety results from repressed, unresolved conflicts (imaginary threat).
10. Even when anxiety is neurotic (imagined), it is still very real to the person.
11. All behavior has meaning.

BIBLIOGRAPHY

Committee on Nomenclature and Statistics of the American Psychiatric Association. *Diagnostic and Statistical Manual of Mental Disorders.* 2d ed. Washington, D.C.: American Psychiatric Association, 1968.

Kyes, Joan, and Hofling, Charles K. *Basic Psychiatric Concepts in Nursing.* 3d ed. Philadelphia: J.B. Lippincott Co., 1974.

Maslow, Abraham H. "Neurosis as a Failure of Personal Growth," in *Psychopathology Today: Experimentation, Theory and Research.* Edited by William S. Sahakian. Itasca, Ill.: F.E. Peacock Publishers, Inc., 1970, pp. 122-130.

CHAPTER 10

Personality Disorders and Sexual Deviations

Ann K. Kirkham, R.N., M.S.

The personality disorders and sexual deviations that are discussed in this chapter correspond to the non-psychotic disorders classified by the American Psychiatric Association in the *Diagnostic and Statistical Manual of Mental Disorders* (Committee on Nomenclature and Statistics of the APA, 1968). Although the *Diagnostic Manual* also includes alcoholism and drug abuse as non-psychotic disorders, these two problems are explored in a separate chapter in this text. Other sex-related topics of increasing importance to the nurse then follow the discussion of sexual deviations.

PERSONALITY DISORDERS

Rather than specific mental or emotional symptoms, personality disorders are pervasive, maladaptive behavior disorders that produce relatively little or no distress to the individual and persist throughout life. These disorders evolve from early developmental stages and are recognizable by adolescence, if not earlier.

The patient with a personality disorder is encountered in many fields of nursing, such as the medical, industrial, community health and administrative specialties. An understanding of the typical behavior associated with each personality disorder enables the nurse to assess and intervene appropriately and effectively.

While personality disorders differ in rather obvious ways from psychoses, the distinction between personality disorders and neuroses is more ambiguous. The major differentiation is the degree of distress. Since personality disorders produce little or no distress, the individual views his symptoms as a desirable aspect of the self. The maladaptive patterns that others describe as symptomatic are egosyntonic to him: that is, the very behavior that causes distress to others brings satisfaction to him and fulfills his needs. In neuroses, however, distress results from anxiety either experienced directly or converted into a defensive symptom picture. The neurotic individual finds his thoughts, feelings and actions to be unpleasant and undesirable. His symptoms are ego-alien, meaning that they are repugnant to the individual's self-concept. Typically, personality disorders do not defend against anxiety, as do neuroses, nor do they result from excessive stress, as do psychoses. Thus, an individual with a personality disorder does not always present a clear-cut symptom picture.

Unlike personality disorders, transient situational personality disturbances result from overwhelming stress. Events such as natural disaster, imprisonment or military combat may precipitate a transient situational personality disorder. If supportive care is provided during the situational crisis, recovery generally ensues.

The personality disorders are defined in the *Diagnostic and Statistical Manual of Mental Disorders* (Committee on Nomenclature and Statistics of the APA, 1968): inadequate, schizoid, cyclothymic, paranoid, passive-aggressive, explosive, asthenic, hysterical, obsessive-compulsive and anti-social disorders. These personality disorders will be discussed in regard to etiology, characteristic behavior patterns and specific nursing interventions. Dyssocial behavior will also be discussed, in order to distinguish it from antisocial behavior. Finally, a case study will be presented, using the nursing process as the framework for planning interventions.

Inadequate Personality

This individual is neither physically nor mentally grossly deficient, yet he manifests inadequate emotional, social, intellectual and physical responses to situations. His behavior is characterized by poor judgment and by a lack of flexibility and adaptability. Motivated by neither rewards nor successes, he acts according to the pleasure principle, since he is unable to wait for or to delay gratification.

The inadequate personality is illustrated by a fictional Russian character named Ilya Ilyitch Oblomov, a man of breeding and promise who lapses into a lazy, emotionless existence, without goals, and concerns himself only with his next meal and nap. After Ilya is denied his request for medical discharge from government service, he submits his resignation, and his days continue to deteriorate:

> Ilya feared them [women] and kept away. His soul was still pure and virginal. . . . Hardly any outside attractions existed for him, and every day he grew more firmly rooted in his flat. . . . As he grew older, he reverted to a kind of childish timidity, expecting harm and danger from everything that was beyond the range of his everyday life—the result of losing touch with external events. . . . With a lazy wave of his hand he dismissed all the youthful hopes that had betrayed him or been betrayed by him, all the tender, melancholy and bright memories that make some people's hearts beat faster even in their old age. . . . (Stone and Stone, 1966, pp. 228-229).

Growing more and more used to his isolation, Ilya decides at last that there is nothing further for him. Although he once dreamed of a poetic existence among the peasants in his native village, he now believes that he has attained his ideal life.

If a person is successful in any aspect of life, the diagnosis of inadequate personality is not appropriate. Frequently a true inadequate personality is considered untreatable, since the patient obviously does not feel distressed by any inadequacy. In such cases, prognosis for change is not positive. Nursing care includes encouragement, comfort and pragmatic advice regarding daily problems of living.

Schizoid Personality

Because the schizoid personality characteristically avoids close relationships with others, he experiences feelings of emptiness, barrenness and chronic loneliness. Despite a yearning for human contact and closeness, he conceals this desire because of a fear of rejection. He attempts to reject others before others can reject him, in order to preserve his self-esteem and autonomy.

A schizoid person often experiences acute discomfort when

others offer him warmth and affection. Because the inability to form satisfying relationships permeates the individual's entire life, many schizoid people never marry; those who do, often experience difficulty in the day-to-day closeness with their mates, and the marriages may end in divorce. The schizoid person may spend a considerable amount of time daydreaming and may substitute daydreams for people-oriented activities. His job is frequently determined by the need for aloofness, since he functions best in solitary work assignments that require minimal direct contact with others. For example, long-distance truck driving, bookkeeping or jobs requiring correspondence rather than direct, face-to-face contact may prove satisfying.

Even though the schizoid person is a "loner," he is very sensitive to the way others treat him. Often, he fears aggression—not only his own, but the aggression of others toward him. He may fantasize that any expression, particularly one with a negative connotation, will lead to an overwhelming outburst of rage from others. In order to protect himself from the emergence of uncontrollable, aggressive thoughts and impulses, he generally reacts to minor disturbances and conflicts with outward detachment. He may become depressed in the face of conflict, since depression is often anger and rage turned inward. He may use drugs and alcohol to find respite from loneliness. For the schizoid personality, withdrawal in many forms serves a protective function.

People with schizoid personalities may seek psychiatric care for diametrically opposed reasons. In some cases, the sudden loss of or inaccessibility to the person's few sustaining relationships may precipitate a crisis. In other cases, a warm, intense interpersonal relationship may prove so threatening that the schizoid person feels psychologically overwhelmed.

The primary objective of nursing intervention is to provide an opportunity for the patient to establish and maintain a satisfying, one-to-one relationship. If the patient is to overcome his fear of others, he must first find pleasure instead of fright in his association with the nurse. Successful nursing intervention requires both patience and an on-going assessment of the patient's ability to tolerate psychological or physical closeness. To enter too closely into a patient's territorial area may stifle the patient and cause him to feel threatened and "back away."

During the establishment of their relationship, the nurse should communicate acceptance as the patient tests new ways to express feelings of closeness or aggression. For example, on the day after a lengthy discussion in which Nurse Jones and Mr. D. had carefully examined his fear of rejection, Mr. D. approached the nurse by saying, "You again?" Had Nurse Jones responded, "Yes, who did you expect?" or something similar, she would have conveyed a negative reaction to Mr. D.'s attempt to test the relationship. In contrast, by responding, "Sounds like you aren't eager to talk with me to day," she focuses on the overt message with an awareness that the covert, subtle message may be, "Will you reject me if I am a little caustic?" The nurse may now discuss with Mr. D. the possible impact of similar behavior on other relationships.

It is also essential for the nurse to maintain a safe environment that enables the patient to change at his own pace. In the example above, the patient might reply, "I don't want to talk with you today." In that case the nurse would respond with, "Okay, I'll check with you after lunch to see if you would like to play checkers." In this way, the nurse conveys respect for the patient's need for distance. The nurse also leaves the door open for another attempt at establishing closeness. The use of games and other activities frequently enables the patient to tolerate a one-to-one relationship.

Some patients respond better to a group therapy situation, because closeness is diluted by the increased number of participants in the relationship. By observing other patients' experiences in the group, the schizoid patient may discover that the establishment and maintenance of a relationship with another person can be rewarding.

Cyclothymic Personality

Mood swings are the predominant behavior pattern in the cyclothymic personality. This person has chronic highs and lows. As with the hysterical personality, the affect of the cyclothymic personality is labile. But unlike the paranoid personality, reality testing is not impaired, and mood swings do not prevent the person from carrying out responsibilities to job and family. The cyclothymic person is basically friendly and outgoing; he is able to form close interpersonal relationships, prefers to be with others and shuns solitary activities. However, due to rejection and emotional coldness during childhood, the same person also may experience feelings of inadequacy, a hunger for closeness and periods of mild depression. Unable to reconcile these conflicting emotions, the cyclothymic personality has swings in mood caused by forced and overactive euphoria that defends against imminent depression.

The cyclothymic patient is rarely admitted to psychiatric services; however, the nurse may see him in the emergency room, medical-surgical units, university health services and industrial clinics. Although depression is frequently the presenting symptom, evidence indicates that psychotherapy is not particularly helpful. The nurse should be aware that a cyclothymic patient is oversensitive to physical complaints when in the depressive state, yet pays little attention to physical problems when in the euphoric state. Thus, careful assessment of the patient's mood must be made before physical problems are treated.

Paranoid Personality

The paranoid personality primarily exhibits a rigid, pervasive and unwarranted suspiciousness. Additional characteristics include hypersensitivity, jealousy, envy and excessive self-importance. An individual with a paranoid personality disorder may be shy, seclusive, stand-offish, arrogant or aggressive. Whatever the symptom pattern, the individual spends considerable energy attempting to confirm his paranoid ideation that most or all people want to harm or betray him. His personality characteristics interfere with his ability to develop and maintain satisfactory interpersonal relationships.

The most widely held theory regarding the etiology of all types of paranoid states is that chronic hostility builds up in early life and causes the paranoid person to project hostility onto others. Having endured much emotional coldness and loneliness during childhood, the paranoid has considerable pent-up anger by adolescence and is unable to form close relationships. As this pent-up hostility is projected onto others, the person feels that "everyone is against me."

The primary objective of the nursing intervention is to create a safe and trusting relationship with the patient, so that he can forfeit some of his psychological isolation. The nursing management thus includes avoidance of inadvertent rejections, oversights or slights.

For instance, if the nurse always gives medications alphabetically and a paranoid patient's last name begins with Z, the patient may react as though he has been personally affronted. The nurse, in this situation, would matter-of-factly explain her system and would ask the patient if he would prefer that she alternate through the alphabet, beginning with Z. This intervention presents reality to the patient and also allows him an opportunity to contribute to the solution of the troublesome situation. Such nursing action enhances the patient's feelings of esteem and provides a new way of dealing with an old problem.

When possible, the patient's freedom of movement and choice should not be stifled. The nurse should stringently avoid situations in which the patient feels that he is trapped or that his autonomy is threatened.

Due to impaired reality testing, a patient with paranoid ideations may ignore evidence that conflicts with his perceptions. Therefore, arguing the patient out of paranoid perceptions may precipitate an array of paranoid behavior. The nurse might anticipate such reactions as inappropriate anger, threats of revenge or accusations that the nurse is "like all the others."

Another objective of the nursing intervention is to remind the psychiatric team that inadvertent rejections, oversights and slights can be handled in a therapeutic way. If a nondefensive attitude pervades the staff, the patient may begin to trust: defensive retorts by the staff only reinforce the patient's paranoia. Maintaining a nondefensive attitude requires insightful, perceptive analysis. It is helpful for the nurse to allow time to assess an appropriate response by asking simply, "Will my reply help the patient?" This "double thinking" process discourages non-therapeutic statements.

Passive-aggressive Personality

Probably the most common psychiatric disorder is the passive-aggressive personality, which is characterized by deep dependency and morbid resentment. For the person with this disorder, the two major difficulties are fulfilling dependent needs and responding to authority. Characteristic behavior includes pouting, stubbornness, failure to keep appointments, procrastination, intentional inefficiency and tardiness.

Overdependency is a complex need that can give rise to anger at the very authority on which the person depends. Although the mentally healthy adult feels neither compelled to rebel against authority nor afraid to oppose it if necessary, the person who is overly dependent on a person or institution may be unable to respond realistically for fear of jeopardizing his position. As a result, anger and frustration complicate the problem. For example, the head nurse tells the staff to attend a meeting regarding changes in a policy manual. A particular nurse does not want to waste her time at a meeting, when she feels pressured to care for an overload of patients. Because the authority figure dislikes excuses, the nurse feels too threatened to be direct and honest about her reasons for not wanting to attend. Therefore, she arrives ten minutes late, unprepared and stubbornly attempts to put down any ideas that are proposed by others. Although she complies with the head nurse's request, she manages to disrupt the meeting by indirectly expressing her hostility.

Because the individual's responses reflect an inability to express hostile feelings directly, openly and maturely, passive-aggressive behavior is usually self-defeating. For example, after a wife repeatedly asks her husband to help her wash the dishes, he begrudgingly assists her. But by doing a sloppy job, he indirectly expresses his hostile feelings. When the wife lets the husband know that she is not pleased with his inefficiency, the husband experiences only the disadvantages of and none of the advantages of compliance. In contrast, the mentally healthy adult would say directly, "I really don't want to help you right now, because I'm working on a project. If you will wait till later, I'll help then."

Some theorists speculate that the etiology of passive-aggressive behavior is closely tied to society's restrictions upon aggressive activity. Others maintain that the problem begins in the oral stage of psychosocial development.

The passive-aggressive personality tends to become more pronounced as the patient grows older. The more persistent the passive-aggressive behavior, the more likely the person is to be socially isolated or unemployed. Frequently, loneliness or joblessness is the motivating factor in bringing the passive-aggressive patient to therapy.

For effective theraputic intervention, the nurse assists the patient to:

1. identify the maladaptive aspect of his behavior

2. relate the consequences of the maladaptive behavior to the behavior itself
3. recognize a need for change
4. identify the goals of the maladaptive behavior
5. identify workable alternatives for reaching these goals.

Through these five steps, the nurse helps the patient understand and resolve his particular behavioral problem.

Since passive-aggressive behavior is often antagonizing and difficult to control, the nurse must work at keeping an accepting attitude toward the patient. It is helpful to anticipate that therapeutic efforts may be thwarted by behavior such as stubbornness, helplessness or failure to keep appointments. To avoid initiating this behavior, the nurse might eliminate unnecessary requests or demands of the patient.

Explosive Personality

The explosive or epileptoid personality is characterized by uncontrolled outbursts of rage. This rage is the only presenting symptom of the patient's deviation from normal limits. Etiology is unknown; however, the five nursing interventions listed for the passive-aggressive personality serve equally well in the nursing care of the explosive personality.

Asthenic Personality

The characteristic behavior pattern of the asthenic is lack of enthusiasm, lack of energy and fatigue. Unlike the inadequate personality, the asthenic person adjusts adequately to many aspects of life. However, he is typically self-pitying and tends to project the blame for his problems on others. Nutritional status should be evaluated, since oversensitivity to physical and emotional strain, apathy, increased irritability and loss of spontaneity can result from semistarvation or chronic vitamin and mineral deficiencies. Because of the idiopathic etiology of asthenia, nursing interventions vary. Assessment of sleep, work and recreational habits may be helpful in assisting the patient to direct more of his limited energy and enthusiasm into satisfying activities. Since stimulants might be prescribed for the asthenic patient, the nurse must be aware of any anticipated side effects that could occur during the treatment of this life-long disorder.

Hysterical Personality

The characteristic behavior pattern of the hysterical personality (also known as the histrionic personality) contains several apparent paradoxes. This person is lascivious and coquettish but usually sexually frigid. Although affect is labile and emotional outbursts are part of the behavior pattern, the person is emotionally shallow and cannot feel empathy, loyalty or sensitivity to others. Since this person is also vain and egotistic, a dramatic, exhibitionistic personality pattern is predictable. These characteristics, coupled with a strong need for dependency, present a complex pattern of immaturity.

Although men demonstrate the hysterical personality pattern, the female hysterical pattern is frequently the pattern described in the psychiatric literature. The characteristics of the hysterical personality are more frequently displayed in Western cultures than in other parts of the world.

Due to lascivious and provocative tendencies, the hysterical person will compete with a member of the same sex in situations involving the opposite sex. That is, the female hysteric often competes with female nurses and behaves seductively toward male nurses; the opposite tends to be true for the male hysterical patient. In either case, the objective of the nursing intervention is to provide support and even maternal responses to competitive behavior, or to provide nonsexually oriented caring responses to seductive behavior. For example, if a female hysteric displays competitive behavior toward a female nurse, the therapeutic response might be, "I've been noticing how pretty your hair is today." It is imperative, however, that this nurturing, non-competitive remark be genuine if it is to be therapeutic. A patient who "sees through" a phony compliment loses trust in whatever else the nurse may say. If the female hysteric displays seductive behavior toward a male nurse, the therapeutic response might be, "I enjoy hearing you play the piano. Would you play for me?" Again, it is important for the male nurse to make a sincere request and to plan to take time and listen, if the patient plays. It is also important that there are no sexual overtones in the nurse's request.

Nurses need to be aware of their own emotions, as well as those of the patient, if the relationship is to be therapeutic. For example, if the nurse feels that a patient's behavior is disgusting, it is wise to think through the reasons for this reaction. What causes the nurse to view the patient's behavior in this way? Often, it is helpful to discuss personal reactions with a trusted member of the therapy team. By understanding the meaning of both the patient's behavior and the nurse's own negative reactions, the nurse can achieve the objectivity necessary for effective problem-solving. Because the person with a hysterical personality usually suffered severe maternal deprivation in early childhood, competitive and seductive behavior is considered a sexually masked request for caring and nurturance. Thus, it is vital for the nurse to understand the reasons behind the patient's behavior. It is essential to keep in mind that each person's behavior is purposeful: the provocative patient is seeking to meet his own needs through his actions. If the nurse were to say that the patient's seductiveness toward the opposite sex was ridiculous and embarrassing, the nurse would be saying exactly the opposite of what the patient needs to hear.

Two defense mechanisms used extensively by the hysterical personality are dissociation and denial. Dissociation is the psychological segregation of an emotion from an idea, object or circumstance. Denial is the dismissal of undesirable or intolerable thoughts, wishes and feelings. Denial also may be the rejection of unendurable external reality, a mechanism often depicted by the ostrich that hides his head in the sand. Both dissociation and denial cause the individual to have difficulty functioning in unpleasant situations. By failing to associate or to accept the negative aspects of reality, the hysterical person is sometimes unable to act responsibly. The nurse should keep this in mind when counselling such patients regarding desirable employment.

Obsessive-compulsive Personality

The obsessive-compulsive personality is manifested by an excessive concern with conformity. Major personality traits include rigidity, perfectionism, ambivalence and a critical and self-righteous vindictiveness. Other traits such as neatness, orderliness and punctuality are often constructive, if not exhibited in extreme degrees. Banking, scientific research, accounting, library work and other occupations that require meticulous attention to details are well suited for people with obsessive-compulsive personalities.

When obsessive-compulsive traits become overemphasized, they prove ineffective and become liabilities. For example, the drive to complete one task and launch another makes rest and relaxation difficult. In addition, ambivalence may be so severe that it interferes with the individual's ability to make decisions and take action. This ambivalence can be extremely frustrating and annoying to others, who consistently find themselves waiting for the obsessive-compulsive person. Moreover, a severe conscience and a strong need to be in control of the self, as well as the environment, tend to limit spontaneity and creativity.

Two defense mechanisms are frequently called into service by the obsessive-compulsive person. The first, "undoing," is the ego-defense mechanism by which a person attempts to undo or negate his own act or communication. By the ritualistic performance of the opposite of what the obsessive-compulsive person has done or said, he tries to cancel out the evil or vice of his behavior. This defense mechanism operates at the unconscious level and comes into existence through unconscious conflicts. If these unconscious conflicts are allowed to emerge into consciousness, this person experiences overwhelming anxiety.

The second defense mechanism, "isolation of affect," is the separation of an emotion from a thought or situation. For example, a student in the operating room for the first time may hold at bay the emotion evoked when observing the initial incision and accompanying blood. An air of pessimism seems to pervade the obsessive-compulsive person's attitude toward life. Seldom experiencing spontaneous joy and enthusiasm, this person has a high risk of depression, especially involutional melancholia. In the middle years, he may discover that his dreams and aspirations have not and may never be realized; postponed gratifications were not in fact postponed, but denied. The inability to fantasize leaves the person with no way to rectify this self-denial. He thus experiences a feeling of barrenness and impoverishment. Depression, anxiety or an exacerbation of obsessional symptoms may result from the patient's inability to maintain control over his feelings, actions and environment.

The primary objective of the nursing intervention is to help the patient regain control over his world. The nurse offers herself as a non-judgmental listener, as the patient describes his overwhelming feelings and impulses. By verbalizing these feelings and impulses, the patient may be able to regain control and avoid acting unrealistically. The nursing approach includes helping the patient learn new, more effective modes for directing his compulsions. The nurse continually assesses the environmental context in which the compulsion is carried. The charting should include the precipitating event, the patient's thoughts and actions and the response of others to the compulsive act. As this information is validated with the patient, assessed and recorded over a period of time, a pattern of precipitating events and effective therapeutic interventions should become evident.

Consistency between the approaches of the nurse and the psychotherapist regarding the treatment of compulsive acts is essential. Some therapists prefer to ignore the compulsive act, whereas others choose to place limits on the compulsive behavior. If the patient is to be permitted to carry out his compulsion as frequently as he requires, the nurse must be accepting and non-critical. It only increases the patient's anxiety if the nurse points out the ridiculousness of the act. For example, the compulsive hand-washer complains to the nurse that his hands are dry, cracked and bleeding. The nurse provides protective cream but does not allude to the fact that the problem is self-inflicted. If the compulsion interferes with the patient's ability to meet basic needs, certain restrictions should be established. The patient who washes his hands so often that he is unable to eat requires immediate nursing intervention. Snacks and finger foods should be made available, while the patient is excessively anxious.

A second objective of nursing intervention is to anticipate, assess and prevent social isolation. The patient's interaction with others is severely restricted by his obsessions and compulsions. The nurse non-critically encourages the patient to be aware of the price he is paying for his preoccupation.

Since the obsessive-compulsive patient has a prevailing pessimism, the nurse can anticipate a resistance to change. It is important not to push or hurry an obsessive-compulsive patient. New ideas or suggestions are more successful if made indirectly. A new idea has a better chance of being considered if it is offered by a nurse who has established a trusting relationship with the patient. An onslaught of suggestions and new ideas will generally be met with considerable resistance.

As the patient proceeds in his treatment, the previously repressed hostility begins to present itself. The nurse should expect repeated hostile outbursts as the patient improves. Since the obsessive-compulsive patient fears uncontrollable anger and views it as undeniably destructive, his eventual verbal attacks on the therapist provide an opportunity for him to become aware of his misperceptions regarding anger. Sullivan (1956) states that the therapist must be able to tolerate repeated angry outbursts, because this is how the patient gets well. These angry releases also free the patient from some of his rigidity, for he learns that anger can be expressed in a manner that is not overwhelming to himself or others. The nurse should consistently encourage and assess spontaneous behavior. She should problem-solve with the patient, so that he can learn the consequences of his expressions of anger. He should learn that hitting and kicking the nurse are unacceptable expressions of anger, while verbalizing or engaging in strenuous activities are acceptable.

The maintenance and reestablishment of the patient's self-esteem is also a component of the nursing intervention. One of the main things to remember is that the obsessive-compulsive patient rarely has a sense of humor. Teasing or joking are generally contraindicated. Any attempt at leading the patient to an awareness of his behavior must be done with preservation of self-esteem.

The nurse can anticipate dependency-independency conflicts, which often are frustrating to handle. For example, a patient might ask the nurse for advice on a particular subject and then choose the completely opposite course of action. This apparent ambivalence regarding the need to be dependent or independent may indicate the patient's fear of becoming involved with or obligated to the nurse. Patience, as well as a clear understanding of the dynamics of this struggle, make it easier for the nurse to cope with the ambivalent behavior. The nurse should consistently support the patient in his attempts to problem-solve. The consequence of each type of behavior should be examined, and alternative approaches for future use should be assessed. If the patient is to function effectively, he must become aware of his behavior and must be willing to give up the causes of his anxiety and discomfort.

Antisocial Personality Disorder

In the past 60 years, three different terms have been applied to patients who demonstrate behavior that is now described as an antisocial personality disorder. In the first part of the twentieth century, the term "psychopath" was used; this term was later replaced by "sociopath," and in 1968, the American Psychiatric Association adopted the term "antisocial personality disorder." (Committee on Nomenclature and Statistics of the APA, 1968, p. 9.) Therefore, the three terms are sometimes used interchangeably to describe the most expensive and the most destructive form of abnormal behavior.

An antisocial personality disorder is apparent in an unsocialized individual whose behavior consistently results in conflict with society. He is amoral and unable to demonstrate or feel a sense of loyalty to a group, a culture or another person. Moreover, his behavior is often impulsive and irresponsible, and he can rarely endure frustration. The primary goal of an antisocial individual is the narcissistic satisfaction of his needs, with little or no concern for the consequences. Attainment of this goal—however selfish—is accompanied by minimal, if any, anxiety or guilt.

A compilation of research studies indicates the following common factors among individuals with antisocial personality disorders:

1. Frequently intelligent, spontaneous and likeable on first acquaintance
2. Emotionally immature, irresponsible, impulsive and lacking in judgment
3. Unable to attain a sense of loyalty to another person or group
4. Unable to defer pleasure, operating similarly to a newborn infant: "I want what I want when I want it"
5. Inadequate conscience development with a marked difference between intelligence level and ability to incorporate a moral code
7. Unable to profit from mistakes or learn from past experiences
8. Devoid of close friends or alliances
9. Unable to accept authority or discipline
10. Skillful at rationalizing and blaming others for personal mistakes and shortcomings
11. Lacking in anxiety and guilt

The antisocial person's inability to defer pleasure is due to an intolerance for frustration and anxiety. Operating by the pleasure principle, this individual frequently abuses alcohol and drugs, has a poor work and school history and feels very little, if any, guilt regarding his actions. Despite the complete absence of a life plan, he has little anxiety about the haziness of his future. Neither experience nor punishment alters this defective judgment. The coping patterns most frequently observed in antisocial patients are rationalizing, placing blame on others and minimizing situations.

The person suffering from an antisocial personality disorder frequently comes to psychiatric attention because he has caused or has threatened to cause harm to himself or others. The combination of low tolerance for delayed gratification and lack of superego makes this person an obvious candidate for prison. Studies have delineated demographic data or commonalities in people with antisocial personality disorders. They are predominantly male, come from a low socioeconomic group and often have a history of a similar disorder in a parent, parents or sibling. Illegitimacy or parental deprivation, usually desertion by the father, are frequently found. These individuals are accident-prone, due to poor judgment and relentless operation on the pleasure principle. Conversely, motor activity, attention span and intellectual ability are all within normal limits. Research indicates that there are institutional or psychological commonalities, such as a tendency toward a mesomorphic or "he-man" body build.

EEG tracings, which record brain waves in the frontal lobe, are frequently found to be abnormal in antisocial patients. The possible genetic etiology of this disorder is the subject of much research. Specifically, researchers hypothesize that an antisocial disorder is due to a defect in the XY chromosome, since antisocial individuals frequently have an extra Y chromosome (XYY).

In considering the etiology of antisocial personality disorders from a psychosocial viewpoint, one must recognize that both home environment and parent-child relationship are paramount in influencing early superego development. For example, a child who is moved from home to home often lacks the opportunity to identify with a set of values. The child who is reared by multiple caretakers may become confused about the values he will identify as his own. Although this problem is more common in lower socioeconomic groups, upper income parents can confuse their children by delegating the parenting role to surrogate parents or boarding schools. Further, a child who is reared in an institution, such as an orphanage, is high risk for a superego development problem. This risk is minimized, however, if the staff provides a consistent surrogate parent for each child.

If parents set up an unreasonable value system for the child, an antisocial personality disorder may result. When unreasonable parental standards are at cross-purposes with the child's instincts and peer enviornment, the dilemma may set the child at war intrapsychically and cause him to solve the problem by "walling off" his superego. Sometimes the child will cope with the problem by developing protective devices that hide his disorder. Any incident that breaks through his protection can cause a devastating explosion. Newspaper accounts frequently reveal intrapsychical conflicts in antisocial children. For example, a 13-year-old boy, known as a good student and an active church and Boy Scout member, methodically shot and killed his parents, sister and himself. Although neighbors and teachers agreed that this was an "ideal child " who was "never naughty" and "always did the right thing," clues to the boy's intrapsychical problem emerged during the search of his home. Pictures he had drawn symbolically portrayed his rage at the conflict between what he was and what was expected of him. Hoarding, especially of food items, indicated his extreme need for nurturing and the pervasive fear that it would not be provided. As this evidence was made known, neighbors began to remember the unreasonableness of the father and the passiveness of the mother; one neighbor remembered wondering how the boy stood his home life.

Parental hypocrisy can also contribute to subnormal superego development. If parents make an outward display of a value system that is opposite to the values by which they operate in private, the child's belief in any value system weakens. For example, if a mother punishes her child in the grocery store for taking a stick of candy but then switches price stickers to her advantage, she contradicts her value lesson. This "do as I say, not as I do" message, if pervasive, leaves the child confused and unclear about his developing value system. Another example of parental hypocrisy is the inconsistency between how the family acts at home and how it presents itself in public. If parents are sociable and charming with outsiders but routinely argue and degrade each other in private, the child learns to develop a superficial facade that hides his real feelings. Further, inconsistency in discipline may appear to be hypocrisy, leaving the child confused about his parents' values. If a parent sometimes punishes the child for lying and at other times ignores the lie, the child becomes unsure of what the truth is worth.

Thus, families in which antisocial traits develop tend to be replete with inconsistencies and often controlled by unreasonable standards. Instead of experiencing strong love, shame, approval or disapproval, the child lives his life in an emotional vacuum and learns to react to others with indifference.

Heaver (1943) found in a study of 40 male sociopathic personalities the following characteristics:

1. The mother is often overindulgent, pleasure-loving, frivolous and undermining of the husband's success.
2. The father is critical, stern, distant, obsessional and fear-inspiring.
3. There are marked discrepancies and conflicts in parental attitudes regarding authority, independence and goal achievement.
4. The family attempts to keep up a "front" or illusion of a happy family

Both the severity of the parental pathology and the frequency of the adverse childhood experiences affect the probability that an antisocial personality will develop.

The nurse needs to be acutely aware of the superficial charm that is characteristic of the antisocial patient, for this charm often masks manipulative behavior and inadequate superego development. Typically, the patient will describe his allegiances and goals and will in no way indicate his antisocial outlook. Only by discovering the patient's past conduct and by carefully observing his behavior can the nurse learn to recognize the patient's real intent. If the nurse is to treat manipulative behavior, she must first be aware that she is being manipulated. For example, the patient may begin by telling the nurse how beautiful her eyes are. While the nurse is recovering from this unexpected flattery, he then tells her how good it makes him feel to talk with her, and next he mentions her sensitivity to a patient's needs. Eventually, he slyly slips in a request for a pass out of the institution.

For successful intervention with the antisocial patient, the nurse's responses must be both nonpunitive and consistent. In the above example, an appropriate response would be to say calmly that the pass will not be issued. Further, the nurse should explain the regulation regarding passes, so that the patient has objective data regarding the decision. If the patient persists, perhaps reasoning that the regulation does not pertain to him, the nurse must once again nonpunitively explain that it does. As with other personality disorders, patience is an essential characteristic of the nurse who works primarily with antisocial patients.

Another important aspect of intervention is the nurse's awareness of her own psychological needs. Her basic need for security or self-esteem does not lie dormant when dealing with a patient; if these or other needs are unmet, the nurse's reactions, objectivity and therapeutic value are affected. Unless she is able to meet her personal needs outside the clinical setting, the nurse may be tempted to use the patient for her own gain.

Some situations predictably cause nurses to react unhelpfully to antisocial behavior. For example, when the patient's behavior does not agree with the nurse's expectations, the nurse is likely to react negatively. Conversely, when the nurse's behavior does not live up to the patient's expectations, the situation is negatively charged. In either case, the antisocial personality might be expected to take advantage of the situation and try to motivate the nurse by guilt to "undo" the mistake. For example, if a patient attempts to take another patient's tranquilizer, the nurse might spontaneously exclaim, "I can't believe you would steal Mr. Jones' medication; you don't care about anyone." After thinking over her reaction, she decides on a more therapeutic approach. Realizing that the patient was displaying a characteristic pattern of antisocial behavior, she says openly, "Mr. Smith, I reacted to your behavior without thinking this morning. In order to help you control your behavior, the nurses' medication area will be off limits to you for two weeks." Predictably, the patient now focuses on the nurse's first statement by saying something like, "Well, I'd sure feel better about your bad reaction to me if I could have something to calm me down." The nurse should non-judgmentally point out the patient's manipulative behavior, and then she should examine the facts to decide how to respond to the patient's request.

When dealing with the manipulative behavior of the antisocial personality, the nurse needs to assess carefully patient temptations in the environment. Is money left on night stands? Are narcotics and potentially abused medications left uncrushed before being given to the patient? Are keys dangling on chains about the staff's necks or from belt loops—non-verbally indicating to the patient his loss of freedom and power? If these types of environmental temptations are evident, the nurse would want to point them out to the staff. It would be most beneficial to do this in a staff meeting, where the staff could deal with the underlying motivation. For example, if a staff member thinks wearing keys around his neck indicates a position of authority and distinguishes him from the patients, a name tag with his job title would achieve the same end without creating an unnecessary temptation.

The type of manipulation discussed so far is destructive manipulation: behavior that allows the manipulator to get what he wants from others while creating interpersonal problems and preventing his own improvement. Manipulation, however, may also be constructive. The constructive manipulator applies his own strengths in promoting successful, mutually beneficial relationships with others. Manipulation, constructive or destructive, can occur on a subconscious level.

One of the major objectives of the nursing intervention is to provide the patient with a socially acceptable role model. This enables the patient to identify with and "take on" the superego of one or more staff members. Therefore, the nurse must be adapted to the rules of society. A nurse with poorly controlled antisocial impulses may vicariously enjoy the patient's antisocial acts; thus, she may unconsciously and subtly encourage the patient to act in ways contraindicated by prevailing rules and norms.

Another aspect of the role model superego is that it should be flexible. If the nurse is overly rigid, the patient may view the value system as diametrically opposed to his and, as a result, his identification with the nurse's value system may not even be a viable possibility.

Acting out behavior is characteristic of antisocial personalities, especially of young patients. The hospitalized patient who acts out is indeed a challenge to the staff, since possible violence demands quick assessment of the total situation. An example of acting out behavior is provided by Sally, a teenager who is angry at a patient named Rhonda and is running after her and threatening to "beat her up." When the nurse steps between the two patients in order to help Sally gain control, Sally shoves the nurse against the wall, picks up a chair and throws it at Rhonda. Sally then begins to run toward Rhonda again. Now the nurse must rapidly assess the situation and the consequences of her intervention. She might ask herself these questions:

1. Based on Sally's past behavior, what can I predict her next move will be?
   She will hit Rhonda and yell obscenities.
2. Will she hit hard enough to injure Rhonda?
   Very probably.
3. What coping mechanisms might Rhonda use?
   Last time a similar situation occurred, Rhonda locked herself in the bathroom.
4. How can I predict Sally will react if I block her by stepping between her and Rhonda?
   Predictably, she will hit me or try to push me out of the way. I have known Sally for only one week, and she has been very stand-offish when I have attempted to establish a relationship.
5. If I am injured or pushed around physically, how will this affect the other patients?
   For the patients who are aware of the situation, my injury could have very frightening effects. They could justifiably feel that this is not a safe place, when authority figures can be shoved or hurt.

Having asked herself these questions, the nurse is prepared to act. She decides to subdue Sally by throwing a bedspread over her. This allows time to call for a staff nurse who has a closer relationship with Sally, so that together they can help Sally control herself.

According to Anders (1977) when intervening with a violent patient, the nurse should remember to resist the temptation to rush in and attempt to intercede physically. A violent, frightened patient needs room between himself and others and also needs to feel that he has control of what happens to him. Other important aspects of interventions with violent patients are:

1. Acknowledge the feeling. "You sound as if you are very angry at Rhonda."
2. Encourage verbalization. "Tell me what happened to make you so angry at Rhonda."
3. Propose alternative action. "Let's you and I go in your room and beat on the pillow, Sally."

4. Set limits of behavior. "I will not allow you to hurt Rhonda."
5. Provide reassurance. "I will help you control your behavior."

The assessment process in acting out situations takes only seconds and is based on data that are readily available. Since the nurse does not have time to read the chart or refer to textbooks for alternative interventions, the continuous assessment and reassessment of patients is essential.

A movement is beginning which views the person with an antisocial personality disorder as a person with a health problem rather than as a criminal. The nursing division of the New York prison system has made great strides in approaching comprehensively and therapeutically the problems of both the patient and his family.

Since antisocial citizens are a costly problem to society, in terms of human suffering and expensive law enforcement programs, the control of this personality disorder is of utmost importance. For several reasons, the most logical means of control is prevention rather than apprehension and punishment. First, antisocial personalities do not learn from punishment. Further, this disorder is difficult to treat, and the prognosis is poor. Prevention of antisocial personality disorders depends upon early detection. Through a massive study of delinquency, the Gluecks (1950) found that the average age of onset of delinquent behavior is 8.35 years.

Based on the *Bristol Social Adjustment Guides* (1969), by Stott and Sykes, six categories of behavior considered to be predelinquent are observable in 5- to 16-year-olds:

1. lack of concern for adult approval
2. hostility toward peers (inhuman attitude)
3. uncontrolled, habitual hostility toward adults
4. defensive withdrawal, such as avoidance of eye contact
5. continuous depression and neurophysical exhaustion
6. overdemand for attention, caused by fear of adult rejection.

The nurse, especially the school nurse, is in a position to identify these early warning signs. By recognizing and referring young children who demonstrate predelinquent behavior, the nurse might help to correct causal conditions, before the disorder becomes firmly established.

Dyssocial Behavior

Dyssocial behavior is mentioned here primarily to emphasize the ways it differs from behavior characteristics of antisocial personality disorders. Dyssocial behavior is classified under "Conditions without Manifest Psychiatric Disorder and Non-specific Conditions" in the *Diagnostic and Statistical Manual of Mental Disorders* (Committee on Nomenclature and Statistics of the APA, 1968, p. 52). This classification recognizes that people do seek therapeutic assistance for problems that are not indicative of psychiatric illness.

While an antisocial is socially irresponsible and cannot conform to the prevalent norms of society, a dyssocial individual actively counters society by associating with a subculture that holds conflicting values. Unlike the antisocial person, a dyssocial person is able to defer pleasure, tolerate frustration, form close and lasting relationships, experience guilt feelings and modify his behavior in response to undersirable consequences. Because of strong relationships with significant others in childhood, the dyssocial is capable of trust by the time he reaches adolescence and adulthood. There is often a strong sense of loyalty within the group in which the person becomes attached.

An example of dyssocial behavior is organized crime, vividly portrayed in the book and movie, *The Godfather*. In this subculture, there is "honor among thieves." The superego of individuals is oriented toward group ethics, in contrast to personal values and conscience development.

The dyssocial person regularly finds himself in conflict with society. When motivated to change his behavior through therapy, he is much easier to treat than the antisocial personality. Treatment of dyssocial behavior consists primarily of abandoning the cultural group whose value system so sharply conflicts with that of the larger society.

SEXUAL DEVIATIONS

Defining deviant behavior is a formidable task, because society's expressed sexual standards often differ from the behavior of society's members. In other words, what we say and what we do can be inconsistent. Nevertheless, a significant variable in distinguishing between normal and deviant sexual behavior is the accepted value system of a given culture or subculture. With over 2,000 subcultures in the United States, each with its own unique sexual norms, it is not surprising that a definition for deviant sexual behavior is unworkable.

Because of this great variety of sexual practices, several definitions of sexual deviation form the basis for the discussion in this chapter. Bruno Cormier (Resnik, 1972) defines sexual deviation as a sexual act that is harmful and that is performed without the mutual consent of the sex partners. Eaton (1976) refers to sexual deviation as sexual behavior that is a source of worry, displeasure or disagreeable consequences to the person or persons indulging in it. The *Diagnostic and Statistical Manual of Mental Disorders* (Committee on Nomenclature and Statistics of the APA, 1968, p. 44) defines sexual deviation as sexual behavior that is carried out under bizarre circumstances or that is usually not affiliated with coitus. It is inappropriate, however, to apply this latter definition to people who are deprived of their normal love objects, as in the case of prisoners of war or penitentiary inmates.

In this chapter, the following sexual deviations are discussed: fetishism, pedophilia, voyeurism, exhibitionism and sadomasochism. Etiological theories, characteristic behavior patterns, dynamics and therapeutic interventions are described. Since the same nursing interventions are appropriate for each of these deviations, the descriptions of therapeutic techniques are grouped in the section on sadomasochism. Following the discussion of the five sexual deviations, three other sex-related topics of increasing importance to the nurse are considered: homosexuality, transsexuality and rape. When working with patients who exhibit the behavior patterns discussed in this chapter, the nurse must assess the recurrence of the aberrant behavior, noting whether the pattern is episodic, incidental or persistent. Whatever the type of deviation, the sexual deviate displays a persistent pattern of sexual practices that almost entirely exclude normal sexual behavior as defined by the group.

Fetishism

Fetishism, sexual interest focused on an inanimate object, is a type of avoidance deviation (as are voyeurism and exhibitionism), in which a person fears sexual contact. In an effort to avoid a sexual relationship, the individual seeks sexual stimulation and gratification through an object that, to others, may seem to have no sexual significance. In severe cases, this object, or fetish, becomes the primary means by which the person can achieve orgasm. For example, one man found sexual gratification by looking at the undented exhaust pipes of cars with idling engines.

More males than females are fetishists, and the inanimate objects that most frequently serve as fetishes are women's undergarments. However, if a man has made an otherwise satisfactory heterosexual adjustment, the sexual arousal he might obtain from viewing black lace panties is not considered fetishism. Often, an object must meet specific criteria before it becomes a fetish: generally, it is owned by, used by or stolen from a member of the opposite sex. Since the person who steals a fetish object or snips a lock of hair from a stranger runs counter to societal norms, fetishism at times brings the individual in contact with legal authorities. Unlawful fetishism varies in degree and significance, for even pyromania (deliberate and compulsive fire setting) is a fetish when it is done for sexual gratification.

Although the etiology of fetishism is unclear, one causative factor is the repeated association of an object with sexual pleasure. An experiment by Rachman (1966) demonstrated that a mild fetish can be created from a neutral object under laboratory conditions. In this experiment, male subjects were simultaneously shown pictures of provocative nude women and women's boots. The stimulation was repeated until sexual arousal could be elicited by pictures of the boots alone; finally, the response was generalized to other types of female footwear.

When fetishism becomes the sole or preferred pattern of sexual gratification, this deviation indicates uncertainty about masculinity and potency. Further, fetishism, to this degree, indicates a fear of rejection or humiliation by members of the opposite sex and is a mechanism to protect low self-esteem and compensate for feelings of inadequacy. It is not unusual for the apprehended fetishist to be embarrassed and remorseful; he is frequently anxious to deny the sexual implications of the act.

Behavior therapy is the most commonly practiced and most effective treatment for fetishism. Initially, the sex object is paired with a negative stimulus until the fetish disappears. (This aversive conditioning is the opposite of the process by which Rachman created the boot fetish.) A desensitization process then deals with the patient's fears and anxieties regarding heterosexual relations. Through therapeutic association with members of the opposite sex, the patient can desensitize his fear of rejection at his own pace. Supportive coed discussion groups, which share ideas about sexuality and mutual experiences of rejection, enable the patient to realize that he is not alone. Also, group members can suggest new ways of coping with the fear of sexual inadequacy.

The quality of nursing care depends upon the nurse's ability to understand the defensive characteristics of the fetishistic patient. A non-judgmental attitude, as well as clear communication with team members involved in the behavior therapy, is essential to the patient's progress. If the nurse is female, the male patient may use her to test out his newly discovered masculinity during the desensitization phase of treatment. The nurse should encourage the patient to test new ways of relating to women, and she should remain supportive as they work together to assess these attempts. Also, the nurse should ensure that the patient's new behavior is kept within conventional or socially acceptable bounds. A trusting nurse-patient relationship and self-awareness on the nurse's part are essential to the success of nursing care.

Pedophilia

The person who uses a pre-puberty child as a sex object is a pedophiliac. Studies have shown that the child is usually known to the patient and is either his own child or the child of a friend. Most pedophiliacs are male and are personally immature; that is, they have never been able to establish and maintain satisfying relationships with others.

One type of pedophiliac is considered regressive. This offender has a history of relatively normal sexual experiences in adolescence but regresses in adulthood to selecting helpless, youthful sex objects. A common precipitating factor for the regressive pedophiliac is the discovery that his wife or girl friend is having an affair. Another type of pedophiliac is the aggressive offender, who has a history of hostile aggressive acts and selects a child unknown to him as the victim of his impulsive sexual attack.

For the aggressive offender, imprisonment appears to be the only method of protecting society. For the immature and regressive pedophiliac, however, behavior modification techniques and group therapy have demonstrated effective changes in behavior. Nursing interventions described in regard to sadomasochism are also effective in treating pedophilia.

Voyeurism

The voyeur receives sexual gratification from a pathological indulgence in viewing sex organs and sexually oriented nudity. Usually timid and almost always male, the voyeur is heterosexually maladjusted and has a strong need to prove his masculinity and potency. A person with this deviation is plagued by an underlying immaturity. According to Freudian theory, the voyeur attempts to observe scenes that repeat childhood experiences of castration-anxiety. This repetition of the anxiety-provoking experiences theoretically allows the patient a chance to master the anxiety. Unlikely to demonstrate behavior of other, more serious deviations, the voyeur responds well to group investigative therapy as discussed in the section on sadomasochism.

Exhibitionism

The exhibitionist needs to display his sexual organs to a member of the opposite sex in order to receive sexual gratification. Like the voyeur, the exhibitionist is almost always a male who is unable to maintain a satisfactory heterosexual relationship. He is more a nuisance than a threat and does not go beyond exhibitionism even when encouraged by the "victim." The exhibitionist rarely exposes himself in a setting conducive to culmination by sexual intercourse, and he tends to repeat his deviant behavior in the same vicinity at about the same time of day. Since the exhibitionist seems to want to shock or frighten the victim, his deviation may indicate hostility toward the opposite sex. Appropriate methods of intervening are described in the section on sadomasochism.

Sadomasochism

Sexual sadism is the need to humiliate or to inflict pain on another person in order to achieve sexual gratification. Masochism, on the other hand, is the need to endure pain or cruelty to obtain sexual gratification. These two deviations are interrelated, and most writers indicate that both phenomena are present in a single person. Thus, sadomasochism applies to both sadists and masochists.

Closely associated with sadism and masochism are coprophilia and coprophagia. Coprophilia is an abnormal interest in excrement (urine and feces); coprophagia is a desire to ingest excretions and secretions. The person who becomes sexually stimulated by watching the sexual partner urinate is demonstrating coprophilia. Sometimes the coprophiliac has a masochistic need to be urinated upon by the sex partner. The person exhibits coprophagia by consuming the sexual partner's saliva, urine, vaginal secretions or semen.

Sadomasochism varies in intensity and can be very dangerous. Numerous examples of extreme sadomasochism were reported during wartime and in concentration camps. The infamous Peter Kurten was a sadomasochist who directed his perversions against dogs, squirrels and sheep, and who achieved sexual gratification by murdering men, women and children. Clifford Allen (Ellis, 1961) indicates that persons falsely confessing to murder are latent sadists who may eventually live out their fantasies and actually kill. Extreme masochism, on the other hand, can lead to suicide, as in the case of a man found tied to a ladder in a London sewer. Due to the position of the body and the known history of the man, authorities concluded that the victim tied himself in the gruesome environment to suffer a masochistic death.

When the sadomasochist's behavior becomes disruptive to society, the patient is hospitalized or imprisoned in an attempt to protect society. However, most minor sadomasochistic deviations can be treated in an outpatient setting.

One of the theories of etiology is that sadomasochism is caused by the repeated association of sexual pleasure and traumatic, pain-related stimuli. The association may be coincidental, as in the following case study:

> A 25-year-old male sadomasochist was raised in a very strict boarding school, where punishment was meted out by a school master who insisted on the baring of buttocks for whippings. Later the boy remembered having erections during the beatings, at first from the friction as he leaned nude over the end of the couch. During puberty, he fantasized about these whippings while masturbating. As a sexually active adult, he could only become aroused if his partner beat or whipped him, or if he fantasized the abuse.

A second theory of etiology is that sadomasochism results from a belief that pain must be endured as the price for pleasure of any kind. Applying this theory, Hariton (1973) indicates that women commonly fantasize during intercourse that they are overpowered and forced to participate in a wicked or forbidden act. Supposedly, the fantasy absolves any guilt felt about active participation in intercourse, which the woman has been taught is "bad." This, however, does not mean that all women with these fantasies are sadomasochistic; only when the person depends on the infliction or endurance of pain for sexual gratification is the term appropriate.

A third theory is that fear of impotence may be a motivating factor in sadomasochism. Since the sadomasochistic behavior is the stimulus for gratification, the sexually inadequate person uses the infliction of pain to guarantee his own performance.

A fourth theory of etiology relates sadomasochism to psychopathology. In severe forms of psychopathology, thinking and reasoning ability are disrupted, and sadomasochism may occur. Wertham (1949) describes a schizophrenic who held puritanical views regarding sex, therefore castrating boys and mutilating and killing girls, while achieving full sexual gratification. The puritan's reasoning for these acts was that he saved the victims from immoral adult behavior.

The nursing interventions and treatment modalities appropriate for sadomasochism also apply to voyeurism, exhibitionism, fetishism and pedophilia. Ideally, the objective of the nursing intervention is to enable the patient to overcome the deviation. For the sadomasochist, this means breaking the association between pain stimuli and sexual pleasure. Sometimes long-term investigative psychotherapy is necessary to bring the erroneous association into the patient's consciousness. Since the promotion of healthy sexual encounters is adjunctive to investigative psychotherapy, the nurse should acknowledge and encourage the patient's normal sexual behavior.

Several methods of intervention are effective in mild cases of deviation. One method encourages the patient consciously to restrain deviant behavior and to explore socially acceptable means of meeting sexual needs. Another method, suppressive therapy, promotes the intentional exclusion of desires and thoughts from the patient's consciousness. A third method enables the patient to accept the deviation and to feel less guilty about it. For example, the woman who becomes sexually excited by being bound, pinched or spanked might respond well to the acceptance approach. Conceivably, this approach would require acceptance by the woman's husband as well, for he must understand her need if the patient is to overcome her guilt.

More extreme cases of sexual deviation respond to primal therapy. According to Eaton (1976), primal therapy is based on the theory that unmet infantile needs become repressed and cause frustration in later life. To reach the source of the patient's problem, the primal therapist, usually with a group, regresses the patient to the early psychosexual stages of development. The patient reexperiences the unmet needs and reacts to the experiences as he would have then. By facing the repressed frustration and talking out the accompanying feelings, the patient brings the conflict to the consciousness, where it can be dealt with in the company of supportive others. Because the patient reacts with catharsis (the expression of thoughts and feelings that have been suppressed) and abreaction (the emotional discharge experienced when suppressed or repressed material is reexperienced), this method is sometimes called Primal Scream therapy.

The treatment modality for a particular patient is selected by the psychotherapist or the team and is based on the assessment of available data. Therefore, observations must be objective, clear and comprehensive. The perpetual charting or recording of observations is an invaluable aid in selecting appropriate treatment and in evaluating the effectiveness of the treatment.

Homosexuality

Homosexuality was listed as a diagnosis under the classification of sexual deviations in the 1968 *Diagnostic and Statistical Manual of Mental Disorders* (Committee on Nomenclature and Statistics of the APA, p. 10). However, in 1973, the American Psychiatric Association voted to remove "homosexuality" from the standard official nomenclature and to substitute "sexual orientation disturbance" (Tripp, 1975). This new diagnostic category applies to persons who are primarily attracted to people of the same sex and who are disturbed by, in conflict with, or want to change their sexual orientation. Homosexuality is defined as sexual preference for members of one's own sex. Usually the term "homosexual" refers to either males or females, and term "lesbian" signifies the female homosexual.

The difference between the transsexual and homosexual is that the transsexual actually thinks of himself or herself as the opposite sex, whereas the homosexual does not want to change his or her sex organs. The homosexual does not have a gender identity conflict and does not want to become the opposite sex; rather, this person is simply psychosexually drawn to persons of the same sex.

The incidence of homosexual activity in the United States, as estimated by Kinsey in 1948, was 37 percent of the white male population. Those white males with an exclusive homosexual orientation comprised 4.0 percent of the white male population. It is difficult to assess whether Kinsey's estimates remain valid, for homosexuality appears to be more prevalent in today's society. Some investigators attribute this apparent increase in the incidence of homosexuality to the liberalizing of social values.

Kinsey perceived homosexuality as one extreme on a scale of sexual behavior:

0	1	2	3	4	5	6
Exclusively heterosexual			Bisexual			Exclusively homosexual

Some psychotherapists utilize Kinsey's scale by relating sexual behavior to sexual fantasy. Theoretically, the type of fantasy should parallel the type of sexual activity. If, for example, a person's sexual fantasies rank 5 on the scale while sexual behavior ranks zero, the person is likely to be a latent homosexual. In latent homosexuality, a Freudian term, the individual is drawn to people of the same sex but is not conscious of his inclination.

Although the etiology of homosexuality is uncertain, it is probable that multiple agents cause this sexual preference. The primary etiologic agents presented in scientific literature include biological, parental, genetic and cultural influences.

A growing body of research investigates the relationship of biological determinants to homosexuality. It is possible to reverse the sexuality and sexual behavior of the Rhesus monkey by injecting male hormones into a growing female fetus or by injecting the female baby monkey soon after birth. Apparently, the prenatal hormone affects the brain or the endocrine system, which later alters the sexual development of the laboratory animal. Studies made by

Kolodny (1971) and others verify the effect on the endocrine system. Comparing homosexual and heterosexual urine and blood testosterone levels, they found that the testosterone levels of the homosexuals were lower than those of the heterosexuals.

The impact of the parents' role in the development of homosexuality has been widely discussed. Some researchers theorize that an intimate relationship with an overprotective and seductive mother combined with a negative relationship with a rejecting, weak, detached or absent father, causes the male child to identify with the mother.

Other theories of etiology are based on genetic factors. One study by Kallman (1952), comparing identical and fraternal twins, indicates that among identical twins there is a higher incidence of both twins being homosexual. Since environment is likely to be a constant whether twins are identical or fraternal, genetic influences appear to be the variable.

Cultural studies indicate that homosexuality has occurred throughout history in almost all cultures. According to Opler (1967), the cultures and subcultures that have sanctioned homosexuality include ancient Greece, pre-Meigi Japan, and top echelons in Nazi Germany. Homosexuality is nonexistent in such cultures as the Comanche, Mescaleo and Chiricahua Apache tribes, which are basically hunting and gathering societies that turn male children over to the men after two years of living closely with the mothers. These studies substantiate the relationship between cultural influence and homosexual development.

Dr. Evelyn Hooker's (1956) study, which compares a group of homosexual and a group of heterosexual males, tests the theory that homosexuality is a psychiatric illness. Both groups were given a battery of psychological tests. A panel of experts, who did not know which men were homosexual or which were heterosexual, assessed the psychological adjustment of all the subjects. The results of the study indicated that there were no differences between the psychological tests of the groups; furthermore, the experts were not able to distinguish the homosexual from the heterosexual on the basis of the psychological tests.

To explore some of the myths, problems and dynamics of homosexuality, this writer interviewed a minister from a church whose membership is largely homosexual. The following are a few of the major topics that were discussed, as well as excerpts from the interview.

One of the more prevalent myths regarding homosexuality is that homosexuals actively recruit heterosexuals.

Kirkham: Some books say there isn't solicitation among homosexuals and yet, frequently, people tell me they have been solicited.

Minister: There is solicitation, just as there is with heterosexuals. The idea that we are trying to get across now is that homosexuals do not recruit.

Kirkham: Have you ever heard of a situation in which a homosexual recruited a youngster?

Minister: No, not really. If a person is not inclined to do something, they're not going to do it. I don't think anybody is going to recruit anybody into being a homosexual any more than you recruit someone to be a heterosexual.

Kirkham: You've probably dealt with how many homosexuals?

Minister: Thousands of homosexuals.

Kirkham: With all these people, you've never heard of anyone saying that recruiting from a homosexual was the turning point?

Minister: No, I can't envision anybody changing anybody's sexual orientation. I had a friend, another minister, who had over 100 shock treatments [aversive therapy] trying to change his sex orientation. It did not work.

A common stereotype of the homosexual is that males are effeminate and females are "butchy" or male-like.

Minister: Years and years ago, it was thought that if you were a homosexual, you were effeminate. You were a he-she. Homosexuals acted out that stereotype. In the last fifteen years, the males, especially, say "I don't think I'm a woman. I don't want to be a woman; I'm a man." Now our pendulum has swung the other way, and the image now among gays is super-macho.

Homosexually oriented people seek psychiatric assistance for the same variety of reasons heterosexual people seek help. The presenting problem might be depression, increased anxiety or situational stresses, such as sudden moves away from support systems, grave financial loss or the death of a loved one.

Kirkham: Do you think that homosexuals in our culture tend to be high risks for suicide?

Minister: Probably we are a little higher, especially among teenagers. Teenage homosexuals can't face their parents along with all the other problems they have. ... I don't worry about the suicide rate as much as I worry about the homicide rate. In my experience, I've known of more gay people being murdered by homophobics than of committing suicide. Personally, I've known of a dozen.

Kirkham: What is a homophobic?

Minister: A person who is afraid of homosexuals.

Kirkham: Is the murder in retaliation for, or in conjunction with, some other fact?

Minister: No. For example, in Phoenix last year a young man was in a gay bar. A bunch of young 16- to 17-year-olds were out to get a queer. They spotted him coming out of this bar, jumped out of their car and literally stomped him to death.

Some individuals who seek help have fought homosexual tendencies for years and have finally become so drawn to a person of the same sex that the defense mechanism of denial finally fails. If this person is married, homosexuality creates a triangle that is sometimes difficult for the spouse to accept or understand. The spouse often feels bewildered, angry, rejected and confused. Frequently, the spouse has great difficulty understanding how to compete with a person of the same sex. The nurse needs to assess the total picture and try to discover ways of facilitating problem-solving so as to support each member of the family.

Minister: I've had two calls just this week from men. One 32-year-old man had been married for fifteen years and had begun having an affair with another man. He hadn't told his wife or children yet but was becoming so uncomfortable about the situation that he wanted me to help. I let him talk it out and explore different alternatives. The other man handled it much differently. He sat the whole family down and told them all at once. He said his mother handled it fine, and told him that she had a feeling that he was gay (they [mothers] usually know, I've always said). His kids handled it better than he thought they would. He didn't say how his wife reacted. . . . About 20 percent of our congregation are straight but married to one of our members.

The homosexual, when first consciously aware of the sex preference, frequently displays anger, guilt, fear and shame. Young persons first reckoning with their homosexuality may feel isolated and helpless.

Minister: One night very late I received a call from a 14-year-old boy. He had heard about our church on a late night radio talk-show. He lived in a little town, attended a very strict church where homosexuality was considered a sin, and he didn't feel that he had anyone he could trust to talk to about what he was feeling.

Some of the situations and pressures that are unique to the homosexual are related primarily to the culture's prevailing attitude toward homosexuality.

Kirkham: What do you see as the biggest problem of the homosexual?

Minister: I think the biggest problem that homosexuals face is acceptance. Just general acceptance. This is a hard thing to deal with. We live in a world that is constantly telling us that we are sick—perverts, you know, garbage. That includes acceptance by your parents. While you may be content with yourself—who you are and what you are—your parents or your brothers and sisters may have trouble dealing with it and may have nothing to do with you. Acceptance problems start with the family and go on out into other parts of the world—your job, your church, wherever you happen to be.

Because they doubt that heterosexuals can understand their problems, homosexuals may avoid therapy even when they need it the most.

Kirkham: If you had gone to a therapist when you were dealing with your own homosexuality, what kind of therapist would you have chosen?

Minister: Today, I would say I would choose a homosexual counselor, probably because I have very little trust in heterosexual counselors. I don't feel that they can be sympathetic toward how I feel. I'm beginning to outgrow that, because people are trying to deal with us.

Kirkham: So openness helps? If nurses are open about where they're coming from, it would help?

Minister: The problem with older gays is that you've been battered and beaten so often that when someone says, "I accept you as you are," you have trouble believing them. You have to remind yourself that this person is reaching out to you and is genuinely interested in understanding you. (Metropolitan Community Church, 1977.)

If the nurse feels uncomfortable with homosexuality and is not able to work through the feelings, it is only fair to the individual seeking help that the nurse refer the individual to another therapist. Perhaps in a group therapy setting, the nurse can get to know what the homosexual in this culture endures and can begin to feel comfortable with the topic. Talking out myths and stereotypes associated with homosexuality frequently assists the nurse in dispelling erroneous beliefs. Consulting with another member of the health care team is often helpful in working out the negative feelings and learning new ways of thinking. With the cultural taboo in mind, the nurse must first of all be honest about personal feelings elicited by a homosexual. It is imperative to the success of the therapy that the nurse feel confident about her ability to react therapeutically (Braverman, 1973).

Transsexuality

Transsexuality is frequently confused with transvestism, although the two phenomena are quite different. Transsexuals persistently perceive themselves as actually being the opposite sex; transvestites persistently desire to dress in clothes of the opposite sex. While the transvestite feels sexually aroused by cross-dressing, the transsexual feels relaxed and right in the opposite sexual role.

Transsexuals suffer from a disorder in gender identity. Although the male transsexual is anatomically male, he perceives himself as female; the female transsexual is anatomically female but perceives herself as male. The pain and frustration that transsexuals tolerate and the enduring patience that they demonstrate while undergoing sex-reassignment therapy indicate the finality of their identification with the opposite sex. Errors in gender identity are, at best, difficult to change; in most instances, change is impossible. Because gender identity is firmly established by age 14, conventional psychotherapy has repeatedly failed to correct identity errors. Therefore, transsexuals can only resolve their dilemma by changing the body to conform to the mind's perception.

The etiology of gender-identity disorders is, at this point, theoretical (Benjamin, 1973). The theory of neuroendocrine etiology implies definite psychological differences between males and females, supposedly due to the production of fetal androgen and its masculinizing effect on the genetic male hypothalamus. Masculinization will not occur without androgen. Thus, theoretically, the normal environment in utero is critical to gender identity. The genetic female with her XX chromosome make-up lacks fetal androgen and therefore develops typical female gender identity. Should the genetic female experience androgen influence upon the hypothalamus at a critical prenatal time, the result would be an anatomically female transsexual.

Other theorists believe that behavior patterned at crucial times in the early years of development, as well as significant social interaction, has an indelible effect on the child's gender identity. Histories of female and male transsexuals indicate a common childhood experience of feeling different from children with the same anatomy as their own. As these persons entered puberty, they became upset with the onset of secondary sex characteristics; some were attracted to adolescents of their same anatomical sex. With some patients, cross-gender behavior was reinforced by significant others in the environment. For example, the female transsexual might have been encouraged to continue being the "tomboy" by a grandfather who wanted a grandson.

When a determination has been made that the patient is a suitable candidate for sexual reassignment, the patient is first feminized or masculinized by the use of hormones. During this one- to two-year preoperative period, the patient begins or continues to live and work in the new sex role. While the desired secondary sexual characteristics start to develop and the undesired characteristics to disappear, this hormonal therapy period gives the patient a chance to experience the social, economic and familial consequences of sex reassignment. Since it is during this period that the patient usually meets the indignation and anger of the family, any conflict must be as completely and successfully resolved as possible, in order for the patient to make a satisfactory postoperative adjustment.

The hormonal therapy period also allows the patient time to adjust to new physical characteristics. For the anatomic male, this means experiencing breast development, reduced body hair, softened skin and diminished erections. At this point in the therapy, the changes are still reversible. By simply stopping the hormone treatments, the feminization or the masculinization process ceases, and the male or female hormones take charge once again. If the patient continues to believe that surgery is necessary, the anatomic male patient may remove his beard by electrolysis and take lessons to feminize his voice before major surgery is performed.

The surgical procedure is the final step in sex reassignment. In anatomical males, surgery includes orchidectomy and vaginoplasty; in anatomical females surgery consists of hysterectomy and closure of the vagina. Although the artificial vagina has proved to be very functional, the results of the artificial penis have been disappointing.

Postoperatively, each patient needs to resolve feelings of doubt and to work toward acceptance of a new body. To facilitate this objective, the primary nursing intervention is to listen non-judgmentally to the patient's fears and needs. By offering sincere answers to questions, the nurse indicates concern for the patient. For example, if a newly feminized patient worries that her voice remains too low, the nurse may explain that voice change takes time and sometimes doesn't change as much as desired. Moreover, the nurse may accentuate the patient's more feminine traits, thus providing support and positive reinforcement. Nurse Joyce Strait (1973) applied this technique while providing nursing care for four transsexual surgery patients. Noting that heavy makeup, low-cut tops and sheer nightgowns were initial attempts at femininity, Nurse Straight found that offering herself as a role model enabled the patients to ask some very basic questions. Usually, if patients are afforded the opportunity to express themselves in the desired sex, they can resolve most of the other problems themselves.

Canary Conn (1974), a vocal transsexual who underwent a sex change operation, described to television audiences the discrimination she suffered because of the condemning attitude of the nursing staff. Unable to have surgery in the United States, she was hospitalized in Tijuana, Mexico, where neglect led her close to death. The night following her surgery, she was ignored by the nurses, and only an unexpected visit by the physician prevented her from massive hemorrhaging. When infection resulted, Canary Conn came closer to committing suicide than at any time during her long struggle to resolve her gender-identity crisis. Prejudice or immaturity can cause the nurse to jeopardize therapy and endanger the patient. Only if the nurse's own gender is secure is it possible to accept the transsexual patient and to provide the support necessary to the patient's successful assumption of a new sexual role.

Rape

Rape is legally defined as natural or unnatural sexual intercourse forced upon an unwilling person by threat of bodily injury or loss of life. Usually, the rapist is a male whose victim is a child, female or another male; however, some cases of female rapists have been reported. Although rape is not listed by the American Psychiatric Association as a sexual deviation, research indicates that this form of intercourse would unequivocally be classified as deviant sexual behavior. The long-held belief that rape is motivated by a need for sexual gratification has been disproved. It is now clear that rape is performed to satisfy pathological nonsexual needs.

Since nurses may have contact with both rapists and victims, the etiology and dynamics of each rape pattern and the therapeutic management of the rape victim are discussed here.

Focusing on the rapist, Burgess and Lazare describe four patterns of rape in *Community Mental Health Practice: Target Populations* (1976). In the first pattern, the rapist uses sex as a means of expressing his anger and rage toward women. Aggression is an integral motivation of this pattern of rape. In some cases, the rapist brutally beats, kicks and chokes the victim far beyond the amount of force needed for sexual entry. In fact, often the rapist exhibits no sexual excitation during the beating of the victim and requires masturbation to obtain an erection. Displacing his hatred for significant women in his past, the rapist sees the victim as a symbol of the females who rejected, humiliated or somehow wronged him during his life. He usually chooses as his victim a stranger who is older than himself. Often, the attack is later described as the result of an "uncontrollable impulse," precipitated by an unresolved conflict with a significant woman in his life.

In the second pattern of rape, the rapist uses sexual assault as a means of proving his manhood, potency, competency and strength. His insecurity about his masculinity is frequently accompanied by a terror of homosexuality, with the rapist reporting a history of female domination by a mother, sister or wife. By forcing a female into submission, the rapist assumes power and control, and he attempts to deny his homosexual anxieties. Rape to prove masculinity is not generally accompanied by violence; on the contrary, the rapist hopes that the woman will enjoy the attack, thereby reinforcing his image as a virile, sexually skillful male. This type of rapist tends to fail in his rape attempt, and he is frequently convicted of "assault with intent to rape." His failure and humiliation only drive him toward repeated attempts.

The third pattern of rape is the most dangerous, for the rapist is a sadist who needs to inflict pain on his victim in order to achieve sexual satisfaction. For this type of rapist, the victim's struggle, terror and protests are erotic stimuli. Through the use of projection, the offender perceives the victim's actions not as a refusal but as an expression of her excitement and pleasure. A vicious circle results, which can provoke the sadistic rapist into committing "lust murder."

The fourth pattern of rape is impulsive and opportunistic, and it is sometimes carried out in conjunction with another antisocial act, such as burglary. The rapist has an antisocial personality disorder and "takes what he wants when he wants it"; thus, rape is another form of stealing.

These four patterns of rape can be interwoven in a single assault. However, one pattern is usually predominant. For example, the rapist may become sexually aroused by the victim's struggle, feel powerful and manly, yet have the predominant drive of the antisocial personality to take whatever he wants.

The primary objective of nursing intervention is to help the rapist develop a more acceptable and effective method of coping with the demands of living. Rape is a symptom of abnormal psychological development, particularly regarding impulse management, identity and interpersonal relationships. Therefore, each patient requires a comprehensive program (including physical, educational, psycho-social, spiritual and vocational aspects) uniquely geared to his individual pathology. Individual therapy and group therapy enable the patient to recognize forces operating within him, to discover the origin of his problem, to reexpose himself to experiences and to develop mature ways of coping with stress. Little information is available regarding the effectiveness of therapy, since rapists are usually processed through the criminal justice system and sentenced to penitentiaries.

Victims of rape experience trauma that upsets their lives and causes long-range effects. Based on a two-year study of more than 300 sexual assault cases, Holmstrom and Burgess (1975) describe the rape trauma syndrome as consisting of an acute phase of disorganization that lasts up to three weeks and a long-term reorganization process. The following were the most common problems reported to the researchers by victims during the acute phase:

1. overwhelming fear of physical violence and death (the predominant emotion of the acute phase)
2. phobias of the indoors, outdoors, solitude
3. strong motivation to change life style by moving, getting an unlisted phone number, seeking out family members for support
4. gastrointestinal upsets, anorexia, nausea, stomach pain
5. sleep disturbances, nightmares
6. tension headaches, jumpiness, increased startle reaction
7. genitourinary disturbances.

Emotions during the acute phase ranged from fear, humiliation and embarrassment to self-blame and the desire for revenge. The means of expressing these emotions ranged from sobbing, tenseness and restlessness to the display of a calm, subdued and flat affect.

The primary objective of nursing intervention throughout the rape syndrome is a return of the patient to her previous level of functioning as quickly as possible. Especially important to the attainment of this objective is the attitude of the staff who care for the rape victim in the first few hours, usually in the emergency room. Terri Clark, in her article, "Counseling Victims of Rape" (1976), describes the resistance she and her volunteer nurse-counselors met at the Yale-New Haven Hospital, where the staff held the false notion that women provoke their assault. Clark believes that the persistence of this myth is due to a fear of admitting that rape can happen to anyone. In other words, if the rape victim didn't do anything to provoke the attack, then a wife, daughter, even oneself is vulnerable. Burgess and Lazare (1976) explain that the persistence and pervasiveness of the myth is related to the misconception that rape is primarily motivated by sexual gratification.

Upon the rape victim's admission to the emergency room, the first nursing intervention is to assure the patient that the nurse will remain with her. The nurse answers any questions the patient may ask about the physical examination, venereal disease and pregnancy, and she assists the patient in working out a way to tell family and friends about the rape. The nurse continues to provide support throughout the police interrogation and the physical exam.

The therapeutic approach during the acute phase is based on crisis intervention. According to crisis intervention theory, the nurse should assume that the patient functioned within normal limits before the rape and should actively deal with immediate problems identified by the patient. For psychiatric problems that predate the rape, the patient is referred to a psychotherapist. Crisis intervention is not psychotherapy but is preventive in nature. Patients who react to rape with depression, suicidal behavior, alcoholism and other compounded responses are referred to a therapist, with the nurse-counselor continuing her supportive role.

During the reorganization phase of the rape syndrome, the rape victim begins to realize that the sexual assault was just the beginning of her ordeal. The nursing interventions during this phase vary according to the individual needs of the patient. Whether the patient needs to find a new home or job or talk out her fears and anger, the nurse in all cases would:

1. provide a community resource list, including names and phone numbers for medical and legal assistance
2. provide her own home phone number, so the patient knows where to reach someone in case of panic

3. provide written information regarding test results and medications received in the emergency room (the patient usually is in shock and is unable to remember what occurred at the hospital)
4. document what the patient says and what the nurse observes (for use in court, if necessary)
5. continue checking on the patient by phone or visit, until both patient and nurse agree that the patient has recovered or needs a referral to a mental health agency.

Due to an increased awareness of and sensitivity to the ordeal of the rape victim, many emergency rooms are now establishing a management plan to provide follow-up care in the weeks after the rape.

SUMMARY

This chapter deals with personality disorders and sexual deviations. In the first part of the chapter, personality disorders are identified as pervasive maladaptive behavior disorders, usually apparent by adolescence and persistent throughout life. Ten personality disorders are defined and discussed in terms of etiology, characteristic behavior patterns and specific nursing interventions. Initial focus is placed on the antisocial personality disorder, emphasizing the variety of theoretical causes and the nurse's role in treatment. Examples of acting out and manipulative behavior are provided to illustrate proposed interventions. Also, a description of dyssocial behavior is included to clarify its distinction from antisocial personality disorders.

In the latter part of the chapter, five sexual deviations are defined and discussed. Pedophilia, voyeurism, exhibitionism, fetishism and sadomasochism are considered in regard to characteristic behavior and etiology. Because of the similarity of treatment modalities and nursing care for these deviations, therapeutic interventions are discussed at the conclusion of the sadomasochism section. Due to the increased frequency of nursing care provided for homosexuals, transsexuals and rape victims, these topics are also discussed. It is noted that recent research regarding the rape syndrome and the need for crisis intervention has increased the nurse's ability to prevent psychopathology of the rape victim.

Finally, the case study of an antisocial personality disorder portrays the assessment, planning of care, therapeutic interventions and evaluation of the nursing action. Both the problem-oriented method of charting and the standards of nursing practice are illustrated as the nursing process is applied to this particular case.

CASE STUDY

Jean, a 17-year-old female, was admitted to a locked adolescent unit. On admission, she was agitated and combative, verbalizing anger and resentment toward her mother for "putting her away." During her first two weeks on the unit, Jean was accused of taking a nurse's cigarette lighter, disrupting the ward by verbally antagonizing other patients and consistently violating rules. Once Jean became oriented to the unit, her combative behavior subsided.

Jean's mother was in her third month of pregnancy when the marriage took place. Neither parent desired children. The week following Jean's birth, her father refused to visit the hospital or to name the child. For the first year of life, Jean's paternal grandparents were essentially her parents. Jean's mother continued to express her dislike for children, and she openly told the patient that she did not want her, that she did not like being "tied down."

Although Jean walked at nine months and talked at a year and a half, her social development was slow. Since she lived in a rural area, she spent her early years without playmates. Throughout her childhood and adolescence, she had difficulty making and keeping friends, usually forming only one close friendship at a time. With this one friend, Jean was excessively possessive.

During her grade school years, Jean's father frequently demanded that she play outside or "get lost," so he could entertain his friends; he consistently ignored or rejected her attempts to get attention. The mother felt sorry for Jean and gave in to many of the child's demands. During the admitting interview, the mother stated repeatedly that she continues to give Jean "anything she wants." Because of the parents' disagreement about Jean, they fought frequently.

By the time Jean was 11, her father was not in the home on a regular basis. He abused alcohol and drugs and lived a free-wheeling life style. About the same time, Jean also lost the paternal grandparents who had been like parents to her during her infancy. When her grandfather died, her grandmother began to date and go to social events, thus totally ignoring Jean.

Jean's parents divorced when she was 15 years old, and her mother soon remarried. The new family further frustrated and angered Jean. She resented this marriage and talked about how nice it would be "if Mom and I lived by ourselves." Unable to accept her stepfather, Jean told her mother that he made sexual advances toward her during her mother's absence. Although the mother believed this story at first, she now "sees things differently" and holds Jean responsible for her recent separation from Jean's stepfather. Jean and her mother have fought frequently and angrily about Jean's attempt to break up the marriage, and the mother is considering reconciliation with her second husband.

Recently, Jean refused to go to school and began dating a 30-year-old man. About two months ago, Jean told her mother that she might be pregnant; however, the physician who examined Jean told the mother there was no evidence of sexual relations. This situation, coupled with truancy, frequent trouble-making and angry attacks on members of the family, motivated Jean's mother to seek psychiatric help for her daughter.

I. OBJECTIVE DATA
    A. General Appearance, Attitude and Activity
        1. Appearance: no makeup, long stringy hair, skin-tight blue jeans, and a T-shirt that states, "Sure I raise hell—so what?"
        2. Attitude: answers nurse's questions briefly and abruptly. Swears frequently, smiles infrequently
        3. Activity: smokes almost constantly, does not maintain eye contact while conversing with others
    B. Communication Patterns
        1. Content of communication is centered around her hospitalization: that she does not want to be or need to be here. Angry statements are levelled at mother and hospital authority figures, especially nurses and her psychiatrist
        2. Communication is usually clear and understand-

able; when challenged, however, she accelerates her speech and changes the subject

C. Contact with Environment
1. Oriented to time, place and person
2. Easily distracted by people in the environment. While being interviewed, frequently made faces at or made remarks to other patients and personnel

D. Sensorium and Intelligence
1. Memory of remote and recent events is accurate, as far as can be determined
2. Frequently inattentive
3. Refers to current events she has read about in *Time* and newspapers, uses good grammar and is able to transfer an idea from one situation to another except when it involves punishment
4. Patient is able to think abstractly and concretely

E. Thought Processes
1. Tends to change the subject frequently when trying to strike up a conversation with a stranger, or when her statements are challenged
2. Thinks in logical sequence
3. Answers questions spontaneously

F. Thought Content
1. Almost continually dwells on anger toward mother or boyfriend
2. No delusions evident or hallucinations reported

G. Social Assessment
1. Education, socioeconomic status, religion: high school dropout. Lower middle class. No religious affiliation
2. Family: mother and stepfather separated, three stepchildren and patient live with mother. Biological father divorced mother when patient was 15. Paternal grandmother lives in distant city
3. Family's understanding of illness: mother states that she is relieved the patient is out of the home for a while, and that she can't understand why "Jean has always been such a trouble-maker"

4. Habits: chain smokes, drinks beer and hard liquor "on weekends" and tries "lots of different kinds of street drugs"
5. Visitors: patient's mother came once but hurriedly left when she and the patient began to fight. No other visitors noted in first two weeks of hospitalization

H. Medical Assessment
1. Complains of severe headaches (frontal and temporal, no time pattern). Patient states, "It will take a strong pill to relieve it"
2. Appetite is fair. Patient skips breakfast, so she can "sleep in." No recent weight loss
3. Insomnia; patient frequently requests sleeping pills
4. Physical examination by Dr. Mox two months ago

II. SUBJECTIVE DATA

A. Present Illness
1. Patient was involuntarily committed for 90 days by mother. Mother states the patient verbally attacks the family and sometimes throws chairs and heavy pots and pans
2. Precipitating event: Jean states that her stepsister, mother and she had such a bad fight about her mother's reconciliation with her stepfather that "somebody called the cops"
3. No previous treatment for emotional illness. Patient states she has a police record for shoplifting and driving while intoxicated
4. Jean states, "I haven't done much right in my whole life"

III. STATEMENT OF THE PSYCHIATRIC PROBLEM

A. Antisocial personality

B. Problem list
1. Disrupted interpersonal relationships
2. Frequent verbal attacks on others
3. Nonsupportive relationship with mother
4. Interrupted education

5. Headaches
6. Insomnia
7. Violation of rules and laws
8. Decreased self-esteem

IV. PLANNING PHASE

A nurse who had established a relationship with the patient held a conference with the patient to begin planning the nursing actions and overall treatment. When the patient did not acknowledge "disrupted interpersonal relationships," "frequent angry verbal attacks on others" and "violation of rules and laws" as problems, the nurse listened to the patient's rationale. Then the nurse explained that limits on behavior were set and that breaking rules or verbally assaulting others were not within these limits. Following a lengthy discussion, the patient and nurse mutually decided that "disrupted interpersonal relationships" already included the problem of dealing with angry verbal attacks on others. Thus, the nurse and patient revised the problem list in the following order of priority:

A. Violation of rules and laws

B. Nonsupportive relationship with mother

C. Disrupted interpersonal relationships

D. Decreased self-esteem

E. Headaches

F. Insomnia

G. Interrupted education

The nurse then presented the patient's problem list at a team conference. The team prepared the following overall plan. The psychiatrist would initiate one-hour therapy sessions, three times per week, with a long-term goal of moving the patient to a group. Because of the history of drug abuse, no medication orders would be included. Behavioral limits would be carefully defined and consistently upheld. The problems and plan were charted on the patient's chart.

A. Violation of rules and laws

1. *Plan:* The nurse will give a printed copy of the hospital rules to the patient and will clearly explain the consequences of breaking these rules. Then the nurse will request the patient to reflect (repeat back what she hears), so that the nurse can clarify any misconceptions. After explaining that choosing to violate a rule also entails accepting the consequences for the violation, the nurse will assure the patient that limits will be enforced consistently, and that destructive behavior will not be allowed. The nurse will then give the patient an opportunity to verbalize how she would like to violate the rule, thus granting in fantasy what cannot be done in reality.
2. *Expected outcome:* The patient will know and understand the rules of the hospital. She will equate the breaking of a rule with the consequences. Verbalizing what she would like to do will become a substitute for the behavior itself. The patient will display self-control and will find satisfaction in avoiding the consequences of breaking rules.

B. Nonsupportive relationship with mother
   1. *Plan:* The primary nurse assigned to the patient on each shift will provide a non-judgmental atmosphere, in which the patient can ventilate and explore her feelings and ideas about her mother. The primary nurses and the psychiatrist will then work with the patient to arrange family therapy sessions with the mother.
   2. *Expected outcome:* By expressing the built-up resentment and anger regarding past "wrongs" she perceives her mother has committed against her, the patient will be more receptive to attempts to arrange a dialogue with her mother. Within a "safe" environment, the mother and daughter can explore new ways of disagreeing, can find points of agreement and can come to a more realistic perception of one another.

C. Disrupted interpersonal relationships

1. *Plan:* The staff will encourage the patient to interact with others through participation in games or group activities. Since group activities are less intense than one-to-one interactions, the patient will be assigned to a discussion group. There she will have an opportunity to share ideas and differences of opinion in an accepting atmosphere where feedback regarding interpersonal skills is offered therapeutically, honestly and openly. Closed-circuit TV tapes of these groups will enable the patient to gain insight into behavior that impedes the building of satisfying interpersonal relationships. If the patient directs angry verbal assaults on the staff or other patients, this behavior will be extinguished by substituting an activity such as hitting a pillow, punching a bag or participating in an active occupational therapy, such as pounding clay.
2. *Expected outcome:* The patient will recognize behavior that impedes interpersonal relationships. In the discussion group, she will find satisfaction in relating to others. Support and feedback provided by other group members will enable her to learn how to manipulate constructively. When the patient is tempted to attack another verbally, she will vent her anger in a socially acceptable manner.

D. Decreased self-esteem
   1. *Plan:* The nurse and patient will agree upon a list of the patient's assets, including such traits as a sense of humor, attractive facial features, pleasant singing voice and high energy level. The nurse will encourage the patient to develop these assets further by:
      (a) encouraging her to try different makeup ideas
      (b) complimenting her when she looks well-groomed
      (c) encouraging her to tape her singing, so she can hear the beauty in her voice
      (d) redirecting her energy from irritating or disruptive activity to authority-role activity, such as refereeing a volleyball game

(e) ignoring caustic humor, encouraging appropriate humor

To reinforce the patient's belief that she is a person of worth, the nurse will genuinely accept the patient as she is, will talk with and listen to her and will stay attuned to her nonverbal expressions of feelings.
2. *Expected outcome:* Although the patient will frequently test the nurse's sincerity in the early weeks of therapy, eventually she will perceive that the acceptance is genuine. Then the patient will begin to experience positive feedback for assets that are uniquely hers. She will also begin to repeat behavior that is supported and to cease behavior that is not supported. This continual reaffirmation of her worth will increase her self-esteem.

E. Headaches
1. *Plan:* The nurse will assess and chart the following in regard to the headache: preceding event, time of onset and patient's behavior and request for pain relievers. No pain relievers will be given; instead, the nurse on duty will encourage the patient to lie down in a dark, quiet room, to drink juice or to participate in a diversionary activity. After three weeks, any pattern will be assessed, the etiology will be discussed and the plan will be reevaluated.
2. *Expected outcome:* The patient will complain less frequently of headaches, once she realizes that no pain reliever is going to be given to her. She will learn that using headaches as a method for getting drugs will not be successful. If the patient's headaches are not a manipulative device, then the precipitating conditions and the appropriate therapeutic interventions will be defined.

F. Insomnia
1. *Plan:* Primary nurses on the 3:00 p.m. to 7:00 a.m. shifts will assess and chart the sleep status of the patient every two hours to establish a sleep pattern. No sleep-inducing medication will be given. Instead, warm fluids, soft music and back rubs will be offered.

2. *Expected outcome:* The assessment of sleep patterns will verify if insomnia exists or if sleeplessness is due to frequent napping. If insomnia does exist, the nursing interventions will decrease the requests for sleep-inducing medication.
G. Interrupted education
  1. *Plan:* The nurse will consult with a social worker and with the patient's school counselor to determine the academic requirements necessary for the patient to complete her high school education. Also, the nurse will assess the feasibility of the patient's being tutored in the hospital setting. Whether or not tutoring is feasible, the nurse will encourage the patient in her educational endeavor and will provide guidance and help when needed. Any of the patient's attempts to entice the staff into doing the lessons will be firmly stopped.
  2. *Expected outcome:* The patient will continue to progress toward high school graduation even though hospitalized. This will increase both her self-esteem and her chances at independence through increased job opportunities.

Evaluation, a frequently neglected phase of the nursing process, includes a mutual assessment of the problem, the plan and the therapeutic interventions. Although evaluation might be carried out weekly, it is essentially an on-going, continuous process, in which the patient and nurse decide what problems have been resolved and what new problems have been added. For any problems that remain unresolved, the nurse and patient assess the validity of the expected outcome and the feasibility of the plan. Any changes are then made in the appropriate area on the patient's record.

PRINCIPLES

1. Constructive manipulation is the application of one's own capabilities and strengths to promote successful personal relationships with others.

2. Destructive manipulation is the wielding of others for one's own purposes, thereby causing difficulties in interpersonal relationships and inhibiting individual growth.
3. A common manipulative device is to play on the sympathy or guilt of others, so that they feel compelled to cooperate.
4. The person who manipulates others has difficulty in forming relationships, because his selfish motivation precludes any genuine regard for other individuals.
5. One person's expectations can influence another person's behavior.
6. The purpose of limit-setting is not to control the patient. It is to provide the patient with consistent expectations and guidance toward self-control.
7. In setting limits, the nurse must know what she is limiting. Generally, she is limiting varied forms of excessive dependency and destructive forms of aggression.
8. Acceptance of the patient is communicated by relating to the patient in a non-judgmental and non-punitive manner, conveying direct and indirect interest, recognizing and reflecting the patient's feelings, talking and listening to the patient and permitting the patient to express strong emotions.
9. To accept a patient as a person, it is not necessary to sanction undesirable behavior.
10. Acceptance can be conveyed by the simple act of staying with the patient.
11. Identifying the patient's attitudes and feelings becomes difficult if emotions are confused with the intellectual content of the patient's conversation.
12. Vicarious and symbolic methods of releasing negative emotions should be provided until the patient is able to bring his anxiety or hatred out into the open.
13. The degree of consistency in feelings, thoughts and actions demonstrated by the nurse affects her therapeutic potential.
14. Tension that has mounted is sometimes discharged through indulgence in ritualistic behavior, though the relief gained is only transient.
15. Intervention that prevents the ritualistic act may result in the patient's terror.

BIBLIOGRAPHY

Anders, Robert L. "When a Patient Becomes Violent," *American Journal of Nursing*, Vol. 77, No. 7 (July, 1977), 1144-1148.

Benjamin, Harry, and Ihlemfeld, Charles L. "Transsexualism," *American Journal of Nursing*, Vol. 73, No. 3 (March, 1973), 457-461.

Braverman, Shirley J. "Homosexuality," *American Journal of Nursing*, Vol. 73, No. 4 (April, 1973), 652-655.

Burgess, Ann Wolbert, and Lazare, Aaron. *Psychiatric Nursing in the Hospital and the Community*. Englewood Cliffs, N.J.: Prentice-Hall, Inc., 1976.

――――. *Community Mental Health Practice: Target Populations*. Englewood Cliffs, N.J.: Prentice-Hall, Inc., 1976.

Clark, Terri Patrice. "Counseling Victims of Rape," *American Journal of Nursing*, Vol. 76, No. 12 (December, 1976), 1964-1965.

Committee on Nomenclature and Statistics of the American Psychiatric Association. *Diagnostic and Statistical Manual of Mental Disorders*. 2d ed. Washington, D.C.: American Psychiatric Association, 1968.

Conn, Canary. *Canary: The Story of a Transsexual*. Los Angeles: Nash Publishing Co., 1974.

Eaton, Merrill, Peterson, Margaret, and Davis, James. *Psychiatry*. 3d ed. Garden City, N.Y.: Medical Examination Publishing Co., Inc., 1976.

Ellis, Albert, and Abarbanel, Albert (eds). *Encyclopedia of Sexual Behavior*. New York: Hawthorn Books, Inc., 1961.

Glueck, Sheldon, and Glueck, Eleanor. *Unraveling Juvenile Delinquency*. Cambridge, Mass.: Harvard University Press, 1950.

Hariton, Barbara E. "The Sexual Fantasies of Women," *Psychology Today*, Vol. 16, No. 10 (March, 1973), 39-44.

Heaver, W.L. "A Study of Forty Male Psychopathic Personalities Before, During, and After Hospitalization," *American Journal of Psychiatry*, Vol. 100 (November, 1943), 342-346.

Holmstrom, Lynda Lytle, and Burgess, Ann Wolbert. "Assessing Trauma in the Rape Victim," *American Journal of Nursing*, Vol. 75, No. 8 (August, 1975), 1288-1291.

Hooker, Evelyn. "Preliminary Analysis of Group Behavior of Homosexuals," *Journal of Psychology*, Vol. 42 (October, 1956), 217-225.

Kallman, Franz. "Comparative Twin Studies on Genetic Aspects of Male Homosexuals," *Journal of Mental and Nervous Disorders*, Vol. 115 (April, 1952), 283-298.

Kinsey, Alfred, et al. *Sexual Behavior in the Human Male*. Philadelphia: W.B. Saunders, 1948, pp. 610-666.

Kolodny, Robert, et al. "Plasma Testosterone and Semen Analysis in Male Homosexuals," *New England Journal of Medicine*, Vol. 285, No. 2 (November, 1971), 1170-1174.

Metropolitan Community Church. Minister, March 10, 1977: Personal Communication.

Opler, Marvin K. (ed). *Culture and Social Psychiatry*. New York: Atherton Press, Inc., 1967.

Rachman, S. "Sexual Fetishism and Experimental Analog," *Psychological Record*, Vol. 13, No. 3 (1966), 293-296.

Resnik, H.L., and Wolfgang, M.E. *Sexual Behaviors: Social, Clinical and Legal Aspects*. Boston: Little, Brown & Co., 1972.

Stone, Alan, and Stone, Sue S. *The Abnormal Personality Through Literature*. Englewood Cliffs, N.J.: Prentice-Hall, Inc., 1966, pp. 228-229.

Stott, D.H., and Sykes, Emily. *Manual: Bristol Social Adjustment Guides*. San Diego, Cal.: Educational and Industrial Testing Service, 1969.

Strait, Joyce. "The Transsexual Patient After Surgery," *American Journal of Nursing*, Vol. 73, No. 3 (March, 1973), 462-463.

Sullivan, Harry Stack. *Clinical Studies in Psychiatry*. New York: W.W. Norton & Co., 1956.

Tripp, C.A. *The Homosexual Matrix*. New York: McGraw-Hill Book Co., 1975.

Wertham, F. *The Show of Violence*. New York: Doubleday & Co., Inc., 1949.

CHAPTER 11

Alcoholism and Drug Dependence

Anne Lind, R.N., M.S.

ALCOHOLISM

Alcoholism has been and is considered variously as a social problem, an illegal condition, a symptom and a disease. Controversy as to classification continues today. The World Health Organization defines alcoholism as "a chronic behavioral disorder manifested by the repeated drinking of alcoholic beverages in excess of the dietary and social uses of the community and to the extent that it interferes with the drinker's health or social or economic functions" (World Health Organization, 1964). Alcoholics Anonymous, the self-help organization of alcoholics, states that alcoholics are driven to self-destructive behavior and that they have a disease which can only be controlled, never cured (AA, 1955).

The use of alcohol to the extent described above was traditionally believed to be a condition acquired over a long time and affecting primarily adults. Studies being done internationally show that an adolescent population of alcoholics is now a reality. The adult alcoholic population continues to be present. Many alcoholics consume excessive amounts of alcoholic beverages secretly or at least within the limits of "normalcy." When behavior of the alcoholic causes him to run afoul of the law, his alcoholism becomes a matter of court record.

The legal test for inebriation or intoxication in some states is a blood alcohol level of 0.15 percent or above. A level of 0.2 percent is moderate to severe intoxication, while a blood alcohol level of 0.5 percent may be fatal (Burgess and Lazare, 1976).

Etiology

Many experts have attempted to determine why people become alcoholics and, to date, have been unsuccessful. Some theories are:
1. Nutritional: inability to synthesize food results in nutritional deficiencies
2. Endocrine: disorders or dysfunction of endocrine glands predispose people to alcoholism
3. Heredity: children of alcoholic parent(s) are more likely to become alcoholics
4. Others: allergic response to alcohol requires more alcohol; alcohol itself causes alcoholism when ingested; and metabolism in certain people increases susceptibility to alcohol (Burkhalter, 1975)

Alcohol is consumed by many people in an attempt to decrease tension and encourage social interaction. The amount of alcohol consumed and the effects obtained by the individual vary greatly. What, then, is the difference between the social drinker and the problem drinker? Why is one person able to have an occasional cocktail or beer, while another has a compulsion to drink often and regularly?

The personality of the alcoholic has undergone extensive study. There is no exact pattern, but common characteristics do exist. These include anxiety, social or sexual inadequacy, depression, desire to lower inhibitions, social pressures and a tendency to self-destruction. Many alcoholics have been deprived of affection in childhood and subsequently experience usually heavy stress. The excessive drinking expresses their physical and psychological isolation (Hoff, 1975).

Difficulty with dependency has been studied as a factor in the personality of alcoholics. Some alcoholics are openly dependent upon others for their existence, presenting a passive, childlike reliance upon others. Other alcoholics avoid any type of dependent behavior, striving to exhibit typical masculine characteristics. This latter group, termed counterdependent, has intense dependency needs met by hidden dependency upon alcohol (Blane, 1968).

High tolerance to alcohol intake early in life may set a pattern of drinking which continues over a period of years. In later life, the tolerance lessens and problem drinking, with accompanying social and emotional complications, begins. Studies have shown some characteristics of typical older problem drinkers. These alcoholics fall in the over 55 age group, have high school education, a history of marital problems and are unemployed.

Studies regarding the cause of alcoholism have been done over a long period of time. Much useful data have been collected, but, at this time, it is impossible to specify a definite etiological factor for alcoholism.

Clinical Course

Ethyl alcohol comprises about 50 percent of most alcoholic beverages. Alcohol is absorbed from the stomach, enters the bloodstream and then goes to the brain. The rate of absorption varies, depending upon the contents of the stomach, the type of beverage consumed, the emotional state and the general physical condition of the consumer. The alcohol is partially oxidized, with the remainder eliminated from the body by the kidneys and lungs.

Alcohol acts in the body as a central nervous system depressant. Manifestations may be expressed as stumbling, lack of coordination or slurred speech. These result from depression of various parts of the brain. As inhibitions disappear with intake of alcohol, the person feels clever, stimulated and excited. In contrast to his own impressions, to others he seems awkward and slowed down. As the effects increase with more alcohol intake, motor impairment becomes more severe, loss of consciousness ensues and perceptions become dull. Further drinking may result in coma and death.

As alcoholism becomes a way of life, some predictable phases and systems ensue. These are described by Kogan (1970).

The first phase begins with an initial blank period. The person begins to sneak drinks, is preoccupied with drinking and gulps drinks to hide the amount consumed. This is followed by a second period of amnesia.

The second or crucial phase follows with loss of control of drinking. The person becomes aggressive and extravagant. He makes elaborate alibis for his drinking and has periods of remorse followed by intervals of abstinence from alcohol. Loss of friends, job and outside interests increase his self-pity and preoccupation with alcohol.

Loss of sexual desire and feelings of jealousy and resentment are common. Malnutrition may result from limited or no food intake. The alcoholic may be hospitalized at this stage. Inability to face another day without an alcoholic drink becomes a reality.

The final or chronic stage is characterized by prolonged intoxication. The alcoholic now loses social and ethical values and drinks anything, anywhere, anytime and with anyone. Drinking becomes an obsession and any alcohol is acceptable, whether it is found in the wine bottle, aftershave lotion or a bottle of food flavoring. Tolerance for alcohol decreases during this time. The person is fearful, has tremors and needs alcohol in order to perform any task. The alcoholic at this time is a defeated, self-admitted failure (Kogan, 1970).

Another approach to classification of alcoholism in phases is the categorization of alcoholic persons. Two broad categories described by John Ewing (1967) are reactive and addictive persons. Reactive alcoholic persons are those who turn to alcohol for relief from some stress. They generally have good life adjustment, with alcohol used as a crutch to blur perceptions or break down psychological barriers. The individual is able to terminate the alcoholic period with much effort of control. The addictive alcoholic person demonstrates gross disturbances in adjustment and interpersonal relationships. Job and marital instability are common. A self-destructive personality component is evidenced by repeated bouts of drinking, which continue until he is physically unable to keep going (Chafetz 1967).

Whatever the description of phases or classification of alcoholism or alcoholics, the physical deterioration that accompanies alcoholic intake is well-known. Nutritional disorders range from gastritis to malnutrition and esophageal varices. The liver is affected by the nutritional problems and the direct effect of the alcohol. Cirrhosis is the classic example of liver damage due to prolonged alcoholism. The nervous system is often involved, the most severe effect being Korsakoff's syndrome, with its memory and thought disorders. Painful peripheral neuritis causes difficulty in walking.

When the level of alcohol in the blood drops on withdrawal from alcohol, delirium tremens occur. The tremors, hallucinations and convulsions may stimulate a return to drinking to reduce the frightening symptoms (Hoff, 1975).

If the alcoholic progresses to the advanced state of physical and psychological deterioration, friends and relatives are affected, as well as the alcoholic himself. The alcoholic is often admitted to a general hospital, because of physical illness or a psychiatric hospital, because of hallucinations or delirium tremens. The economic burden of caring for the alcoholic in a medical facility and providing financial aid to his family leads to a broad-spectrum effect upon society in general.

Treatment

The patient who is in an acute state of intoxication requires a period of sobering or "drying out" in an inpatient setting before beginning long-range treatment. As the alcoholic undergoes withdrawal or detoxification, he progresses through stages or phases. The mild first stage is marked by psychomotor hyperactivity with tremors, elevated blood pressure, nausea, loss of appetite, nervousness and agitation. This stage lasts about 36 hours and is followed by auditory and/or visual hallucinations, which mark the second stage. Delirium tremens begin 24 to 72 hours after withdrawal occurs. Tachycardia, tachypnea, disorientation and seizures characterize this third phase. Often, serious complications such as aspiration pneumonia, myocardial infarction or traumatic injuries cause further damage (Burkhalter, 1975).

Drug therapy attempts to reverse the depressant effect of alcohol on the central nervous system or control symptoms. Medications which are prescribed are chlordiazepoxide (Librium), chlorpromazine (Thorazine), chloral hydrate, paraldehyde and diphenylhydantoin (Dilantin).

Fluid and electrolyte imbalances, if present, are corrected by intravenous fluids. Multivitamins, especially vitamin B complex, are administered. Maintenance of adequate diet—liquid progressing to regular as tolerated—alleviates some of the nutritional deficiency symptoms. Laboratory tests include blood work, kidney and liver function and isolation of agents of infection.

The detoxification process may last two to three weeks. As the acute symptoms subside and the immediate distress is eliminated, the client may be treated as an outpatient.

Physiological treatment of alcoholism includes aversion therapy and disulfiram (Antabuse) therapy. In aversion therapy, the patient is given a drug such as emetine, followed by a drink of alcohol. The nausea and vomiting induced by the medication create an aversion for alcohol based on the reflex association between alcohol and vomiting. Antabuse alters the metabolism of alcohol, forming a toxin, acetaldehyde. Therefore, no alcohol may be taken during the treatment.

Psychological treatment includes all types of therapy. Psychotherapy deals with alcohol as a defense. Denial, hostility and depression must be dealt with by the therapist and client (Chafetz, 1967). Group therapy is often more effective than individual therapy. Milieu therapy and family therapy are often used.

The patient may be referred to Alcoholics Anonymous, a self-help group whose members are arrested alcoholics. This organization encourages growth and spiritual awareness on the part of the individual. Members are on call at all hours to provide personalized one-to-one support and encouragement for those who need help. Regular meetings are held during which the members tell of their personal struggles with alcoholism. The goal of each alcoholic is abstinence, which is accomplished in small steps, one day at a time. AA has been in existence since the 1930s and has an excellent record of helping alcoholics in the community. The organization provides similar groups, Al-Anon and Al-a-Teen, for members of the family of the alcoholic.

Whatever the method of treatment selected, the effective treatment results in both abstinence or reduction in alcohol consumption and changes in personality problems. These personality problems previously required the support of the continued use of alcohol and its effects.

Nursing Intervention

The attitude of society toward the alcoholic necessarily affects the attitudes of the nurse who cares for the alcoholic patient. These attitudes may be expressed in the nursing care she gives. It is important, even necessary, that the nurse recognize and examine her attitudes toward alcoholism and alcoholics, changing or correcting any negative attitudes. Once the nurse has dealt with her own feelings about alcoholism, she can begin the nursing process.

Assessment is the first part of the nursing process. Data obtained from the patient include the patient's interpretation of his drinking problem and his attitude toward control of his alcoholism.

While talking with the patient, the nurse notes clues indicating that the patient is oriented and alert.

The patient's general physical condition is assessed, especially regarding signs of withdrawal, hygiene and nutrition. The central nervous system is responsible for many symptoms presented by the alcoholic and is evaluated carefully.

The amount of alcohol usually consumed by the patient is determined. How much the amount has increased over time is questioned. The usual situations under which the person drinks is important information. The behavior the alcohol intake causes and the effect of this upon the family, friends and employment is discussed. Recall of this information may be painful for the patient, so the nurse is observant of any distress evoked by her questions. This assessment may span several conferences, as deemed necessary by the nurse. In all contacts with the patient, the nurse consistently maintains a non-judgmental attitude, as in all other nursing care situations. Alcoholics are accustomed to criticism from others and themselves, and any judgmental actions on the part of the nurse adversely affect a trust or therapeutic nurse-patient relationship.

The nurse continues to add to the data base by conferring with family and significant others. Information gathered from the patient and others, plus her own observations, form the basis for the list of problems. Priorities on the list of problems are established, dependent upon the needs of the patient. If he is in the stage of withdrawal, his needs differ widely from those in the stage of intoxication.

Once the problem list is begun and subjective and objective data collected, planning of nursing care can be completed. In cooperation with the patient, as well as other medical personnel, acceptable plans for patient care are established. Medical needs are met first, as well as correction of nutritional deficiencies. Tranquilizer therapy helps prepare the patient for further treatment.

Nursing interventions at this time include maintenance of adequate fluid intake, both intravenous and oral. Careful recording of intake and output is essential. Since the alcoholic patient is often in poor physical condition, thorough nursing care and observation of the skin and mouth are indicated. Symptoms of complications indicate cirrhosis, diabetes or pneumonia. Provision of tranquilizer therapy, including safety precautions, aids the tolerance of the patient for treatment during this phase. Supportive emotional care helps to restore self-worth. Acceptance by nursing personnel is ongoing.

When the alcoholic person's physical problems are under control, emotional treatment can begin. Various methods of therapy are used, but some type of psychotherapy or behavior therapy is usually prescribed. The nurse participates in one-to-one counseling or group therapy. The caring attitude of the nurse is demonstrated, regardless of the treatment method used.

As the patient improves, the nurse continually evaluates progress toward solution of the problem list. New problems are listed and those resolved are marked inactive. During the evaluation period, the nurse often makes referrals to agencies. The patient is usually being seen on an out-patient basis, and referral to agencies can aid him in his return to active participation in society. Maintaining contact with the nurse often facilitates the transition to a successful life in the community.

The alcoholic must be involved in the evaluation phase of care as much as he was in the planning phase. Both patient and nurse reexamine each plan and gauge progress toward the goal. The goal for the alcoholic is generally absence of dependence upon alcoholic intake in order to cope with life.

DRUG DEPENDENCE

Drug abuse is a problem that cuts across all cultures, educational levels, economic and age groups. The drug abuse problem attracted major concern during the 1960s, and it continues to be a major problem today. Part of the difficulty in discussing the problem is in the multitude of terms or definitions used in the literature. The World Health Organization has proposed the term *drug dependence* as a substitute for *drug addiction* and *drug habituation*. Drug abuse has been defined as the "non-medical use of chemical substances in the form of drugs . . . including the general misuse of drugs—alcohol, narcotics, amphetamines, sedatives, inhalants, etc." (Burkhalter, 1975).

Psychological dependence upon a drug with the desire to continue the drug use is habituation. Addiction, on the other hand, implies physical dependence accompanied by withdrawal symptoms upon cessation of drug consumption. Recognizing that many stages or degrees of drug habituation may exist, for purposes of this discussion, the term *drug dependence,* as defined above, is used.

An estimate of the number of drug addicts is difficult to obtain. The Federal Bureau of Narcotics reports about 50,000 active addicts. The incidence of drug dependence is higher in males, about three or four males to one female addict. More than half the drug users are Negro, between 21 and 30 years of age and live in slum areas of large cities. In this type of environment, drugs are easily available, and adherence to law and order is limited. Family relationships are often disrupted, and the delinquency rate is high (Wikler, 1967).

Etiology

A description of the personality of the person dependent on drugs includes characteristics such as loneliness, lack of direction, poorly defined values and distrust of authorities. Desire for immediate gratification, expression of rebellion, a need to conform to peer pressure, or an attempt to gain escape or affection precipitates drug use by adolescents or adults. Some young drug users have adopted their parental example of tranquilizer or stimulant use, as a prelude to their own drug habit.

Once a person has an initial drug experience, he either stops immediately or continues drug use. Reasons for continuing drug use include development of physical dependence; having a pleasant, satisfying experience; withdrawal symptoms, if discontinued; or adoption of the drug culture as a life style (Burkhalter, 1975).

In order to obtain drugs, once dependence develops, the drug user must employ dishonest or devious methods to obtain the drugs and/or money to buy them. Efforts to conceal his drug dependence from family and friends compound the deceit. The drug user often becomes involved in criminal acts in order to finance the increasingly expensive drug habit. Such behavior is harmful to the individual, his family and society at large.

People, such as physicians, pharmacists and nurses, who have legal access to drugs are especially at risk to become drug users. The R.N. who works the night shift only, who changes jobs often and who charts many medications for pain relief is a likely suspect for illegal drug use. She may administer partial or "watered-down" doses to the patient and accumulate the other partial doses for herself.

If a person suffers from a medical condition accompanied by much pain, drugs usually are prescribed. A young woman hospitalized with third degree burns of the face, chest and hands is an example. She required plastic surgery in stages to correct deformities of the hands and face, which were caused by scar tissue formation. She received meperidine to relieve the pain. After many hospitalizations over a period of a year, the hospital staff realized that increasing dosages at more frequent intervals were required by this patient. She was addicted to the meperidine, which had been prescribed to meet a very real need. Either improper or extended use of the prescribed medication may lead to drug dependence.

Clinical Course and Treatment

The variety of substances which may be used is endless. The expression of the dependence upon the drug necessarily relates to the substance used. A few of the more common drugs, their manifestations and signs and symptoms are described in Table 11-1.

To describe further the effects of one of the groups in Table 11-1, narcotics will be discussed. Narcotic drugs have a depressant effect on the central nervous system, which gradually becomes tolerant of the narcotic substance. The drug has a sedative effect, as the result of the central nervous system depression. In an attempt to invalidate this sedative effect, nervous energy is discharged by the central nervous system. This means that the drug user requires increasing amounts of the drug to gain the desired effects or condition, once drug dependence has been established. If the drug is discontinued, the discharge of nervous energy continues, causing the anxiety, stomach cramps and shaking hands associated with withdrawal.

If a person is dependent on drugs for a long time, he may develop many physical complications. Intravenous injections of drugs may cause bacterial endocarditis, affecting aortic, mitral and tricuspid valves. If oral drugs are injected intra-arterially, the extremity distal to the injection may become gangrenous, requiring amputation. Contaminated injections may cause thrombophlebitis, lymphedema and gangrene. If foreign particles are introduced into veins, either with the drug (as talc) or alone (as peanut butter), pulmonary emboli may result. Since many drug users are in poor general health, they, like the alcoholic, are especially susceptible to respiratory infections (Burkhalter, 1975).

TABLE 11-1
Selected Drugs Causing Dependence, Manifestations and Treatment

Drug	Manifestations — Early Effect	Later Effect	Withdrawal	Treatment — Overdose	Withdrawal
Narcotics, e.g., Morphine	Feeling of well being Confusion	Lethargy	Restlessness Discomfort Shakiness Hallucinations Coma	Airway Narcotic antagonist Respiration stimulant	Relief of symptoms Methadone treatment
Hypnotics, Sedatives and Tranquilizers, e.g., Phenobarbital	Drowsiness Relaxation Lack of inhibition	Lack of drive, energy	Insomnia Convulsions Weakness Sweating Anxiety	Maintain respiration, I.V. therapy, medication to raise B.P. Removal of drug—gastric lavage, diuresis, dialysis	Prevent seizures Detoxify, withdraw therapy. Prevent psychosis, D.T.s, panic Drug substitute
Stimulants, e.g., Amphetamines	Tachycardia Euphoria Hyperactivity	Tension Sleeplessness Impotence Anorexia Psychoses	Depression Suicide attempt	Detoxification, Quiet, environment, sedatives, prevent injury	Supportive therapy to combat depression, mild tranquilizer
Hallucinogens, e.g., LSD	Sensation of mind expansion	Impaired judgment Flashback Bad trips	Depression	Orient to reality, Quiet environment, Prevent injury.	Establish communication Reality therapy.

(Eaton and Peterson, 1969)
(Ewing, 1967)

Hepatitis, due to the use of contaminated needles and syringes for injections, occurs very frequently among those with drug dependence. Poor nutrition, weight loss, constipation and hemorrhoids also develop. Skin infections, abscesses and ulcers complicate injections of drugs. Injuries such as burns and fractures occur because of impaired judgment resulting from drug use (Burkhalter, 1975).

Some researchers have evidence to support their theory that drug dependence can result in genetic disorders of children of drug users. Others do not agree that this genetic damage occurs. Addiction of the newborn infants of drug dependent mothers is, however, an established problem. These mothers have a high incidence of abortions, still-births and premature deliveries. The surviving infants show signs of withdrawal soon after birth, depending upon the drug, usual dosage and general condition of the infant. The infant is hyperactive, with a high-pitched, weak cry. The baby will nurse vigorously and vomit the feeding. The child becomes dehydrated quickly, has diarrhea, and death may be the final result. The treatment is mild sedation in decreasing doses.

The drug user comes to the attention of a treatment agency and nurse for any number of reasons related to drug use, or physical conditions unrelated to the drugs. The patient may have one of the complications described above. Often the person comes to the emergency room having taken an overdose, which may be accidental. The patient may wish to stop or decrease his drug use, or be under court order to obtain psychiatric help.

Nursing Intervention

Attitudes of nursing personnel often influence care given to drug dependent patients, much as they affect care for alcoholic patients. In a study done by Brink (1973), nurses stated that they believed that addiction provided a way out of reality for people who were not adequate in personality or character. Since many undesirable characteristics are attributed to the addict, the nurse needs to cope with the reality of helping such a person. She can best do this when her own knowledge and skills have developed to a degree sufficient to handle the nursing care of the drug-dependent patient.

The patient may have his first contact with the nurse in the emergency room, general hospital, psychiatric unit or drug treatment center. Wherever the initial encounter occurs, the nurse begins her assessment. If the situation is one of crisis, her data collection involves whatever is essential for immediate care. If the condition is less acute, the information-gathering is the basis for the developing care plan. The patient who comes to the emergency room with an overdose of phenobarbital, extremely low blood pressure, and depressed respiration, has far different needs than the excitable patient in the doctor's office whose prescription for Librium is out-of-date.

Physical assessment includes recognition of overdosage or withdrawal. Each drug has its own set of signs and symptoms of these conditions, and the nurse recognizes the behavioral manifestations. Monitoring vital signs carefully, observing incidence of central nervous system depression such as slow irregular respiration or low blood pressure, recognizing tremors or hyperirritability as preludes to seizures or coma, provide data essential to medical management.

The patient may be unable or unwilling to identify the drug or the amount he is using. The odor of some drugs may be recognized on the patient's breath or clothing. The skin is inspected for cuts, bruises, infection, abscesses, poor turgor, scars, needle tracks and jaundice. Initial assessment provides a baseline for complications developing after admission for care. General nutritional state, hygiene and breath sounds are evaluated.

The nurse determines the orientation of the patient to reality. If he is experiencing hallucinations, he often needs immediate help in recognizing them as drug-induced (Burkhalter, 1975). A history of drugs used and how they have been used is determined from whatever sources are available: patient, family or friends. The reason for seeking help and the kind of help desired are elicited from the patient or concerned others, as soon as possible. Meeting patient-perceived needs cannot be adequately accomplished until this part of the assessment is completed.

When the patient's condition allows, his support system is evaluated. If the patient comes to the health agency from a drug culture, will a return to that situation frustrate his attempt to break the drug habit? If the patient has been involved in criminal activities in order to buy illegal drugs, what is his legal status? Do the family and friends of the drug abuser show concern for and ability to help him?

As the nurse continues to collect information regarding all aspects of the patient's situation, the problems are identified and listed. Those of immediate priority, such as withdrawal, are alleviated first. Information is added to each problem listed to complete the data base.

Goals are set and nursing plans made for attaining the goals. As soon as the patient is able to participate in these plans, he is encouraged to do so. Protection for the patient from the effects of overdosage or alleviation of symptoms of withdrawal necessarily precede any long-range plans or interventions.

Careful and continuing observation of the patient is inherent in nursing care for the drug-dependent patient. Recognition of symptoms and provision of appropriate medical relief for these symptoms is needed. Excellent skin care to prevent further deterioration or complications is required. Any cuts or abscesses should be gently, thoroughly cleaned and topical medications and/or sterile dressings applied. The nurse assists with gastric suction, if the contents of the stomach are emptied.

These patients have little interest in eating and are often nauseated. Adequate nutrition for nourishment and tissue repair is a challenge. The nurse consults the dietary department so that appetizing meals, considering special preferences of the patient, stimulate eating. Dietary supplements in the form of extra, small feedings and vitamins are given to the patient.

While the immediate and sometimes devastating physical effects of drug dependence are being treated, psychological treatment is also begun. The nurse participates in individual or group therapy. Her attitude of honesty, support and acceptance is evidenced in all contacts with the patient. He oftentimes needs to relearn social skills and interpersonal relationships, and therapy may assist with these skills.

The patient may see himself as worthless, a discard of society. An interaction with the nurse might be as follows:

Nurse: I'd like to spend some time with you each day. Is this a good time to plan?
Patient: Look for someone worth your time. I'm a lost cause. The only time I feel like living is when I'm zonked out of my mind. Got any magic for that?
Nurse: You have had a rough time, but you are important, and I care about you. Could we set up an hour to talk today?

The regard shown by the nurse for the patient is essential, but only if she really means what she says.

When the patient shows improvement psychologically, as well as physically, he may be discharged to a half-way house. The nurse participates in therapy in this situation or in an outpatient or methadone clinic. As the patient gradually assumes responsibility for his own rehabilitation, the nurse and patient continue to evaluate his progress toward established goals. Nursing plans and approaches are revised appropriately. Problems become inactive, and new ones are identified. As drug dependence becomes less of a problem, the need for a job and acceptance into the family situation becomes more important.

Optimism and continued acceptance and regard for the patient are characteristics of the successful nurse who works with the drug-dependent patient. It is not unusual for a patient to be treated physically and emotionally, return to society as a participating member and then resume a drug habit. The acceptance by the nurse, in spite of repeated episodes, is of great value to her effectiveness as a part of the plan of therapy.

When an all-too-familiar patient returns to the emergency room with the same diagnosis—toxic reaction to overdose of tranquilizers and alcohol—support and concern of the nurse are as important in the patient's treatment as they were in the first episode indicating drug dependence.

CASE STUDY

Steve B. has been assigned to the Day Hospital of a Veteran's Hospital. He was treated in the detoxification unit of a hospital 50 miles distant and referred to the outpatient unit in the city where his sister lives. During his first week at the Day Hospital, Steve did not socialize with the other members, remaining apart from group activities, exhibiting little interest in his surroundings.

Steve, now 34 years old, was the youngest in a family of four children: two brothers, twenty and eighteen years older, and a sister thirteen years older. His birth was unplanned and somewhat of a surprise to his parents. His father was 50 and his mother 43 when he was born. His brothers considered his birth an embarrassment and ignored him. His sister, Mary, however, enjoyed playing with him and carried out much of the mothering which his mother did not enjoy.

Steve's father owned a neighborhood grocery store where he worked long hours. He paid little attention to his youngest child, asking for "just a little peace and quiet." Steve's mother helped in the store and often left Mary in charge of Steve. Mary graduated from high school when Steve was 6. She married and moved to a nearby town, soon becoming a mother herself.

Steve's father died from a heart attack the following year. Steve's mother continued to operate the grocery with intermittent help from her sons. Steve made grocery deliveries in the neighborhood when he was 8. He maintained above-average grades in school but participated in no extracurricular activities, due to his work responsibilities.

The grocery was sold when Steve was 12, and his mother managed to live on a small investment pension and occasional financial help from the older children. Steve had a regular job after school in a supermarket. He was thought to be a hard worker, serious and a loner.

Steve continued to live at home with his mother, who spent most of her time watching television and attending church-related activities. She complained that none of her children cared about her, although the older ones continued to give her money, and Steve gave her part of his weekly salary. Steve maintained a close emotional relationship with his sister, who had three children and an unemployed husband.

When Steve graduated from high school, he joined the Navy, hoping to find a way to attend college. He was soon shipped out for an extended cruise. His mother wrote long letters to him asking for help. Steve, away from home for the first time, found that he was able to make friends and have a good time. He particularly liked shore leaves, when he and some buddies would go ashore, have some drinks and "raise hell." He was never in serious trouble, but did develop a habit of relaxing with some friends and drinks whenever possible.

Though he adapted to Navy life and gained promotions, he did not reenlist when his tour of duty was completed. He took advantage of his G.I. benefits and enrolled in a business course in college. He had a part-time job, studied and relaxed at a friendly bar at the edge of the campus. He often met friends there for a few beers.

Steve dated occasionally but had no lasting romantic relationships—studies and job occupying most of his time. His mother, unable to live alone after a serious hip fracture, moved to a nursing home. He visited her once a month and felt guilty and depressed for several days afterwards.

Upon graduation from college, he worked as an accountant. He took additional courses, eventually becoming a Certified Public Accountant. He continued to "pal around" with his friends at work, meeting them on Fridays after work for drinks. He lived alone in a furnished apartment. He met, dated and married the sister of one of his co-workers. Two years later, their son was born. His mother died soon after the birth of his son. Steve marked both events—his son's birth and his mother's death—with a drinking spree lasting about twelve hours.

His work responsibilities and tensions increased. Steve liked the idea of being a father and husband but found the demands of his wife and infant son to be very irritating at times. He often stopped off for a drink to help him relax before going home after work. His drinking increased as did the marital tensions. His wife moved to her parents' home, taking their son with her. She filed for divorce, which Steve did not contest. When the divorce was granted, he went on a binge, waking up in a strange room, with no memory of the preceding 24 hours. Frightened, he returned home. He was fired, due to his unexplained absences.

Steve obtained work as a clerk in a department store, drinking on weekends and "only a few beers." He communicated with his sister a few times each year. She voiced her disappointment with him, her husband and children. Steve had no contact with his ex-wife or child. His drinking bouts occurred more frequently. Jobs were increasingly hard to find. He lost his appetite, gradually lost weight and became "seedy" in appearance: hair disheveled, clothes unpressed and dingy. Steve was admitted to the hospital four times in a state of intoxication, stayed about a week each time and was discharged only to return within a few more weeks.

During Steve's last hospitalization, he was treated in the detoxification unit of the Veteran's Hospital. In a group conference, the staff explored with Steve the possibility of maintaining abstinence from alcohol on a long-term basis. For the first time, Steve talked about his sister and expressed a desire to be near her. Arrangements were made to transfer Steve to the Day Hospital Unit in the city where his sister, Mary, lived. Lodging was found in a boarding house run by an elderly couple, who had a real interest in the welfare of their roomers.

Steve was admitted to the Day Hospital Unit.

I. OBJECTIVE DATA
    A. General Appearance, Attitude and Activity
        1. Appearance: recent haircut, clean-shaven, wearing clean but wrinkled slacks, knit shirt and tennis shoes
        2. Attitude: answers questions but does not volunteer information, speaks softly and hesitantly; has a sad, withdrawn expression
        3. Activity: chain smokes; keeps eyes downcast; apologizes for smoking, appearance, lack of attention to interviewer
    B. Communication Patterns
        1. Talks about failure he has made of everything: marriage, job, self; communicates hopelessness about changing situation
        2. Communication clear, but soft tones make him somewhat difficult to understand. Tends to drift from topic under discussion
    C. Contact
        1. Oriented to time, place, environment
        2. Not attentive to environment. Stares at floor or looks blankly at others when interrupted
    D. Sensorium and Intelligence
        1. Memory accurate with exception of "blackouts"; has no memory of those
        2. Easily distracted by own activities of lighting cigarette or changing position
        3. Excellent vocabulary; has not read magazines or newspapers recently
        4. Can think in abstractions and concretely
    E. Thought Processes
        1. Hesitates when questioned; has some difficulty in

            phrasing specific answers; somewhat vague
        2. Tends to drift from one topic into another related topic
   F. Thought Content
        1. Lack of ability "to get it together"; "mess he's made of life"
        2. No delusions or hallucinations at this time; did experience auditory and visual hallucinations in detoxification unit
   G. Social Assessment
        1. Education, socioeconomic status, religion: college, 4 years, B.A. in Business; C.P.A.; was upper middle class, now lower class; religious affiliation as child, Presbyterian, none as adult
        2. Family—divorced: no contact with ex-wife or child; siblings—two brothers, no contact for years; sister residing in city, visits often
        3. Family's understanding of illness: sister states she is glad that Steve is getting some real help; hopeful that he can use his brain and return to a productive life; can't understand why "he worked so hard and then threw it all away for booze"
   H. Medical Assessment
        1. Complains of nervousness, lack of energy and ambition
        2. Weight loss over past two years of 30 pounds; appetite has been poor but is improving
        3. Sleeps poorly, waking several times at night to smoke
        4. Physical examination prior to transfer showed no permanent physical effects of alcoholism such as polyneuritis, cirrhosis of liver or Korsakoff's psychosis

II. SUBJECTIVE DATA
   A. Present Illness
        1. Patient transferred to Day Hospital Unit, as decided by detoxification staff and Steve; states he

wants to get off the merry-go-round of drinking
   2. Precipitating events—blackouts following long drinking periods; drying out at detoxification center
   3. Repeated treatment for acute alcoholism; referred to Alcoholics Anonymous in past, attended one meeting and did not return; no long-term or extended psychiatric treatment; arrested twice for driving while intoxicated; has not owned a car for several years
   4. Steve says, "My life is in the gutter of a one-way street."

III. STATEMENT OF THE PSYCHIATRIC PROBLEM

   A. Alcoholism

   B. Problem List: Initial
      1. Chronic alcoholism
      2. Lack of goals
      3. Limited interpersonal relationships
      4. Lack of socialization skills
      5. Chronic smoker
      6. Weight loss
      7. Insomnia
      8. Low self-esteem
      9. Depression
      10. Not employed—limited finances
      11. Anxiety

IV. PLANNING PHASE

A conference was held between Steve and the psychiatric nurse in the Day Hospital. The problem list was reviewed. Steve agreed that all problems existed. The problem list was reworded, combining related problems and placing problems in order of priority.

Revised *Problem List* as recorded on patient record:

   A. Alcoholism, chronic

   B. Goals undefined

   C. Depression

D. Anxiety

E. Insomnia

F. Low self-esteem

G. Socialization impaired due to limited interpersonal relationships

H. Financial need due to lack of job

I. Smoker, chronic

J. Weight loss

Following the patient-nurse conference and revision of the problem list, a staff conference was held to plan Steve's treatment. The nurse was to continue conferences with Steve on a weekly basis. Steve was assigned to group therapy twice weekly with the psychiatrist as leader. For work therapy, Steve was assigned as a messenger for the Central Supply Unit at the main hospital for two hours each afternoon. Activity therapy (crafts) according to Steve's preference was scheduled daily. Steve, as a member of the unit, was expected to attend group government meetings weekly. The plans and expected outcomes were entered in Steve's record.

A. Alcoholism, chronic
   1. *Plan:* In one-to-one therapy and in group therapy, Steve will be helped to gain insight into reasons for destructive use of alcohol. Rules of Day Hospital requiring abstinence from alcohol in order to continue therapy will be carefully explained. Encouraging abstinence and praising continuing abstinence will be consistently done by all staff members. Steve will be encouraged to express any felt need to have a drink and directed to alternate activity to gain effect desired.
   2. *Expected outcome:* The patient will recognize limitation set by Day Hospital upon alcoholic consumption as reason for termination of treatment. Encouraged by staff, he will remain sober, seek to find reasons for drinking and alternate solution to his problems.
B. Goals undefined

1. *Plan:* The therapeutic plan of care agreed upon by patient has a number of short-term goals already established. Participation in the planned activities will be the initial goal-setting. Active participation in the activities will be honestly praised by staff, as the patient succeeds in each one. Steve will be allowed to progress at a reasonable rate in assuming additional tasks, as he successfully accomplishes another. Praise and encouragement will be offered, but tension and signs of stress will be recognized and alleviated to avoid additional pressure or failure. The goal of sobriety expressed in plan A1 will relate to this problem also.
2. *Expected outcome:* The patient will gain satisfaction and sense of achievement in accomplishment of pre-set goals. This positive situation will provide atmosphere conducive to future planning, first with help and eventually on an individual basis.

C. Depression
  1. *Plan:* Involvement of patient in worthwhile activities, such as work assignment and productive crafts, will put patient in contact with others and increase feelings of self-worth. Stimulation in group therapy will involve other patients in therapy and provide additional encouragement to that given by staff.
  2. *Expected outcome:* Patient will show signs of optimism, as he recognizes reasons for living and possibilities to become a productive person.

D. Anxiety
  1. *Plan:* Inclusion of patient in physical activities, such as daily exercise sessions and baseball games, to provide outlet for nervousness. Staff will observe for signs of increasing tension and provide activities or interaction to alleviate this.
  2. *Expected outcome:* Patient will recognize warning signs of own increasing tension and handle by regulating activities, such as taking a walk or seeking out a friend to visit.

E. Insomnia
  1. *Plan:* No medications will be offered, since another dependence is discouraged. Instead, patient will be directed into increased physical activity in the evening: walks, exercise,

jogging. Activity then will be followed by pattern of relaxing warm bath, light snack, quiet activity of reading or listening to music. If sleep is interrupted, patient will be instructed to use relaxation techniques to gain additional rest and not to smoke or eat if awakened.
   2. *Expected outcome:* Steve will develop a pattern of behavior leading to restful nights. As other problems or depression and anxiety decrease, it is expected that this one also will improve.

F. Low self-esteem
   1. *Plan:* The staff will convey respect for patient as a person at all times, recognizing his worth. The staff will help him to become aware of his own positive abilities and characteristics: pleasant appearance, intelligence, ability to organize, developing relationships with other members and staff.
   2. *Expected outcome:* Patient will be slow to recognize that he is worthy of trust or praise, since self-esteem has been low for so long. With continued positive feedback and honest regard from others, Steve will gradually become cognizant of abilities and assets and continue to gain confidence and self-respect.

G. Socialization impaired due to limited interpersonal relationships
   1. *Plan:* Structured situations will be arranged, gradually increasing number of people involved. Steve was, at one time, able to maintain such relationships, but only with the aid of alcohol. Social successes, while sober, in contacts in group therapy, work assignment and government meetings will reinforce social skills. Visits from his sister will be encouraged, since she maintains an active "civilian" life. Progress will be determined and new activities planned, as old ones become easier.
   2. *Expected outcome:* Lack of interest in social activities will decrease as social skills are revived, this time using the determination of the patient without the help of alcohol. Simple conversations will improve progress to discussions of current events, then participation in monthly parties at the Day Hospital.

H. Financial need due to lack of job
  1. *Plan:* Patient will continue in work assignment program. Difficulty in tasks will be increased, so long as it does not risk discouragement or anxiety that is immobilizing. Praise will be given freely for good performance, especially in regular attendance and promptness. Vocational counseling will begin, when appropriate, to determine if he wishes to return to accounting work, or if he wants a change of job preparation.
  2. *Expected outcome:* Success in simple job with increasing responsibility will encourage him to return to employment. Process will be gradual, considering stress and the demands of the position and his ability and desire to meet these.

I. Smoker, chronic
  1. *Plan:* This long-standing problem will be dealt with following solution of many others. The desire to stop smoking will be explored with the patient. Decision will not be criticized, if patient decides to continue. Possible increase in stress is considered, if smoking abruptly discontinued while other problems of high priority are still in acute stage.
  2. *Expected outcome:* Patients will be educated to the effects of smoking and will decide to stop smoking or to continue.

J. Weight loss
  1. *Plan:* The staff will encourage regular well-balanced meals. Prescription of a therapeutic multivitamin will supplement nutrition from meals. Breakfast and evening meal are eaten at the boarding house, where the landlady does provide attractive, well-planned meals. The noon meal is a brown bag lunch or hamburger, fries and milk. Will encourage fruits as snacks. Encourage physical activities as described in Problems 4 and 5.
  2. *Expected outcome:* Since appetite is improving, he will continue to eat meals and will regain weight needed to maintain health.

Evaluation

Progress toward desired outcome is a process shared by staff and patient. All people involved in therapy are involved in the assessment of its effectiveness. This evaluative process is done regularly at certain intervals and changes are made in 1) problems, indicating those resolved or changed; or 2) plans, increasing scope when initial ones are met; or 3) interventions, discarding those which are ineffective, improving those which are helpful. Progress is noted in the record, so that all persons involved will continue to be informed and better able to assist the patient as he moves toward achievement of goals.

PRINCIPLES

1. All people experience anxiety, which is reduced through action.
2. Unsuccessful attempts to interact with physical and social environment will result in protective withdrawal.
3. Withdrawal from problems relieves discomfort but does not solve problems.
4. Manipulation is an attempt to control the actions of others.
5. Complete objectivity is impossible to attain.
6. Socialization is a process that is reciprocal.
7. Awareness of judgments about others and their behaviors is basic to the nurse-patient relationship.
8. Setting limits allows a person freedom to gain control of self.
9. Support provides strength until independence is attained.

BIBLIOGRAPHY

Blane, Howard T. *The Personality of the Alcoholic*. New York: Harper & Row Publishers, 1968.

Brink, Pamela. "Nurses' Attitudes toward Heroin Addicts," *Journal of Psychiatric Nursing and Mental Health Services*, Vol. 11 (March-April, 1973), 7-12.

Burgess, Ann W., and Lazare, Aaron. *Psychiatric Nursing in the Hospital and the Community*. 2d ed. Englewood Cliffs, N.J.: Prentice-Hall, Inc., 1976.

Burkhalter, Pamela. *Nursing Care of the Alcoholic and Drug Abuser*. New York: McGraw-Hill Book Co., 1975.

Chafetz, Morris E. "Addictions III, Alcoholism," in *Comprehensive Textbook of Psychiatry*. Edited by Alfred M. Freedman and Harold I. Kaplan. Baltimore: Williams & Wilkins Co., 1967.

Eaton, Merrill, Peterson, Margaret, and Davis, James. *Psychiatry*. 2d ed. Garden City, N.Y.: Medical Examination Publishing Co., Inc., 1969.

Ewing, John. "Addictions II, Categories of Alcoholics," in *Comprehensive Textbook of Psychiatry*. Edited by Alfred M. Freedman and Harold I. Kaplan. Baltimore: Williams & Wilkins Co., 1967.

Hoff, Ebbe C. *Alcoholism: The Hidden Addiction*. New York: The Seabury Press, 1975.

Kogan, Benjamin. *Health: Man in a Changing Environment*. New York: Harcourt, Brace & World, Inc., 1970.

Wikler, Abraham. "Addictions I," in *Comprehensive Textbook of Psychiatry*. Edited by Alfred M. Freedman and Harold I. Kaplan. Baltimore: Williams & Wilkins Co., 1967.

World Health Organization, Expert Committee on Addiction-Producing Drugs. *Thirteenth Report*. (WHO Technical Reports Series, No. 273.) Geneva: WHO, 1964.

CHAPTER 12

Psychoses

Frances K. Richardson, R.N., M.S.

"Reality, for the individual, is the world as that person perceives it, not necessarily as it exists."

Mary Almore (Almore, 1976).

INTRODUCTION

With the possible exception of the sociopathic personality, the psychoses constitute the most serious psychiatric disorders with which the nurse has to deal.

A psychosis is traditionally defined as a subtotal disorganization of personality, in which the individual loses contact with reality. However, the latter part of this definition frequently leads to misinterpretations and sets off specters in the layman's perception of psychosis, which are themselves unrealistic. Perhaps it would be most accurate to say that in a psychosis, the individual moves in and out of reality for, characteristically, the "loss" of reality does *not* involve the totality of the individual's life, at least not for protracted periods. In fact, sometimes the psychotic is sufficiently in contact, that he can maintain himself in society without hospitalization or even without treatment. In such cases, of course, the effectiveness of that person's overall adjustment is minimal. His personality is disorganized, and his behavior tends to be psychologically, if not physically, damaging to those close to him. In any event, no matter how bizarre the behavior of the psychotic may be at times, psychoses may also be seen as an attempt to adapt. What one calls the psychotic's "loss" of contact with reality may be seen as a restructuring of that reality on his own terms, as it were. In effect, these are the best, or only, terms he sees as available and reinforcing to him at the time.

An example of the latter would be the schizophrenic who cuts himself for the reassurance that he is still real because he bleeds and, possibly, hurts. This should not be interpreted so much as a symptom of his "craziness," as it should be interpreted as an indication that he is attempting to structure a less "crazy" world.

Professional treatment, then, ideally becomes a matter of permitting and encouraging the person's redefining of his terms in a more realistic and effective way. In another way, one opens up new options, enabling and reinforcing the person's behaving in a more normal way. This is not a simple process, however, and too often the helping profession settles for no treatment at all beyond custodial care or for removal of symptomatology classified as "sick"—without going on to deal with behavior and without really attempting to encourage growth orientation.

While characteristically more disabling, psychoses follow the same developmental sequence as do neuroses:

1. An increase in anxiety, stress and/or frustration
2. Threat of ego disintegration (e.g., feelings of unrealness, inadequacy or lack of selfhood)
3. Some regression in behavior
4. Reactivation of previous conflicts
5. Transformation and secondary elaboration (i.e., failing accurately to perceive present conflicts, transforming them instead into unrealistic perceptions and developing additional symptoms)
6. Emergence of psychotic behavior

We have mentioned regression or returning to developmental or earlier behavior patterns. The Freudian would explain this regression in terms of the individual's returning, as it were, to a previous developmental period in which he or she was fixated. Fixations are possible at any of the Freudian stages (oral, anal, phallic or latency) and are thought to be able to exist at more than one of these stages.

While not using the term regression, in all probability, the learning theorists would contend that the individual falls back on responses which have been strongly reinforced in the past, but which are now inadequate to cope with the problems at hand. Also, the person may have simply learned maladaptive behavior, which becomes exacerbated under current stress.

The labeling theorist would point out that each of us has acquired some notion (usually through the media) of how "crazy" people act. Once people in the environment begin to label us as crazy, we tend either to seek to refute their allegations—which is frequently taken by others as a sign of our supposed "sickness," even though it may not be—or we adopt the role assigned to us.

Each of these three approaches has important treatment implications. If we follow the Freudian route, treatment becomes largely a matter of seeking to bring into consciousness unconscious conflicts unresolved at some developmental level. If one follows the learning approach, treatment becomes a matter of reinforcing more adaptive behavior and failing to reinforce maladaptive behavior. This may also mean helping to teach the individual coping skills which, for one reason or another, he never had an opportunity to learn. Thus, ignoring "crazy" behavior and expressing our intent to talk with the individual only when he is acting "uncrazy" is sometimes the most effective approach. The labeling theory points out that society often makes it difficult for people who have been negatively labeled to escape that label. Nurses on psychiatric units too frequently view the patient about to be discharged as someone who will inevitably return. Family and community members tend to do the same thing, making effective adjustment that much more difficult. Thus, one may be setting up a sort of self-fulfilling prophecy by viewing the individual as incompetent or potentially so. In the face of such perceptions on the part of others, the individual may come to believe it himself and, as unpleasant as a psychotic state may be, find such a state more rewarding than attempting to cope with the real world.

There are two basic classes of psychoses: functional and organic. Organic psychoses, such as paresis and senile dementia, are those which are clearly physiological in origin. Functional psychoses are those which are thought to be psychogenic in origin, that is, precipitated by intrapersonal conflicts and environmental stress.

There are those who contend that when there is sufficient knowledge, we will discover that all psychoses are, in fact, organic. It is known that all psychoses can be treated by chemical or other somatic intervention. However, this does not, in itself, prove that they are organic in origin, since treatment comes after the diagnosis rather than before. It is also known, though frequently not practiced, that persons with organic psychoses can function more effectively through appropriate learning techniques.

There are three general classes of symptom or behavioral manifestation in psychoses, classes which may exist predominantly singly or in some combination:

1. *Hallucinations:* Perceptual experiences which occur in the absence of any appropriate sensory stimulation. They should not be confused with illusions, which are misinterpretations of sensory experiences.
2. *Inappropriate affect:* This is the display of no apparent feeling when feeling would be appropriate (often called "flatness of affect"); the display of a feeling tone or response which does not seem to fit the situation, e.g., may cry at a happy time or laugh at a tragedy.
3. *Delusions:* Delusions are strong beliefs which are contrary to reality. They are commonly subdivided into three classes:
    a) Delusions of grandeur. Here, the individual may believe that he is some famous figure, or he may believe that he possesses power or money which he does not actually have.
    b) Delusions of persecution. As the term implies, the individual believes that he is the potential victim of a plot being conducted by one or more persons ranging, for example, from a spouse to the Communist Party.
    c) Delusions of reference. In this case, the individual believes that environmental events are directed toward him in some way when, in fact, they are not. An example would be a patient watching some nurses laughing in the nursing station and believing that they are laughing at him, even though he is not even the topic of conversation.

While these three general types of behavioral manifestation are found in psychoses, obviously, each differs in degree or in specific content to the extent that it is manifested at all. Such degree and/or content in the individual's concomitant behavior generally form the basis for the classification or labeling of the psychosis. But it is important to remember that such classification, which follows, is largely a matter of custom and convenience. "Textbook" cases are rare, at best. Contamination by symptoms or behavior associated with other disorders is common.

The psychoses to be considered include: paranoia, affective disorders, involutional psychotic reactions and schizophrenia.

PARANOIA

Paranoia is generally considered to be the least regressive of the psychoses or, put another way, the one representing the least personality disorganization. In contrast to the subtype of schizophrenia called paranoid schizophrenia, true paranoia is characterized by a commonly strong, well-organized delusional system. These delusions (whatever their specific form) are generally grandiose or persecutory, usually with components of delusions sometimes found in other psychoses. The paranoiac, however, does not come to believe that portions of his body have metamorphosized in some bizarre fashion, nor does he come to believe that he is someone other than who he actually is (such as a famous historic or contemporary figure).

Further, he sees himself, but in a delusional context, for example, exaggerating his own importance or attractiveness, as in delusions of grandeur or believing himself the real or potential victim of some plot, as in persecutory delusions. When persecutory delusions predominate, the individual *may* become dangerous, aggressing against others to prevent (as he perceives it) their aggressing against him.

Typically, the paranoic fearing persecution constructs what is called "pseudo-community." That is, he identifies a group of people (not all of whom he necessarily knows) whom he sees as playing a role in the plot against him. Such a pseudo-community may be seen as serving adaptive functions. For example, its construction helps bind tension-produced energy, while it provides a focal point for the individual's projections; and his having to keep watch and be on guard vis-a-vis this group helps maintain reality contact for the paranoic who, characteristically, is hypersensitive to the verbalizations and gestures of those with whom he comes in contact.

An interesting phenomenon, folie a deux, is apparently unique to paranoia. In this case, the second person comes to share the paranoic's delusional system and pseudo-community but, when separated from the paranoic, he readily gives these up. The dynamics of folie a deux are uncertain, but it is commonly thought that identification and dependency are factors. Usually, the paranoic is the dominant individual, though the dominance-dependency relationship may not be clearly or consciously defined. Adding to this may be the fact that paranoic delusions often give the appearance of logic and *may* have some limited basis in reality. For example, Kruschev's "we'll bury you" statement may be translated into a rather personalized, perceived plot carried out by some pseudo-community of often mislabeled "Communists," or a spouse's previous indiscretion may be translated into an ongoing series of extramarital affairs.

Outside his delusional system, however, the paranoic generally maintains realistic relationships with his environment; thus, the common label "in contact paranoid," distinguishes him from the paranoid schizophrenic. Aspects of his behavior may be disturbing or even damaging to those around him, especially to those with whom he has close contact. The paranoic frequently goes virtually unrecognized or at least untreated.

Feelings of guilt and/or inadequacy are common basic components of paranoia, though they are not manifested in consciousness. Rather, they are defended against through overuse of the mechanism of denial (possibly being translated into exaggerated feelings of worth, as in grandiose delusions approaching reaction formation) or through denial combined with projection. Here, as in persecutory delusions, feelings of hatred which are actually directed toward one's self are seen as feelings others have toward the individual; fears of attack or persecution motivation attributed to others are more realistically representations of fear of persecution and derision by the affection component of one's self-concept. Rather than admit these feelings to himself, the paranoic projects them onto his pseudo-community. Such fears are reminiscent of phobic fears, though not identical to them. Similarly, paranoics may exhibit sadomasochistic behavior reminiscent of, but again not identical to, that often found in obsessive-compulsive reactions. In both cases, we see evidence of the symptom contamination mentioned earlier. Thus, while the paranoic is hypersensitive to the feelings of others, he is characteristically insensitive to his own attitudes.

Childhood background commonly includes experiences militating against developing an orientation toward what Erikson (1963) would call "initiative vs. guilt." These experiences typically include such things as the child's not having been adequately protected against anxiety-provoking stimuli or exposure to parents who were themselves sadistic (as manifested in their excessive teasing and their being domineering, or in their letting the child display uncontrolled anger because they enjoy such displays).

AFFECTIVE DISORDERS

As the term implies, the primary (though not necessarily exclusive) behavioral manifestation in affective disorders is significantly inappropriate affect. This is in contrast to the strong, well-organized delusional systems which are the primary behavioral manifestations in paranoia. Also, in contrast to paranoia, affective disorders are commonly thought to represent a deeper regression or, put another way, somewhat greater personality disorganization. Several psychotic reactions may be included under the rubric "affective disorders."

One of these is mania. Commonly, mania is preceded by a period of preoccupation, although such preoccupation may not be particularly noticed by others, at least at the time. With the overt onset of the manic reaction, the individual characteristically displays elation, gaiety, hyperactivity and, sometimes, self-aggrandizement. These manifestations may appear to be essentially exaggerations of a normally happy mood, or they may become rather strongly delusional, as in those cases where the person displays an unrealistic picture of his own importance or success, or as he verbalizes unrealistic deals in which he is engaging, or in which he has been, or will be, successfully involved. Such exaggerated or delusional elation and/or self-aggrandizement are inappropriate not only in degree, but also with respect to the manic's actual situation. For example, believing that he is about to be involved in some windfall deal, the manic may actually go on an unwarranted spending spree and go deeply in debt.

Typically, the manic's physical behavior is seemingly tireless and frenetic as he expends a significant amount of energy, often moving from task to task. His verbal behavior is often analagous to his physical behavior. That is, he talks excessively, flitting from one topic to another in a way that is often difficult for the listener to follow, even if the verbalizations are essentially reality related. This verbal pattern is called "flight of ideas."

The manic's defensive posture most notably involves the overuse of denial in reaction formation—more specifically, denial of potentially depression provoking circumstances and conflicts and adoption of a feeling of jollity with concomitantly elated behavior.

Mania may be viewed as basically a defensive posture, with the individual defending against the onset of a psychotic depression. Though his ways of defending or coping are basically childish, they are, nonetheless, an attempt at adaptation. Analagous to the popular conceptualization of dreams, manic behavior may be viewed as the manifest content of the disturbance, while depression may be viewed as the latent content. In a dream, for example, the manifest content might be that a stranger mugged one's spouse. The latent conflict would reflect one's own desire physically to attack one's spouse.

Finally, it might be noted that one sometimes encounters a disorder labeled hypomania. It is, as the name implies, a mild manic reaction, but rather more akin to a neurotic reaction or what could possibly be classified as a personality disturbance.

A second affective disorder is the manic depressive cycle. While the term "manic depressive" is sometimes casually used (especially by the layman), disorders which can correctly be so classified are relatively rare. In the manic phase, the individual characteristically displays the elation, hyperactivity and flight of ideas associated with mania, while in the depressive phase, he characteristically displays hypoactivity, uneasiness and apprehension. What distinguishes the true manic depressive psychosis is its clear and relatively abrupt mood swing, a swing which follows a cyclical pattern though the given "mood" and may persist for a relatively protracted period. A mild form of this reaction is known as cyclothymic personality.

Probably the most frequently seen affective disorder is the psychotic depression. Typically, psychotic depressions have a fairly gradual onset, during which the individual becomes increasingly less absorbed in his environment (though he may, for awhile go through the motions of routine living) and becomes more absorbed in his own preoccupations. Parallels exist between neurotic and psychotic depressions, as well as important differences. For example, while the neurotic depressive commonly projects his conflicts onto somatic complaints, at least for some period of time, the psychotic depressive may become hypochondriacally preoccupied; while the neurotic often has sleep difficulties, the psychotic tends to suffer intractable insomnia. Interestingly, once hospitalized, the psychotic depressive may sleep for unusual periods of time, although it is difficult to tell whether this represents some relief at being out of the usual environment, whether it represents medication frequently given or whether it is a combination of the two factors. Both neurotic and psychotic depressives experience feelings of dejection, self-condemnation and self-denigration, but in psychotic depressions, these feelings reach delusional proportions. The psychotic depressive is not sustained, even temporarily, by others seeking to provide him with narcissistic supplies (i.e., "strokes" or assurances of worth). In fact, he may react angrily to the efforts of others to offer such reassurance, for, to him, his inferiority and guilt are perceived as factual, not debatable. In this context, and in keeping with the nihilistic delusions sometimes found in psychotic depressions, the individual may come to see punishment not only as deserved but also as inevitable. If only to avoid its further delay, he may view suicide as his only recourse (see Chapter 7 for nursing action with the suicidal patient). Thus, psychotic depressions represent a greater personality disorganization, in general, than the classifications previously considered.

While the underlying dynamics remain basically the same, the psychotic depressive's overt behavior may be labeled as either "agitated" or "retarded." In the former instance, he is characteristically hyperactive—moving about, ringing his hands, picking at his body and verbalizing his feelings of bitterness, self-debasement and ultimate punishment. In the latter instance, he is characteristically hypoactive, displaying an apparent decline of mental functioning and withdrawing into essentially silent preoccupation with his feelings of worthlessness and doom; the withdrawal sometimes resembles virtual stupor.

While the paranoic attempts to deal with his guilt or lack of self-esteem primarily through projection, and the manic through denial and reaction formation, the psychotic depressive, instead, depends primarily on the more primitive defense of introjection. This may involve almost grandiose delusions of guilt that are unrelated or distorted out of proportion to the situation. For example, many persons who survive natural or man-made disasters experience delusions of guilt, although often at less than psychotic levels. Also, it often involves the person's introjecting and ambivalently loved and hated significant other. Here, guilt may arise from the ambivalence, per se, while both guilt and feelings of self-derogation may result from taking on as an aspect of one's own ego the disapproval manifested by the introjected significant other.

Not surprisingly, the childhood background of the psychotic depressive typically involves his having had experiences which prevented his developing an orientation to what Erikson calls "basic trust," especially trust that he would not be abandoned. More specifically, significant others (most usually the parents) threaten to withdraw love whenever the child behaves in ways contrary to their desires. In addition to the defense of introjection, then, the psychotic depressive becomes overly dependent on the coping device of appeasement or compliance. [In Horney's (Cofer, 1964) conceptualization, he has become inappropriately locked into a defensive posture of "moving toward others"].

But, while parental attitudes have been psychologically damaging (though not consciously and deliberately so), they have also typically been consistent, and this consistency has lent a certain predictability to the psychotic depressive's life, predictability which can help him to retain or regain a better hold on reality.

Hospitalization is a frequent outcome, if only for the individual's own protection from himself. The treatment is generally fairly successful, no matter what modality is used, at least from the standpoint of improvement.

INVOLUTIONAL PSYCHOTIC REACTION

A third psychotic classification is involutional psychotic reaction, formerly called involutional melancholia. This is a debatable reaction, perhaps better included under the broad rubric of affective disorders than considered separately or, best of all, eliminated from the classification scheme altogether.

Typically, the involutional psychotic reaction is, in fact, a psychotic depression which may be accompanied by rather bizarre somatic delusions. Infrequently, it may manifest itself as paranoia or, rarely, as mania or schizophrenia. Because of its onset at or following middle age, it was once considered to be precipitated by hormonal changes accompanying menopause in women or the supposedly analogous climacterium occurring in men. More objective and informed analysis points to its being psychogenic, arising from the psychological concomitant of changes in body function or appearance (which, as indicated, may be translated into somatic delusions), from threatened loss of important role functions (as when children begin to leave home and establish their own more independent lives), from real or perceived career crises and/or from a second (and severe) identity crisis.

What distinguishes involutional psychotic reactions is not their underlying dynamics or behavioral manifestations, but rather the age at which they occur in the absence of a previous history of psychotic reaction.

An example of this classification would be a 49-year-old female admitted to a psychiatric unit of a general hospital for the first admission, with presenting complaints of feeling worthless, no purpose for "going on," remorse, vague references to not feeling well physically, loneliness and not being able to eat or sleep. The patient's youngest son had recently gone away to college, and her husband's work required his being away from home quite frequently. Objective data would include a rather unkempt appearance; body language much like that seen in the depressive person, such as drooped shoulders, lowered head, sad or forlorn facial expression, no eye contact, slow movements; and, generally, appearing to be a sad, dejected person. Intervention in such an instance would involve a carefully constructed case history and helping the individual establish new growth-oriented goals incrementally.

SCHIZOPHRENIA

The psychosis generally considered to be the most regressive or, put another way, the one representing the greatest personality and behavioral disorganization, is schizophrenia.

This disorder was originally called dementia praecox, meaning youthful insanity, because it is characteristically manifested in adolescence or young adulthood.

In 1911, Eugene Bleuler (Rosen, 1972) gave us the term schizophrenia and identified four primary symptoms, which he said were always associated with this disorder: ambivalence, autism (or fantasy thinking), disruption of affect and disruption of association. By disturbance in association we mean thought disorders manifesting themselves in frequently bizarre body movements or in verbalizations, which the schizophrenic apparently finds quite logical, but which make no sense at all to the person listening.

The term schizophrenia means "split-mind," representing the individual's split from reality. However, it is frequently translated "split-personality" and confused with the neurotic reaction called multiple personality.

Traditionally, efforts were made to classify schizophrenia into nine varieties or subtypes. Some of these varieties are virtual admissions of the inability to make any meaningful distinction (e.g., "acute," "chronic undifferentiated" or "residual"). Similarly, so-called "childhood schizophrenia" is a somewhat questionable label and a manifestation not always clearly distinguished or distinguishable from other disorders.

Among adults (and, as indicated, schizophrenia seems most apt to manifest itself between mid-adolescence and middle age), five fairly distinct varieties are noted. They are considered briefly before proceeding to a more general discussion of schizophrenia, but, here again, it is important to remember that symptom contamination is the rule; and, in fact, the individual may move, as it were, from one variety to another. These subtypes are:

1. *Simple:* Unlike other schizophrenic reactions, simple schizophrenia is not characteristically accompanied by evidence of delusions or hallucinations. Rather, the person's behavior is described as a fairly gradual and, without professional intervention, apparently inexorable decline in adaptive capacity. The person becomes increasingly more idle and withdrawn. In some cases, he may require institutional care. In other cases, he may remain in the community, eschewing virtually all responsibility, or he may drift about aimlessly. He may be employed but, if so, it is characteristically on a sporadic basis and at a level far below his intellectual capabilities. In effect, rather than restructuring a world with which he cannot cope, he remains in it but psychologically apart from it.

2. *Hebephrenic:* The hebephrenic's behavior may best be characterized as silly, disorganized and stereotypically juvenile. It is punctuated by giggling, which seems to the observer to be inappropriate, by posturings and usually bizarre mannerisms, by hallucinations and by delusions—often including delusions of somatic changes. Also characteristic are rather incoherent speech patterns, including expressions of the hallucinations and delusions. There may be episodes of anger or sadness, though such sadness often appears both inappropriate and superficial.

3. *Catatonic:* While delusions and hallucinations are a part of catatonic schizophrenia, probably the most obvious overt manifestations are found in the individual's mode of behavior. This behavior may range from an agitated state not unlike the hyperactivity seen in manic reactions (although it appears more disorganized and bizarre than catatonic reactions) to the mute, immobilized state (comparable to a stupor), which we tend commonly to associate with catatonic reactions. In either case, both the delusions and hallucinations tend to be persecutory and frightening and/or fraught with mysticism. A single individual may display both agitation and immobilization, sometimes shifting from one to the other rather abruptly, in a response to no apparent external stimulus. This potential shift should be kept in mind by treatment personnel.
4. *Paranoid:* As mentioned earlier, this subtype of schizophrenia is similar to true paranoia with its persecutory or grandiose delusions and delusions of reference. However, hallucinations (most frequently auditory) are common in paranoid schizophrenia and, generally, support in some way the individual's delusions. Also, there are differences in the delusions of the true paranoid and the paranoid schizophrenic. Quantitatively, in the latter, they include a larger portion of his time in life; qualitatively, in the paranoid schizophrenic, delusions are more clearly unrealistic, containing more mystical components, and are less well organized.
5. *Schizo-affective:* Again, there are similarities to either mania or psychotic depression, but with the schizo-affective disorders (which may be either *basically* manic or depressive), behavior is typically less well organized, delusions tend to be more prevalent or at least more bizarre and hallucinations are common.

Considering schizophrenia, in general, then, all three classes of behavioral manifestation associated with the psychoses—delusions, hallucinations and inappropriate affect—are found in schizophrenia in varying degrees, with hallucinations having a more permanent role than in any other class of psychosis.

The onset of schizophrenia is usually gradual. Even where it appears to be sudden or acute, the pre-schizophrenic generally has a history of making various attempts at adapting. Such attempts may take a variety of forms and offer an example of what is called symptom contamination. They may include the individual's having experienced feelings of estrangement or depersonalization as in dissociative reactions; his having tended to excessive ritualism or rumination as in obsessive-compulsive reactions; his having displayed phobic reactions (even if to largely imaginary threats); his having expressed or experienced strong feelings of apprehension, hyperactivity or generally vague somatic complaints as in anxiety reactions; or, in some cases, his having exhibited transitory conversion reactions. In some cases, suicide is attempted.

This does not imply that schizophrenia, or any other psychosis, should be represented as an exacerbated neurosis. More accurately, it represents the inadequacy of neurotic efforts to offset psychotic breakdown.

The defenses employed by the schizophrenic are not easily listed, as a variety of mechanisms may be used at different points in the course of his behavioral disturbance. However, excessive and, hence, inappropriate use is characteristically made of denial, projection and introjection. For example, there may be denial of actual conflicts or perceived threats and of greater or lesser amounts of reality, replaced by a reconstructed reality representing, basically, projections of conflictive material and introjection of persons or situations outside one's self.

Separating self from other aspects of the environment is characteristically difficult for the schizophrenic, and his behavioral manifestations may be viewed largely as an attempt to establish and maintain *some* type of selfhood, so as to avoid a threatened plunge into non-identity.

Schizophrenia is not necessarily as hopeless as it is sometimes construed to be. However, its treatment is difficult; in part because of the attitudes and needs some have to deny that something is wrong, thereby treating the pre-schizophrenic's behavior lightly, or allowing it to go seemingly unnoticed or unrecognized (although, of course, this can also be caused by lack of sufficient contact with the person or insufficient knowledge). Treatment is also difficult, because of the degree of personality disorganization involved, as well as present professional knowledge and methodological limitations. With respect to this last limitation, schizophrenia is probably the most written about of the psychological disturbances and, simultaneously, one of the least understood.

There are those who contend that its ideology is biogenic, its roots lying in the brain chemistry changes that are manifestations of inherited, or at least congenital, predispositions. Various studies (including the introduction of such psychomimetic drugs as LSD) have lent credence to the idea of chemical components. However, in evaluating these studies, at least two cautions should be kept in mind. First, they are usually correlational; and, second, they are after the fact (that is, they employ subjects already diagnosed as schizophrenics, so that even where a control group of non-schizophrenics is also used, one cannot be entirely sure whether chemical differences were an effect of the psychosis or vice-versa). In any event, one does not typically find even the avid biogenic theorists arguing for the inevitability of schizophrenia; rather, the contention is that some persons have a predisposition to it, given sufficient environmental stress.

Others contend that its ideology is psychogenic, arising from severe infantile conflicts, the overuse of essentially primitive defenses and the failure to develop other coping devices adequate to meet current stress, anxiety or frustration. Here, any definitively established chemical components need not be denied, but, rather, placed in a somewhat different time frame.

Whatever the *basic* source of its ideology, schizophrenia is seen by quite a few people in terms of its being essentially a perceptual disturbance (analagous to Bleuler's idea of disturbances and associations). Certainly, there is some behavioral evidence for such a view; evidence seen, for example, in the schizophrenic's delusions, inappropriate affect and hallucinations, which typically involve a combination of perceptual narrowing and distortion. Such evidence is also seen in the schizophrenic's verbalizations, which frequently include rhyming, neologisms and indications of a peculiar non-sequitur logic pattern, which may be incomprehensible to a listener.

Finally, again, whatever the basic source of schizophrenic ideology, the schizophrenic's childhood experiences frequently include his having had inadequate opportunities to establish a meaningful sense of autonomy and selfhood, his having grown up in a rather pathological family situation where his early identifications were themselves disturbed and/or where other family members apparently maintained their own rather shaky adjustment by "choosing" this individual as a scapegoat onto whom they could displace their own symptoms. Also frequently found is the schizophrenic's having characteristically been placed in so-called "double-bind" situations where he was the recipient of conflicting messages (sometimes from the same person), so that he would somehow be wrong whatever his behavioral choice. An example of a "double-bind" would be the mother who wants her youngster to grow to be a successful physician, but, at the same time, argues against his leaving the home to attend college for that purpose. Under any of these circumstances, of course, it would be difficult to learn adequate perceptual discriminations.

With repeated situations such as this, and, frequently, a long history of pathological communication of varying types, the individual's feelings of low self-esteem, rejection, ambivalence and lack of identity are reinforced. When he reaches the adolescent stage of psycho-social development, he has a poor foundation on which to resolve his identity crisis. As he moves into early adulthood—the stage Erikson describes as "intimacy versus isolation"—he will probably be very guarded, as he attempts to establish meaningful relationships outside the home. The person with such a history has considerable difficulty establishing a truly intimate relationship, in which he can give as well as accept love. His feelings of loneliness tend to be extreme, and his lack of coping devices leaves him unarmed for alternate ways of dealing with the pain of severe alienation and extreme loneliness.

SUMMARY

These are the major categories of psychotic behavior. Eschewing such clearly inadequate explanations of such behavior as demon possession or deliberate, conscious choice to "sin" in the context of unmitigated free will, an attempt is made to balance both the traditional medical model and the somewhat newer socio-psychological or learning model viewpoints of abnormality.

Perhaps such an attempt tends to be confusing. Hopefully, it provides an opportunity for contrast and comparison, for viewing a field in transition and for thinking through the arguments and implications on your own, rather than simply adopting someone else's particular frame of reference as "incontrovertible fact"—perhaps only to be replaced by a new, equally superficial set of "incontrovertible facts" on any subsequent exposure.

It is not the purpose of this chapter to discuss in any detail the psychoses which are clearly organic in origin. However, a note regarding treatment of these psychoses is appropriate. Characteristically, and unfortunately, these psychotic persons have been relegated to the back wards, receiving only minimal maintenance treatment. However, there have been some exceptions to this rule. Where exceptions have occurred, evidence indicates that providing as normal as possible an environment and rewarding adaptive behavior can increase the individual's ability to cope. Perhaps the increase is not sufficient to permit him to function in the outside community; but it is sufficient to allow him to function more effectively, more humanly and more humanely in the institutional setting. Before proceeding to an example of nursing management, it would be appropriate to mention some basic relevant psychological principles.

Anxiety, stress and/or frustration have been mentioned as precipitating or exacerbating factors in the development of psychoses. Each person is subject to these factors, and each has a different level of tolerance at different times and in varying settings. Following the Yerkes-Dodson (Cofer, 1964) law, these factors produce what is called an inverted U-shaped curve vis-a-vis performance. That is, in the absence of anxiety, etc., performance tends to be at a minimal level. As anxiety, stress or frustration increase so does performance, up to a point. However, as any or all of these factors increase beyond that maximal point (which again varies from individual to individual), the adequacy of performance again approaches a base or minimal level. One's perceptual field is narrowed. That is, one is less capable of seeing behavioral options available to him. In accordance with the empirical law of effect, we *do* tend to repeat responses which are perceived as having been reinforced in the past in comparable situations. Given the narrowing of the perceptual field, situations which are, in fact, not similar may come to be perceived so through a process of overgeneralization. Thus, we seek to use a relatively minimal number of coping devices over and over again. Frequently, these are inappropriate to the situation, and their overuse only worsens matters. The outcome may be a variety of psychological disorders, including a psychotic episode. An important part of treatment, therefore, lies in reinforcing adaptive responses, ignoring maladaptive responses to the extent possible and helping the individual to see that he does have other options—that is, helping to broaden his perceptual field.

NURSING MANAGEMENT

As noted in Chapter 6, nursing management on a psychiatric unit would include collecting a viable data base, identifying problems and preparing a plan of action to care for the patient.

A problem list for a person diagnosed as a paranoid schizophrenic, for example, could include any or all of the following:

1. feelings of loneliness
2. feelings of fear, threat and/or being watched (monitored)
3. feelings of unrealness
4. thoughts that inanimate objects are communicating
5. unpredictability of behavior, affect and/or cognitive processes
6. sleep disturbances
7. reduced food/fluid intake and/or
8. difficulty in maintaining a therapeutic relationship.

Once the problem list has been established, nursing actions are planned. The nurse must remember that both these components—i.e., identifying the problems and making a plan—must be periodically assessed and updated to keep current and appropriate to the patient's behavioral changes. Hopefully, behaviors will be modified, given that the nursing approach is accurate for any given patient.

1. Feelings of loneliness
   Plan: The nurse must be able to accept her own feelings of loneliness, before she can assist the lonely person to begin overcoming such feelings. Be honest with the patient, so that he can begin a trusting relationship. By doing this, the nurse provides a conducive atmosphere which will allow the patient an opportunity to begin feeling more comfortable and to express the painful feelings of loneliness. Also, the art of *active* listening is of utmost importance with the lonely person. The nurse can further convey to the patient that at least one person recognizes his painful feelings by carefully listening to his overt, as well as his covert communication. Again, the nurse should be aware of her feelings, as the patient begins to express his discomfort at feelings of loneliness, abandonment, remoteness, alienation, desertion and/or inability to relate to others.

2. Feelings of fear, threat and/or being watched (monitored)

Plan: The feelings of fear, threat or being monitored may cause the patient to behave as the withdrawn patient or the agitated patient. Since nursing action for the withdrawn patient has been discussed previously, this section will deal with the delusional suspicions and the agitated person.

The highly suspicious patient may be convinced that the nursing staff is involved in a conspiracy with the family, friends and/or doctor to do him harm—that one or more of these persons is "out to get him." In other words, his environment is hostile and threatening as he perceives it. Initially, the nursing care plan would keep staff contact to a minimum. As the patient improves, this approach, of course, would not be applicable. Minimum contact here would involve short interaction, while helping the patient meet the basic human needs in a consistent and matter-of-fact manner. Examples include giving simple and concise explanations of the routine procedures of the unit. Staff would limit physical contact, give direction in terms of what is expected of the patient, allow him a choice of activities and, above all, avoid laughing, whispering or talking quietly where the patient can see but cannot hear what is being said. Again, as with all patients, staff must be honest and keep promises to him. For instance, should the nurse promise to have lunch with him and, for some reason, find herself unable to do so, she must personally tell him this or, if that is impossible, get the message to him by another staff member. The past experiences of this person have reinforced his feelings of not trusting others, so the nurse's actions should help to break this cycle of reinforcement.

Some patients feel sufficiently threatened that they may actually request to sleep in a secure area, such as a seclusion room. Remembering that these beliefs are very real to the patient, the nurse should make every effort to assist him in feeling safe. As discussed earlier in this chapter, the patient may respond to his anxious feelings either by withdrawing from the situation or becoming agitated and hyperactive in an effort to reduce anxiety. The agitated patient can be very challenging for the nursing staff and, perhaps, frightening to the other patients. His behavior would typically include any or all of the following: increased verbal and motor activity, flight of ideas, combativeness, belligerence, short attention span, over-reaction to stimuli, the use of obscene language and/or uninhibited sexual interests, being demanding in terms of attention and giving little attention to physical needs (such as grooming, elimination, nutrition, or rest and sleep which can lead to exhaustion).

The nursing care plan for the agitated person would be essentially to provide a minimally stimulating atmosphere. This would include such things as eliminating bright colors from his environment; reducing loud noises; providing a quiet area; avoiding arguments; being consistent, concise, matter of fact and honest; avoiding detailed and lengthy discussions and explanations; letting the patient know what is expected of him; avoiding hurrying him or getting caught up in his "games"; and preventing his playing one staff member against another. It is oftentimes well to assign one staff person to such a patient to assure a consistent approach in helping to calm him. The patient should be provided with non-competitive activities, which can be accomplished successfully in short periods of time, to reduce his anxiety. Large groups should be avoided, and the nurse should assist and encourage the patient's personal grooming. Finally, so long as the patient is not physically combative, he should be allowed to verbalize his feelings of hostility, fear and/or entrapment without punitive or judgmental reactions from the staff.

3. Feelings of unrealness
Plan: Feelings of unrealness may include a variety of somatic delusions, such as the patient's believing that he has no heart, that his intestines have turned to wood or stone, that he has snakes in his stomach, that he is suffering from mixed gender or any other modification of body parts. Again, it is important to point out that these strong but less well-organized delusional systems are extremely real to this person. Consequently, it is futile to attempt to disprove his delusions at that point in time. Rather, the nurse should plan care for this patient to include ignoring the delusions and instructing him not to discuss them with others. This is a form of limit setting, which he needs at this time. The entire staff needs to be aware of this stretching of limits to assure consistency of approach. Without supporting his delusions per se, it is possible to give the patient support, conveying to him that you care and are aware of his feelings of

discomfort. Another helpful part of the plan for the person experiencing feelings of unrealness is to encourage him to tell you the meaning of his communications, preferably in an "uncrazy way," so that the nurse can better understand what he is feeling and experiencing. Diversionary activities are helpful here, to assist the patient to move from his self-centered position to a more integrated status, where he will begin interactions more appropriate to the environment. At first, one-to-one contacts, moving to small groups are useful; then moving to larger groups, participating in games which are non-threatening with a low competitive profile (such as jigsaw puzzles) are also helpful.

4. Thoughts that inanimate objects are communicating
Plan: For the hallucinating patient, the nurse would also need to reduce sensory stimuli avoiding, for example, loud sounds, psychedelic colors, abstract paintings and the nurses own body language, which might "feed" into the hallucinatory process. A structured environment should be provided, with as little change in routine as possible, and explanations given when deviations from expected routine are necessary. Try to question the patient about what happened just prior to his hallucinations and distract him to something real, if he appears to be hallucinating. Avoid agreeing with him that the voices are real or arguing that they are not real; convey to him that they are real for him, but that you do not see or hear what he does.

Avoid disrespectful comments. Rather, if the "voices" are commanding him to harm himself or others, provide a safe environment. Probably most important of all is to discourage the patient from alienating others or withdrawing from them. This can be done by having staff spend short periods of time with him and at close intervals, at first. As he progresses, more interactions with groups and involvement with real objects, such as are provided in occupational therapy, can be most helpful.

5. Unpredictability of behavior, affect and/or cognitive processes
Plan: Possibly the most important aspect of caring for the patient with unpredictable behavior is the nurse's awareness and control of her own feelings. She should be calm and cautious but not demonstrate overt fright. Also, she should not react with shock or disdain to verbal abuses. Often, these hostile attitudes are not personalized but, rather, are expressions of anx-

iety, fear and hostility actually directed to others. Even where such expressions are personalized, reacting inappropriately only reinforces them.

The plan for these patients would include letting them know when their behavior is *not* appropriate; assisting them to find alternate ways of behavior that are more socially acceptable and personally adaptive; observing behavior so that subsequent outbursts can be predicted and avoided; assisting the patient to gain control as soon as possible by removing him from the situation; diverting his attention by calling his name in a low, firm, calm but authoritative tone; spending time with him, when it is not inappropriate and giving him an opportunity to verbalize his feelings regarding the restrictions imposed on him. In short, redirect his energy toward more acceptable activities. Critical to nursing care for this and all patients, is giving of oneself in terms of time, attention and interest. This does not mean that the nurse must necessarily like the patient as an individual, and, certainly, it does not mean that she needs to accept his inappropriate behavior. Rather, it means to relate to the individual as a human being who has potential worth and growth orientation.

6. Sleep disturbances
Plan: The nurse should keep records of the sleep patterns of all patients, especially of those experiencing or expressing difficulty in sleeping. Obviously, these records are best obtained by an observant nursing staff, who conscientiously observes and records relevant data. The records are important to the attending physician, who has the basic responsibility for determining if sleep medication is indicated. Nursing action includes such physical measures as providing non-stimulating drinks (preferably warm), providing a light snack (such as crackers, toast, or custard), straightening the bed, regulating the temperature and light in the room whenever possible and giving warm baths. The nurse may find it helpful to sit by the patient's bed, assuring him that she will continue to check to see how he is sleeping. As with any suspicious person, provide the patient with as safe an environment as possible. For example, with his permission, lock the door to his room or offer a secluded area where he will feel secure. These measures convey

to the patient that you recognize his psychological state and are willing to assist him in meeting his need for sleep.

7. Reduced food/fluid intake
Plan: The question of lack of nourishment is discussed in Chapter 7, "Depression and Suicidal Behavior." However, the highly suspicious person may become particularly malnourished if part of his delusional system is the conviction that food and drinks offered are poisoned. Again, close surveillance of the patient's eating habits is maintained by the nursing staff in cooperation with the attending physician. The nurse avoids tasting foods and/or medications for the patient. Medication may need to be administered intramuscularly rather than orally, again in collaboration with the attending physician. It is often helpful to sit with the patient, while he eats, to encourage his socialization and to begin a trusting relationship. By spending such time with the patient, the nurse can convey to him that he is a worthwhile person, and that someone does care.

8. Difficulty in maintaining a therapeutic relationship
Plan: This can be the most difficult problem for the nurse to deal with, especially if she is not aware of her own feelings, or if she is uninformed regarding the dynamics of the patient's condition. The effective nurse should be aware of the changing behavior of the patient and, as previously indicated, be able to accept personal verbal abuse appropriately. How the nurse responds to the patient's remarks and behavior is very important. In addition to being in touch with her own feelings, having a sufficient knowledge base and being aware of changes in the patient's behavior, the nurse needs an opportunity to express some of her own feelings of inadequacy, failure and frustration. This can be done by talking with the physician responsible for the patient, by conferring with the supervisor and/or by sharing problems with other nursing staff at regularly scheduled sessions. As suggested earlier, maintaining a therapeutic relationship requires consistency, concern and an authoritative (though not authoritarian or judgmental) demeanor. It also requires an ability to function effectively in an atmosphere of few, if any, immediate rewards. The nurse cannot be expected to carry the burden of a therapeutic milieu alone, but at least for the hos-

pitalized patient, such a milieu cannot be maintained without her intelligent and willing cooperation.

CASE STUDY: PSYCHOSIS

Mary, a 57-year-old white female, was involuntarily committed to the psychiatric unit of a general hospital for a 60-day observation period. Court action was taken by her husband, Glen, following her apparent attempt to poison their youngest child. Glen subsequently sought protective custody from local juvenile authorities. He had initiated commitment proceedings fourteen years prior to this episode, but, even though two psychiatrists agreed that Mary was certifiable, he did not follow through because of concern for the "family image."

Mary, the youngest of four children, grew up outside a small northern city. Her mother died of typhoid fever when Mary was an adolescent, and no information was available regarding the mother's other history or behavior. Mary's father, although an alcoholic, was a good provider and an excellent craftsman. No information was available pertaining to Mary's behavior as a child or adolescent.

After finishing high school, she moved to a large city where she worked as a clerk for two years. In an unknown way, she "got religion" and moved to another large city, where she enrolled in a fundamentalist Bible College. While there, she met and married Glen, a Polish immigrant.

Mary became pregnant almost immediately and gave birth to a son, Ed. Shortly after Ed's birth, the family traveled to Eastern Europe as missionaries. Approximately eighteen months later, a second son, Perry, was born; reportedly, it was a difficult birth for Mary. The family remained in Europe for another year, returning to the United States shortly after the 1929 "crash."

Subsequently, Mary's relatives indicated that she seemed "strange" after the family's return to this country, although no one offered any specific examples of this "strange" behavior.

Glen had difficulty obtaining adequate employment, since (for reasons never expressed) he had decided to leave the ministry. Glen and Mary were reportedly beginning to experience marital difficulties and decided to have another child to help "cement" their relationship. This child was a girl named Helen.

When Helen was about 2 years old, the family relationship seriously deteriorated. The eldest son, Ed, had already gotten into difficulty with the authorities and had been placed in a foster home. Later, he was to get into even more difficulty, spending some time in a reform school and eventually being placed in another foster home setting. At about the same time, Perry (the second child), ran away from home following a severe beating by Mary. Perry was also placed in a foster home.

Glen, who was basically a passive personality, left home after the boys had been placed and after he had failed to follow through with Mary's commitment. The daughter, Helen, was left with the mother.

Helen remained in the home until she was 16 years old. Ed married and left the area. Perry was killed in World War II. Glen attempted to maintain contact and, unrealistically, rebuild the family unit. This meant fairly frequent contacts with Mary and Helen, each contact culminating in a public display of verbal and/or physical abuse to either Glen or Helen on the part of Mary.

Over the years, Mary had developed a pseudo-community of attackers. This pseudo-community was comprised primarily of Glen, Helen and Perry, who were somehow a part of an alleged "Communist conspiracy." Since she was basically an in contact paranoic, Mary also tried to involve other people in her delusional system. To some extent, she was successful, at least in garnering both sympathy and money—especially from her older sister, local merchants and churches.

Somewhat typically, Mary maintained a strong religious orientation while, at the same time, exhibiting extreme obscenity. For example, regarding Glen, she would frequently threaten to "cut off his Jesus and stuff it in his mouth." While these periods of mixed religion and blasphemy were somewhat unpredictable, they invariably occurred during the Christmas and Easter seasons. Mary remained a constant church-goer and was particularly fascinated by a popular evangelist. At the same time, she would strike the daughter for making "unholy" remarks on the way to church and would make such comments as, "Godammit, shut up! The Holy Spirit is coming!" during evangelistic meetings. It was unclear whether this simultaneous blasphemy and religious affiliation exemplified virtually complete compartmentalization on Mary's part or whether it represented deliberate manipulation. She never spoke in an obscene way in front of religious representatives, and, as noted, she had been successful in gaining financial assistance from them.

At the time of her hospitalization, Mary was physically belligerent, convinced that she was the target of her "Communist" pseudo-community and vacillated between religious or quasi-religious behavior and lascivious verbal communications.

Much of the background information on Mary came from Helen, who even though having undergone some trauma, was evaluated as competent and objective by both psychologists and a psychiatrist, after turning to the juvenile authorities. Once Glen had followed through on the commitment, he withdrew from further cooperation. For whatever reasons, Ed and other members of Mary's family refused to become involved.

Nursing Management

In a case such as this, nursing intervention is predicated on the acknowledgment of several factors. For example, each individual— no matter how strange, offensive or unpredictable his behavior may be—*is* an individual with potential strengths, as well as demonstrated weaknesses. Too often, helping professionals tend to concentrate on the weaknesses. Relatedly, it is important to be able to accept the person as an individual, which does *not* necessarily mean accepting or condoning his behavior. This is a vital, yet for many, a difficult, distinction.

Also, in a case such as this, it is important to remember that the patient may not be hospitalized beyond the 60-day period. This possibility carries with it several implications. The medical staff cannot depend on any meaningful "insight" on the patient's part. This is true, because of the relatively short time-frame and the patient's history of a basically strong delusional system. Consequently, there is a need for a more "now" oriented intervention effort.

Finally, the nurse must recognize that her endeavors may best be aimed at helping to maintain a current, even though inadequate, level of functioning. The nurse must also be prepared to accept the fact that she may never know the ultimate outcome of such potentially short-term intervention.

Nursing Problems

Problems potentially attendant to Mary's involuntary commitment as an apparent paranoic could include any or all of the following, and, as indicated previously, these problems and plans for Mary's care should follow general basic principles in order to modify behavior of the psychotic patient.

Problem List

1. Manipulative behavior
2. Abusive or violent physical behavior
3. Obscene or abusive verbal behavior
4. Persecutory delusions
5. Relative lack of knowledge regarding historically relevant socio-psychological dynamics (e.g., childhood and adolescent experience, as well as experiences while in Eastern Europe)

1. Manipulative behavior

Plan: Mary had a propensity for involving others in her delusional system by exploiting others, playing one person against another, using self-pity, finding others' weaknesses and being charming and convincing, when necessary.

This type of behavior, at best, is challenging to the nursing staff and requires consistency, firmness and open communication among staff members. The initial approach would include such actions as: being alert to the fact that Mary's behavior may be an attempt at manipulation, while avoiding reading such attempts into her behavior; letting Mary know you are aware of what she is doing (*if* you are); helping her examine what she is doing and what she is getting from that behavior; accepting no favors or gifts from her; being aware of your own feelings regarding the patient's behavior, including anxiety, discomfort and/or hostility; letting Mary know what is expected of her in a matter-of-fact and concrete way, without being judgmental; giving her both verbal and nonverbal reinforcement for appropriate behavior; and, finally, helping her give up old behavior by learning more adaptive ways of dealing with her environment.

2. Abusive or violent physical behavior

Plan: The abusive or violent patient can be frightening to personnel on a psychiatric unit, and the initial response to such behaviors is often punitive or authoritarian. This is not therapeutic for the patient. Helpful approaches to the agitated patient include the following: redirect rather than control violent behavior (e.g., provide punching dolls or batik sticks to allow a release of physical aggression); encourage rather than demand cooperation, yet be able to provide non-punitive solitary restraint when or if necessary; help the patient learn alternative ways of reaching out for attention; allow her opportunities and encouragement in verbalizing angry, lonely, stressful or hostile feelings, so long as she does not talk "crazy" or threateningly; recognize one's own feelings of fear, anger, frustration or inadequacy; and finally, be explicit in defining boundaries to insure safety of others.

3. Obscene or abusive verbal behavior

Plan: Again, a very important aspect of dealing with behavior of this type is that the nurse recognize that this may be the patient's way of expressing feelings, often related in the paranoic, towards himself. However, such language may also, or alternately, reflect the linguistic environment in which the patient grew up and may be more socially offensive than psychologically pathological. Also, the patient may well have found reinforcement from her use of such language to the extent that it appeared to intimidate others or, at least, made them uncomfortable. The staff must further be aware that the comments directed toward them are not always personalized; rather, they are forms of behavior the patient has learned which have worked for him in the past.

Things to remember when working with a patient such as Mary could include: letting her know what is expected in terms of acceptable behavior; attempting to identify clues which trigger such behavior; encouraging opportunities for verbalization of feelings without being judgmental; being explicit in expectations of her; and refusing to spend time with her when language is unacceptable or inappropriate. The staff should refrain from giving verbal or nonverbal cues that they are upset (e.g., shocked or threatened) by such language. If the patient's obscene or abusive behavior has been previously reinforced, for whatever reasons, non-emotional reactions tend to extinguish it more than any other single response on the part of the staff.

4. Persecutory delusions

Plan: As previously discussed in this chapter, these false beliefs are difficult for the patient to give up and from her perspective are real. However, this type of behavior can be somewhat effectively dealt with, although it does take considerable time and skill. Some of the following can give guidance to the nursing staff in dealing with the delusional patient such as Mary: within reason, give the patient the opportunity for making as many decisions for herself as possible; make it clear that these decisions are her responsibility, and that intervention will occur if their results are significantly deleterious to herself or others; avoid whispering and incomplete explanations; avoid argumentative discussions, even if this means terminating the conversations if noncontroversial redirection is not possible; respect the intellectual ability of the patient as you would any other patient; assist her in accepting the responsibility for her own behavior; be matter-of-fact, honest, sincere and show an interest in her as a worthwhile individual; attempt to avoid over-interpreting or under-interpreting potential relevant feelings that may be, or seem to be, obscured in the overt content of the message; assist her in developing feelings of security by being consistent; and, finally, avoid being caught up in her delusional system.

5. Relative lack of knowledge regarding history

Plan: The biggest problem in having inadequate information lies in the possibility that the nursing staff may actually further reinforce the patient's maladaptive behavior (e.g., by failing to recognize delusional aspects of the cognitive system and being overly attentive and/or sympathetic to them).

In Mary's case, and it is not an isolated one, it is unlikely that substantive historical information will become available, at least during a 60-day period. However, some of the following guidelines could be initiated: depending on the setting, the patient-care coordinator might confer with the examining psychologist and share this information with the staff, although the results of psychological testing are frequently more accurately indicative of current conditions than of past situations; similar conferences might be held with the attending psychiatrist; additionally, personnel attending change of shift report could share with one another any historical information provided by Mary. *However,* this would be done not in any real effort to discover the "truth" but rather to determine under what circumstances the patient "shared" particular types of information.

The staff could use this in an effort to identify attempted manipulation and/or inappropriate reinforcement—but, again, confabulation on the staff's part should be avoided.

An important difficulty lies in defining this relative lack of background knowledge as a problem. In medical-surgical settings (e.g., the triage situation), the nurse must frequently make decisions and take actions with little or no medical history. In many instances, the psychiatric nurse must accept a similar situation and the requisite responsibility. This may be discomforting, but it may also have some potential advantages. The staff approaches the patient with minimal preconceptions and must deal with the important question of where the patient is and may be going, rather than with where she is perceived as having come from.

BIBLIOGRAPHY

Almore, M.G. Personal communication. (Classnotes. Univ. of Texas at Arlington. "Deviant Behavior." October, 1976).

Cofer, C.N., and Appley, M.H. *Motivation: Theory and Research*. New York: John Wiley & Sons, Inc., 1964.

Erikson, E.H. *Childhood and Society*. 2d ed. New York: W.W. Norton and Co., 1963.

Rosen, E., Gregory, I., and Fox, R.E. *Abnormal Psychology*. 2d ed. Philadelphia: W.B. Saunders Co., 1972.

CHAPTER 13

Organic Brain Syndromes

Judith R. Lentz, R. N., M.S.N.

INTRODUCTION

The terms "organic brain syndrome" (Pincus and Tucker, 1974; Detre and Jarecki, 1971) and "organic psychosis" (Kyes and Hofling, 1974; Matthews and Miller, 1975) represent disturbances in previously normal or unimpaired mental functioning. These acquired disorders in perceptual and cognitive function can arise in any of six general categories: (1) Organic insult (physical and/or chemical), (2) Sensory monotony, (3) Sensory overload, (4) Sleep and dream deprivation, (5) Immobilization and (6) Overwhelming anxiety (Heller and Kornfeld, 1975). These causes suggest that organic brain syndromes are not necessarily a result of actual damage to brain tissue but can be manifested by functional interruptions or alterations in the individual's relationships or environment. When two or more causes unite, the clinical picture of organic brain syndrome becomes more florid. In fact, more subtle organic brain syndromes are often discovered only after they become compounded. The focus of treatment or management of organic brain syndromes may be directed toward the removal or prevention of compounding causes.

In view of this expanding scope and knowledge, organic brain syndromes are no longer the domain of the neurologists. Psychiatrists, psychologists, internists, nurses, occupational therapists, as well as most other health care givers are beginning to recognize OBS as a factor affecting, even determining, care of numerous physical and psychological anomalies. One prominent psychiatrist suggested that, by far, the majority of hospitalized psychiatric patients not only have psychological and interpersonal conflicts but have some measurable degree of organic brain impairment. Although not systematically studied, Blevler et al. suggest that 30 percent of routinely hospitalized patients suffer some detectable degree of organic brain impairment (Heller and Kornfeld, 1975).

ORGANIC BRAIN SYNDROMES

Diagnosis

Diagnosis of organic brain syndrome involves the evaluation of the following cognitive functions (Pincus and Tucker, 1974): (1) perception, (2) memory, (3) orientation, (4) verbal, spatial and numerical ability, (5) level of consciousness, and (6) changes in personality. Although each of these cognitive functions is dealt with separately, disturbances may involve one or any combination of these cerebral functions. When more than one area of function is involved, the degree of dysfunction in each may vary dramatically in severity.

Perception

Perception is an active intellectual process closely related to sensory components of cerebral function. Perception includes activities necessary to filter, modify and integrate sensations with one another successfully and with the individual's previous experience (Lezak, 1976). Organic perceptual defects can occur indirectly through loss or impairment of primary input or through defects of a specific integrative process. In the organically impaired, sensation and perception become unrelated, each having its own function integrity. This disorganization leads to a group of defects commonly referred to as the agnosias (Lezak, 1976). Examples of agnosias would include the inability to recognize familiar faces or distinguish unfamiliar faces.

Memory

Memory remains an often unappreciated key to human behavior. It frees one from dependency on physiological urges or situational happenstance for pleasure. Memory impairment isolates one proportionately from meaningful contact with the world, depriving him of a sense of personal continuity and rendering him passive, bland and dependent (Lezak, 1976).

Memory is clinically divided into three interdependent components: immediate or recent, recent past and remote past. According to Lezak, registration is the process by which content enters the memory system. It involves the programming for learning sensory response patterns and focusing attention. If the information in the registration process is not quickly transferred to short-term (immediate or recent past) memory, recall of the information quickly fades.

Immediate memory is aptly referred to as the "working memory" (Lezak, 1976). This first stage of memory is concerned with the fixation of information selected for retention by the registration process. By the process of rehearsal, an immediate memory can be maintained for hours (Lezak, 1976).

Recent work suggests that immediate memory is temporarily maintained in self-contained neural networks that sustain the memory in the form of a nerve impulse by channeling it repeatedly through the same network (Lezak, 1976). Longer term memory functions are dependent on conversion into a more stable biochemical organization. If this transformation does not take place, the immediate memory traces spontaneously dissipate, resulting in loss of the memory.

Recent past or short-term memory lasts for a few hours to a few days. Content in this stage of memory is not yet permanently fixed, making it more vulnerable to interference. There appears to be a time factor in the establishment of long-term memories. Recent theories postulate (Lezak, 1976) that longer term memory storage is a biochemical process involving transformation of protein configurations in cortical nerve cells. In conjunction, there is possibly a budding of new cell contact points, creating the transmission patterns between cells that constitute the long-term memory trace. These long-term memories seem to involve neural contributions from many and varied cortical and subcortical centers (Lezak, 1976).

Recent and remote memory are clinical terms used to differentiate memories occurring in the last hours, days, weeks or months from memories initiated years previously. For the normal person, it is impossible to delineate clearly the end of recent memory and the beginning of remote memory. In fact, even the most recent memories are intertwined with those dating to infancy. Only when one is considering organic brain syndromes do the concepts of recent and remote memory assume practical and meaningful aspects. In cases of organic disorder, impairment of the most recent of the remote memories may denote the approximate time of illness onset. In conjunction with various diseases and injuries, part or all of some aspects of memory may be lost, providing clues to both the origin and location of the lesion. In addition, a relationship exists between the severity of the brain disease and the impairment in remote memories. Lezak (1976), Detre and Jarecki (1971) and Pincus and Tucker (1974) report that the more severe the cortical damage, the more disrupted are remotely established memories and habits.

Orientation

Orientation, the awareness of self in relation to one's surrounding, has traditionally encompassed the dimensions of time, place and person. As expected, memory and perceptual functions play a prominent role in orientation. Defects in orientation are among the most frequent symptoms of brain disease.

Orientation for time is concerned not only with date, time of day, month or year, but it also includes the sense of temporal continuity. Temporal continuity deals with the awareness of the passage of time—how long and in what order events occur. Deficits in the ordering of events are often the initial symptoms, when one is experiencing disorientation (Detre and Jarecki, 1971).

Disorientation to place usually occurs as temporal disorientation progresses. Orientation for place includes an appreciation of location, direction and distance. Initially, symptoms are subtle, characterized by difficulty in locating or identifying new places. Progression of disorientation to place is characterized by difficulty locating and identifying previously familiar locations. In severe instances of disorientation, an inability to identify one's own address or present location (home, hospital, church) exists.

In extreme instances of disorientation, the realm of person is invaded. Initially, one has difficulty identifying persons around him, particularly "new people." Names are first forgotten, and, thereafter, the disoriented person's relationship to the particular individual. Not until nearly all intellectual function is grossly impaired, does one have difficulty identifying himself or remembering his own name (Detre and Jarecki, 1971). Thus, in terms of orientation, it is anticipated that losses occur in the following sequence: time, place, person (Table 13-1).

Verbal, Spatial and Numerical Ability

Thinking includes the cognitive functions of computation, reasoning, judgment, concept formation, abstracting, ordering, organizing and planning (Lezak, 1976).

> The nature of the information being mentally manipulated (e.g., numbers, design concepts, words) and the operation (e.g., comparing, compounding, abstracting, ordering) define the category of thinking. This "verbal reasoning" comprises several operations done with words; it generally includes ordering and comparing, sometimes analyzing and synthesizing. "Computation" may involve operations of ordering and compounding done with numbers, and distance judgment involves abstracting and comparing ideas of spatial extension (Lezak, 1976, p. 24).

Intellectual functions of abstraction, reasoning, judgment, analysis and synthesis are relatively sensitive to impairment, even when perceptive and memory functions remain intact. Disruptions in these functions are not closely related to specific anatomical lesions; generally, the process of thinking defies localization. However, the quality of intellectual functions depends partially on the degree to which cortical sensory and motor components are intact. Patients with somatosensory perceptual defects are likely to perform poorly on reasoning tasks involving visuospatial concepts. Patients with perceptual difficulties of the visual system are likely to have difficulty utilizing visual concepts (Lezak, 1976; Luria, 1973). Verbal defects tend to be the most obvious defect and have the broadest consequences. Disturbances in verbal systems can disrupt one's ability to follow task instructions, interfere with self-regulation and self-critiquing mechanisms and preclude ideational systems.

Apraxias involve the impairments of voluntary action, even though the capacity for adequate muscle intervention is intact. These dysfunctions or disabilities tend to cluster and are often associated with a particular sensory impairment. Apraxias involving

TABLE 13-1
Organic Brain Syndromes

Symptom	Degree of Organic Impairment		
	Mild	Moderate	Severe
Dysmnesia	Decreased efficiency in absorbing and retaining information	Difficulty remembering events of the recent past but accurate and detailed recall of learning and events prior to onset of illness	
	May appear to be "absent-minded"		
	Compensation with increasingly rigid schedules and routines		
	Notebooks, calendars serve as memory aids	Attempts to compensate increasingly difficult leading to increased rigidity and compulsiveness; decreased intellectual grasp; slowed, more difficult and less effective thinking	Dysmnesia invades patient's past memory, extending further and further into the remote past until global
	Learning more difficult, but this is only evident by comparison with past learning capabilities		
		More difficulty arousing attention	

(Continued)

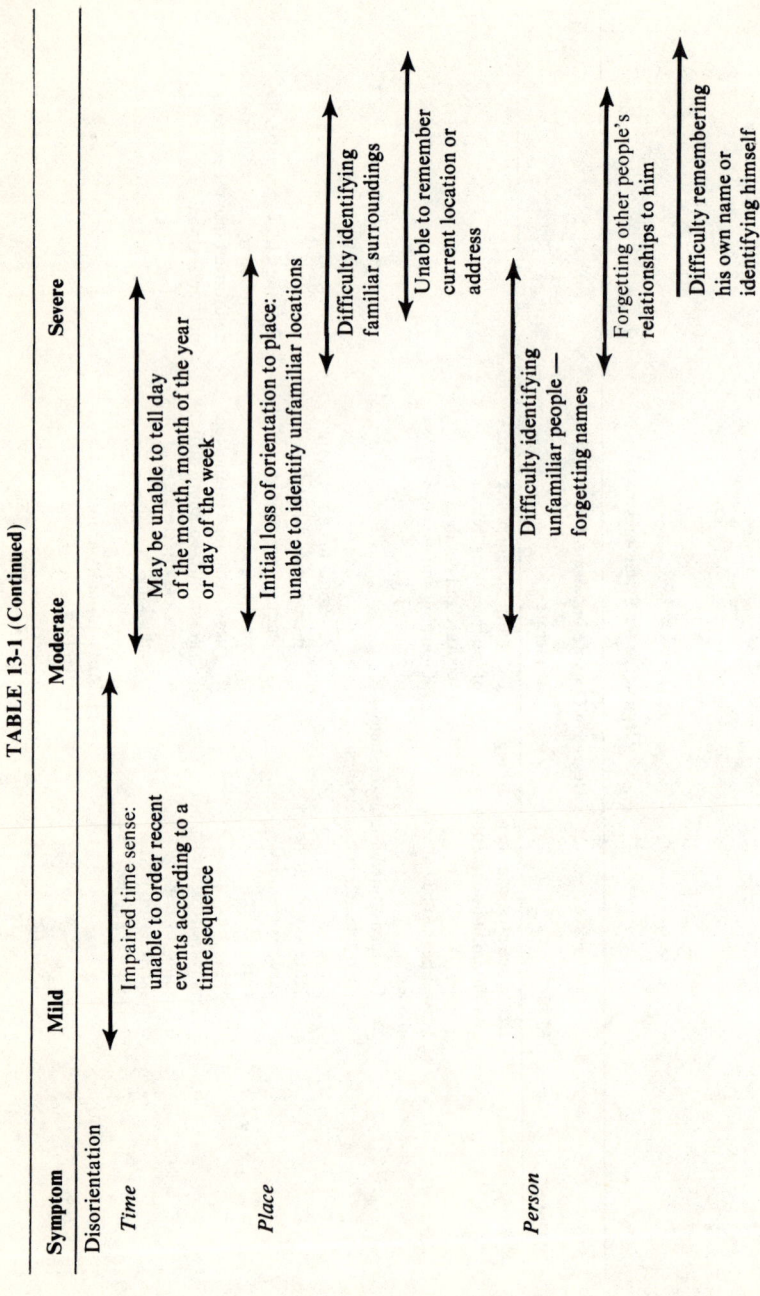

TABLE 13-1 (Continued)

Symptom	Mild	Moderate	Severe
Disorientation			
Time	Impaired time sense: unable to order recent events according to a time sequence ↑↓	May be unable to tell day of the month, month of the year or day of the week ↑↓	
Place		Initial loss of orientation to place: unable to identify unfamiliar locations ↑↓	Difficulty identifying familiar surroundings ↑↓ Unable to remember current location or address ↑↓
Person		Difficulty identifying unfamiliar people — forgetting names ↑↓	Forgetting other people's relationships to him ↑↓ Difficulty remembering his own name or identifying himself ↑↓

Symptom	Mild	Moderate	Severe
Difficulty with Abstract Reasoning	Mild and intermittent symptoms: 1. Inability to bear several factors in mind at the same time 2. Increased difficulty in seeing similarities and differences in similar objects (dwarf and child) 3. Increased difficulty explaining problems	← Only capable of concrete reasoning →	
		← Overlooks the obvious, judgment becomes suspect and decisions increasingly unreliable →	
		Behavior increasingly inappropriate which is often reflected in: 1. Deterioration of grooming 2. Deterioration of eating habits and manners 3. Neglected personal hygiene 4. Decreased ability to manage financial affairs	Unable to care for himself

(Continued)

TABLE 13-1 (Continued)

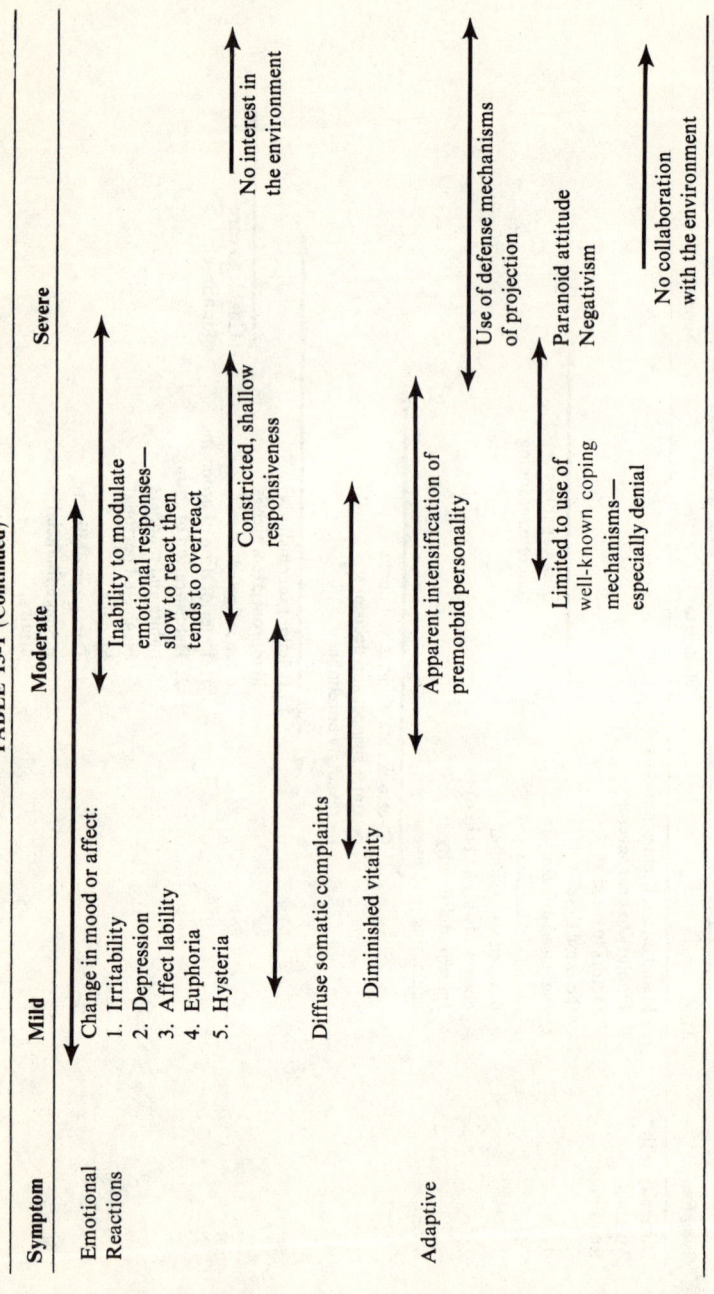

Symptom	Mild	Moderate	Severe
Emotional Reactions	Change in mood or affect: 1. Irritability 2. Depression 3. Affect lability 4. Euphoria 5. Hysteria	← Inability to modulate emotional responses—slow to react then tends to overreact →	
			Constricted, shallow responsiveness
	← Diffuse somatic complaints →		
	Diminished vitality →		No interest in the environment
Adaptive		Apparent intensification of premorbid personality	Use of defense mechanisms of projection
			Paranoid attitude Negativism
		Limited to use of well-known coping mechanisms—especially denial	
			No collaboration with the environment

the inability to use objects appropriately at will are commonly associated with lesions near or overlapping speech centers and are often accompanied by communication deficits (Luria, 1973; Lezak, 1976). Constructional apraxias are often associated with lesions in the non-dominant hemisphere and may be accompanied by defects of spatial perception (Lezak, 1976).

Aphasia is the term presently applied to defects of symbol manipulation and concept formation at central integration levels that interfere with communication (Lezak, 1976). They usually appear in clusters of related dysfunctions. Agraphia and alexia are typically associated disturbances and appear as dysfunctions (dysgraphia, dyslexia) rather than total loss of function. Again, these disabilities are associated with specific anatomical lesions (Luria, 1973).

Level of Consciousness

Levels of consciousness, attentional activities and activity rate comprise a group of closely related behavioral characteristics that do not comprise intellectual functions; yet, they are intimately involved in those intellectual operations. Disorders of attention may arise from lesions anywhere in the brain. Frequent symptoms of impairment are decreased attention span, distractibility, susceptibility to confusion and unpredictable performance (Lezak, 1976).

Levels of consciousness must be seen in terms of a vertical continuum ranging from hyperalertness to coma.

↑ Mania
Highly alert
Alert
Relaxed
Drowsy
Transition states
Dreams
Light sleep
Moderate sleep
Deep sleep
Very deep sleep
↓ Coma

Changes in one's state of alertness significantly alter his intellectual efficiency, causing tiredness, inattentiveness or slowness.

Activity rate involves the rapidity of performance of mental activity and the motor response speed (Lezak, 1976). Slowing of mental activity is observable in the symptoms of delayed reaction time and slowed total performance time, when there is no specific motor disability. Motor response slowing is even more detectable and is often associated with weakness or poor coordination.

Changes In Personality

Like intellectual functions, personality and emotional capacities and characteristics are altered by brain dysfunction or damage. The most common effects are emotional dulling, decreased inhibitions, diminished anxiety with associated emotional blandness, or mild euphoria and decreased social sensitivity. However, increased anxiety, depressed mood, hypersensitivity and irritability are also widely reported (Slater and Roth, 1969; Lezak, 1976). This apparent contradiction of symptoms suggests that, often, changes in personality and emotional characteristics are not so much changes but exaggerations of the premorbid personality and emotional characteristics.

> Direct effects are fairly obvious since premorbid personality characteristics are generally not so much changed as exaggerated by brain injury. Tendencies to dependent behavior, hypochrondriasis, passivity, perfectionism, irresponsibility, etc., can be major obstacles to the patient whose rehabilitation depends on active relearning of old skills and reintegration of old habit patterns while he copes with a host of unrelenting and often humiliating frustrations (Lezak, 1976, pp. 163-164).

Behavioral changes, the visible and measurable aspect of personality change, can seldom be explained solely by the presence of brain dysfunction or destruction. Instead, these changes are viewed in light of complex interactions involving primary and secondary brain impairment, current social and vocational demands, family and interpersonal relationships, community cultural realities and previously established behavior characteristics.

> Although most brain injured persons tend to undergo adverse emotional changes, brain damage seems to have beneficial effects for

a few. These effects are most striking in those emotionally constricted, anxious, overly responsible people who become more easygoing and relaxed as a result of a pathological brain condition. While life seems to be more pleasant for some of the patients who experience release from anxiety and emotional disinhibition, their families may suffer instead (Lezak, 1976, p. 29).

Although diagnosis of organic brain syndromes involves evaluation of all six cognitive areas, it is important to remember that disturbances may involve any one, any combination or all areas. When more than one area of cognitive functioning is involved, the degree of dysfunction in each may vary in severity.

VARIABLES AFFECTING THE EXPRESSION OF BRAIN DAMAGE

Like all psychological phenomena, the behavioral changes that follow brain injury or dysfunction are multi-dimensional. Three classical factors are identified as determining the manifestations of organic brain syndromes (Pincus and Tucker, 1974):

1. The amount of tissue destroyed
2. Location of the lesion in the brain
3. Nature of the disease process

Other identified variables include the duration of the condition, age at the time of onset, pattern of cerebral dominance, life situation and intrapsychic make-up of the individual (Lezak, 1976).

TISSUE DESTRUCTION

There is seldom any question that considerable insult to brain tissue results in marked and undeniable loss of function or even coma and/or death. However, the classical study of Chapman and Wolff, correlating the amount of brain tissue (removed secondary in surgery for tumors) and resulting impairment, demonstrated that adaptive capacities were decreased following tissue losses of less than 120 grams of cortical tissue (Pincus and Tucker, 1974). Symptom patterns fall into four major categories:

1. Expression of needs, appetites and drives
2. Capacity to adapt for the achievement of goals

3. Integration of socially appropriate reactions of defense under stress
4. Capacity for immediate recovery from the effects of stress

Closely related to the actual amount or weight of destroyed cerebral tissue is the nature of the lesion. When the loss of cortical tissue is "clean," leaving little or no necrotic tissue, secondary repercussions of the lesion are minimized, anatomically unrelated functions tend to be minimally disturbed and the prospects for successful rehabilitation maximized.

The presence of necrotic tissue alters the neurochemical and electrical status of the brain. Behavioral changes, more extensive and severe, can involve distortions in other cerebral functions located far from the site of insult (Lezak, 1976). This helps explain why the individual who has experienced an insult to the motor cortex may also demonstrate marked and unpredictable personality changes.

LOCATION OF THE LESION

Subcortical Involvement

The subcortical regions of the brain are those below the cerebral cortex proper. These subcortical structures are phylogenetically ancient, and they are anatomically similar in most mammals, especially primates. Included in these subcortical structures are those anatomical structures which comprise the reticular activating, hypothalamic and limbic systems. These systems regulate basic survival functions, such as appetite, sexual drive, respirations and heart rate. They also have an important integrative function, correlating the function of subcortical structures with the cortex.

A cortical lesion involving subcortical areas compounds and alters behavioral correlations. The depth of a lesion is related to the severity of the impairment of verbal skills (Lezak, 1976). Anosognosia, especially those associated with right parietal lobe damage, illustrates the effects and degree of subcortical involvement. When a primary parietal lesion involves the right optic region of the thalamus, the individual may have a vague awareness of disability but more generally ignores the paralysis. On the other hand, when the lesion is limited to the parietal cortex, symptoms such as confabulation and delusions are more likely to occur (Lezak, 1976).

Since subcortical lesions may cut or disrupt cortical pathways, they are particularly capable of producing atypical symptom patterns. Such lesions can simulate cortical involvement, even when there is none.

Geschwind (1965, 1972) analyzed a case in which a patient with normal visual acuity suddenly could no longer read, although he was able to copy written words. Post mortem examination revealed that an occluded artery prevented blood flow to the left visual cortex and the interhemispheric visual pathways, injuring both structures and rendering the patient blind in his right visual field. His left visual field and right visual cortex continued to register words which he could copy. However, the right visual cortex was disconnected from the left hemisphere so that verbal information was no longer transmitted to the left hemisphere for the symbol processing necessary for verbal comprehension and therefore, he could not read (Lezak, 1976, p. 156).

Lesions of the Cerebral Cortex

The cerebral cortex has traditionally been divided into four lobes: frontal, temporal, occipital and parietal. Although these lobes are considered separately, there is a tremendous functional overlap; the actual separation or anatomical distinctiveness of these areas is not as specific as their separate labels indicate. Numerous daily activities such as reading, following instructions and rearranging the closet require the cooperation of two or more portions of the cerebral cortex for adequate performance.

Secondly, the cerebral cortex is asymmetric; the right and left halves of the cortex in the adult differ slightly anatomically and markedly in function. Recent works indicate (Lezak, 1976; Slater and Roth, 1969) that in 90 to 96 percent of adults, the left cerebral cortex is dominant and responsible for analytical functions, such as language and mathematics (see Figure 13-2 on p. 457). The right cerebral cortex serves more synthesizing functions, such as geometric or spatial construction and intuitive thinking. Although cerebral dominance has classically been associated with handedness, the recent evidence is that the left hemisphere is dominant for most left-handed as well as right-handed individuals. Only when there has been childhood cerebral trauma to the left hemisphere can right hemisphere dominance be readily assumed.

Frontal Lobe

The frontal lobes are the largest of the neocortical divisions. Destruction or removal of much of the tissue anterior to the motor region need not interfere with motor or sensory functions, nor are disorientations and dysmnesia particularly evident. Instead, bilateral frontal lobe damage results in subtle dysfunction in the individual's highest integrative functions. The "frontal lobe syndrome" is characterized by the following symptoms (Pincus and Tucker, 1974; Lezak, 1976):

1. Problem of slowing which appears as decreased spontaneity or loss of initiative. In mild forms, the patient seems to lack initiative and ambition; in more severe forms, he appears unresponsive or mute.
2. Difficulty in making behavioral or mental shifts in attention, movement or attitude. This is often referred to as perseveration and is seen in the patient's inability to suppress an ongoing activity. He is unable to change his response in light of altered circumstances or continues it beyond an obvious and proper end point.
3. Deficient self-awareness results in an inability to perceive one's effect on others or critically to judge a social situation. The individual is likely to be euphoric, self-satisfied, experience little anxiety and be impulsive. Social conventions are of less importance, due to decreased awareness.
4. Concrete attitude is seen in the person's inability to disassociate himself from the immediate environment. He responds in a literal or concrete manner, so that objects, experiences and behavior have only face value of meaning. Thus, the patient is decreasingly or completely incapable of planning, foresight and goal-directed behavior.

Lateralization of cognitive functions appears less marked in the frontal lobes. However, less verbal fluency and impoverishment of speech are more likely to occur with left frontal lesions. Constructual apraxia is more likely to occur with right frontal lesions. Concrete attitude is equally evident, but those with right lesions who are able to utilize verbal cues are more able to compensate in making shifts in behavioral response.

When the dominant motor cortex and subcortical connections

are disturbed, paralysis is a likely occurrence. Other motor symptoms associated with lesions of the motor cortex include (Pincus and Tucker, 1974):

1. Increased muscle tone manifested by a semivoluntary resistance in passive movement of the limb
2. Forced grasping in response to tactile stimulation of the individual's palm
3. Gait disorders, apraxia
4. Disturbances in voluntary conjugate eye movements.

Parietal Lobe

Generally, individuals with lesions in the parietal area suffer from a large group of non-specific but disabling symptoms characterized by poor observation and lack of awareness of deficits. Daily task performance can vary markedly. Lesions in the left hemisphere tend to result in language disturbances and functions, such as an inability to name objects and numbers. Alexia, agraphia, acalculia and aphasia often result, when the lesion overlaps in the temporal and/or occipital lobes of the dominant hemisphere. If the lesion involves the occipital lobe, the individual is more likely to have difficulty reading or writing. If the temporal lobe is primarily involved, the deficits are likely to be noted in speaking and/or understanding.

Lesions in the right parietal hemisphere produce gnostic deficits, faulty corporeal awareness and defective visual spatial conceptualization. The individual is apt to neglect space on the side opposite the lesion, does not recognize faces, easily becomes lost and has difficulty dressing.

Occipital Lobes

The occipital lobes constitute the cortical center of the visual system. Lesions in this area give rise to disturbances in processing visual information. Primary areas of the occipital cortex are those areas where the fibers from the retina terminate. Because of the unique arrangement of the optic pathways a lesion in the R occipital lobe interrupts vision in the L visual field, while a lesion in the L occipital lobe interrupts vision in the R visual field (see Figure 13-3 on p. 458). Neurologically, this is referred to as contralateral homonymous hemianopia.

When lesions are confined to the primary projection areas of the occipital lobe not directly concerned with reception of impulse from the eye itself, the symptom picture changes dramatically. Since these areas of the occipital cortex play a major role in synthesizing visual stimuli, lesions found here are more likely to give rise to reccognizable visual hallucinations, such as images of flowers, animals or familiar faces, rather than the flashes of light, color or spots typical of primary zone lesions.

Although the individual is not blind, he is unable to perceive accurately what he sees. Such deficits are commonly referred to as visual agnosias. Although the affected person looking at a pair of glasses sees separate features such as circular lenses, cross bar and shafts, he is unable to put these components together and may misidentify the glasses as a bicycle, which has similar components. This individual also has difficulty if he is asked to draw a pair of glasses. His drawing represents part but not the whole, and, is, therefore, not recognizable. Such a deficit, while severely limiting, remains a partial deficit and does not affect other intellectual processes, thereby enabling the person to recognize objects by touch, perform calculations and understand the meaning of stories (Luria, 1973).

As the lesions's location comes closer to overlapping other areas of the cortex, the symptom picture becomes more complicated. More integrated cerebral functions such as reading, writing or identifying complex pictures are likely to be disturbed. Secondly, lesions in the left or dominant hemisphere are more likely to cause difficulty in recognizing letters, particularly those with similar outlines (N and M, O and Q, b and d) or those with complicated construction (G and B, g and q, k). This difficulty leads quite logically to difficulties in reading. If, however, the lesion is on the right side, the individual is more likely to experience difficulty recognizing faces or establishing ownership of objects. He is also less likely to be aware of his deficits, making no effort to identify a picture or to correct the most glaring mistakes. Luria (1973) reports one patient with an extensive lesion in the right occipital region, who identified a picture of soldiers on a tank as her family: "... My husband, sons and sisters."

Temporal Lobes

Functionally, the temporal lobes play two important and probably related roles. Most commonly associated with the temporal lobes are the auditory functions of hearing and differentiating groups of simultaneously presented acoustic stimuli. The temporal lobes, in conjunction with the subcortical structures of the limbic system, play a role in memory function and the emotional mood and sexual life of the individual. Anatomical structures of the limbic system project deeply into the cortex of the medial portions of the temporal lobe. As might be expected, there are innumerable neural connections, which, in part, may explain the concomitant memory loss, psychosis, depression, sexual dysfunction and even episodic violence associated with lesions of the temporal lobes (Pincus and Tucker, 1974).

Auditory Perception.—The auditory cortex occupies the convex portions of the temporal lobe. Similar to the occipital lobe, this section has both an area where the acoustic impulses arising in the organ of corti (ear) are first heard as tones and sounds of varying pitch and an area where these varying sounds are interpreted into simple, recognizable sounds or words.

Unlike the occipital organization, however, there is incomplete representation of each ear in the opposite hemisphere.

> The fibers of each organ of corti are represented in both projection zones of the auditory cortex, and they are merely represented predominantly in the opposite hemisphere (Luria, 1973, p. 129).

Thus, central deafness is rare, because there would have to be lesions in the auditory cortex of both temporal lobes. Unilateral lesions in the primary projection areas seem only to produce an increase in the threshold of auditory sensation in the opposite ear (Luria, 1973).

Lesions further inward in the cortex do not cause actual loss of hearing but interfere with differentiation between combinations of sounds, as human speech involves the combination of various simple sounds. For spoken language to be understandable, the areas of the left temporal lobe must be functional. Closely associated is the audio-verbal memory. The individual with a lesion in the left temporal area experiences difficulty retaining even a short series of sounds, syllables or words in his memory (Luria, 1973). Thus, several psychological processes become severely disturbed, including disorders in understanding speech, naming objects, recalling words, alienation of the meaning of words and disorders of speech. The latter disturbance is manifested in "word salad."

> Characteristically, the patient is not clearly aware of the defects in his own coherent speech and cannot of course correct them, so that his speech becomes converted into what has been called a "word salad," in which the nominative components (the substantives) are almost completely absent, and all that are left are either interjections or habitual expressions such as: let me see . . . how does it . . . confound it all . . . I know but I can't . . . and so on (Luria, 1973, p. 139).

The individual described can also be expected to have difficulty writing words requiring complex combinations of sounds. With the exception of familiar words such as his signature, this individual's attempts to write usually end in frustration. It must be remembered, however, that he may be able to copy what he cannot write from hearing, in that different cerebral functions are involved.

Lesions similarly located on the right side are less disorganizing, since speech and language functions remain intact. However, there is some indication that the non-dominant hemisphere plays a major role in musical hearing (Luria, 1973). An individual with such a lesion is expected to have difficulty recognizing songs, reproducing rhythms or identifying such everyday sounds as the clatter of dishes, rustle of a newspaper or rumble of a train.

Temporal Lobe and Limbic System.—Lesions involving the medial, deep portions of the temporal lobe involve at least some of the subcortical structure of the limbic system, a ring of gray matter and tracts bordering the hemispheres (see Figure 13-4 on p. 458). Observing patients suffering from rabies, Papez demonstrated this system's relationship to emotion, behavior and visceral reactivity (Pincus and Tucker, 1974).

Portions of the limbic system are located in the anterior and medial portions of the temporal lobe. Three of the major temporal limbic structures are the amygdala, hippocampus and the uncus. Although *all* portions of the limbic system are to some extent associated with memory, learning, emotional states (anxiety, rage, placidity and alertness,) visceral and endocrine responses, (particularly aggressive, oral and sexual activity), disturbances in recent memory and mood are especially associated with temporal lobe lesions (Pincus and Tucker, 1974).

Bilateral hippocampal destruction leads to recent memory loss with the future prevention of all new learning. Stimulation of the amygdala results in rage reactions and feelings of fear. Chewing; gagging; licking; retching; swallowing; bladder contractions; respiratory, pulse and blood pressure increases; and increased ACTH production have also been associated with amygdala stimulation. Bilateral removal of the amygdaloid nuclei and overlying hippocampal cortex has produced docility and loss of natural, protective fear (Pincus and Tucker, 1974). Thus, lesions of the temporal lobe can produce a confusing picture which, at least initially, closely resembles emotional disorders.

> Malamud (1967) studied 18 patients with intracranial neoplasms which involved limbic structures. All had originally been diagnosed as having psychiatric disorders. Ten were thought to be schizophrenics, four were depressed, one was manic and others severely neurotic. Eleven of the patients had psychomotor seizures (Pincus and Tucker, 1974, pp. 49-50).

NATURE OF THE DISEASE PROCESS

Age of Onset

Age at the time of incurring a non-progressive brain injury is probably the greatest single factor in determining how much recovery of psychological function can be anticipated (Lezak, 1976). After about age 30, recuperative functions tend to diminish. Severely injured young adults, late teens to early twenties, are more likely to display greater recuperation of specific functions, as well as the ability to live independently.

Time—Progressive vs. Non-Progressive Brain Disease

Progressive

Progressive brain disease is characterized by progressive behavioral deterioration. The course, often bumpy with waxing and waning of symptoms, is generally downhill. The pertinent question refers to *when* rather than *if* further deterioration will occur. The most accurate clinical rule of thumb for predicting the course of mental decline is that conditions which are progressing rapidly will continue to do so; conditions which are progressing slowly will continue to do so (Lezak, 1976). Thus, the rate of deterioration in the early stages of the disease gives the best indication of whether further disabilities are likely to occur in a few weeks, months or years.

One major exception to the previous discussion is the prediction of the behavioral effects of a brain tumor. The rate of progression can be assessed by the identification of the brain tumor. Degree of symptoms is also directly affected by the type of tumor, amount of accompanying edema and the direction of tumor growth.

Non-Progressive

In single event or non-progressive brain disorders, the date of onset of the causative event is critical in determining a patient's psychological status (Lezak, 1976; Slater and Roth, 1969; Detre and Jarecki, 1971). Consciousness may be impaired for days or weeks post-insult, and the duration of altered consciousness generally bears a direct relationship to the speed and extent of ultimate recovery (Lezak, 1976). Much of the individual's behavioral or psychological reintegration usually takes place in the first months following the initial injury. Intellectual functions, especially those of immediate memory, attention, concentration and impairments directly associated with the site of the lesion, usually continue to improve substantially during the first six to twelve months. Further improvement, although less dramatic, has reportedly continued to a decade, post-insult. Despite the amount or speed of improvement, total or full recovery is rare, even in instances of relatively minor insult. Once a neuron is destroyed, it is gone; recovery of function is dependent on secondary neurons assuming the function of those destroyed.

Functions which appear intact immediately post-insult may deteriorate over succeeding months or years. Such deterioration usually involves the highest levels of intellectual activity, mental flexibility, reasoning and judgment. The picture is often compounded by a decrease in inhibitions, which leads to deterioration in personal habits and performance standards. These long-range psychological alterations are manifested by the build up of scar tissue, secondary nerve fiber degeneration, changes in blood supply and tissue metabolism (Lezak, 1976). In addition, the initial injury renders the individual increasingly vulnerable to other brain disease, such as a stroke.

DELIRIUM

Delirium is a principle feature of organic brain syndromes and is used synonymously with the nonspecific term, acute brain syndrome. Keynote symptoms of delirium have historically included clouding of consciousness and failure of attention and recent memory, leading to disorientation of time and space. Violent emotional disturbances characterized by fear, misinterpretations of the environment and visual hallucinations are often present. However, delirium can run the gamut from a slight reduction in alertness to coma. Many individuals pass through a sequence of symptoms in both directions during the course of an illness.

The complex of symptoms known as delirium has been recognized since the time of Shakespeare and has historically distinguished acute, reversible brain symptoms from those of chronic mental illness. Delirium was initially associated with psychological manifestations of terminal illness. Later, physicians recognized that the same complex of symptoms occurred in the presence of infection, intoxication, malnutrition, surgical procedures and other physical conditions. Freud identified that the content of delirium is related to the individual's experiences. Delirium was then conceptualized as a syndrome of cerebral insufficiency and defined as any acute reversible syndrome of cerebral insufficiency. In past decades, the conceptualization and, therefore, the definition of delirium assumed the dimension of a psychosomatic condition (Heller and Kornfeld, 1975). This redefinition formalized the view that physical and psychological factors interact causally in the symptom complex of delirium.

Delirium, although historically thought of as acute in nature, may occur in either acute or chronic brain syndromes. It tends to occur more frequently and floridly in acute brain syndromes but is no longer considered the hallmark of acute brain syndromes. Instead, reversibility, not delirium, per se, is the distinguishing factor between acute and chronic brain syndromes (Matthews and Miller,

1975). Acute implies reversible, whereas chronic implies irreversible.

The use of acute vs. chronic brain syndrome as diagnostic categories is increasingly disputed. Some argue that chronic brain syndromes refer only to those disease conditions which have not been accurately identified or treated. On the other hand, others argue that any insult to the brain leaves permanent damage; thus, there are no truly acute brain syndromes. Too, the reversibility or irreversibility of a brain syndrome is often better assessed in retrospect. The clinical picture is used in an attempt to bring some order to the classification of generalized organic brain syndromes.

In the following discussion of organic brain syndromes, the three somewhat overlapping categories identified by Doctors Detre and Jarecki (1971) are utilized. According to the authors, these syndromes are based on the most severe or dramatic expression of clinical symptoms:

1. Dementiform is characterized by memory impairment, disorientation, personality changes and impairment of intellectual functioning and adaptation
2. Deliriform is characterized by memory impairment, disorientation and dysattention, as well as delusions, hallucinations, excitement or apathy
3. Epileptiform is characterized by episodic disturbances of consciousness. Included in this category are the psychological disorders associated with grand mal, petit mal and psychomotor seizures. Syndromes of narcolepsy and somnambulism, though not strictly epileptiform, share the paroxysmal occurrence of symptoms.

DEMENTIFORM SYNDROMES OR DEMENTIA

Dementia refers to a global deterioration of mental functioning. The clinical picture is usually dominated by intellectual disintegration, with affect and motivation also affected. In fact, the key to understanding dementia is that it is evident not only in what an individual says and thinks but in his behavior, as well. Intellectual deterioration is most striking in the impairment of recent memory, which is the initial symptom and leads to the individual's difficulty with abstract reasoning and ultimate disorientation (Detre and Jarecki, 1971; Slater and Roth, 1969). The following is a list of the disease entities and syndromes which are most likely to manifest themselves in a dementiform syndrome (Matthews and Miller, 1975):

Primary:
   Huntington's Chorea
   Jakob-Creutzfeldt disease
   Picks
   Alzheimer

Secondary:
Early changes will allow at least some reverse of symptoms and will avert further deterioration.
   Syphilis
   Vitamin B-12 deficiency
   Cerebral tumor
   Metabolic disorders

Static form:
   Gross cerebral trauma
   Severe, prolonged anoxic states, i.e., secondary to cardiac arrest, carbon monoxide poisoning, asphyxia
   Post encephalitic states
   Hypertensive cerebral disease
   Poisoning by heavy metals
   Alcoholism
   Disturbed Protein Metabolism, i.e., chronic liver failure and chronic renal failure

Clinical Picture

The mildest form of dementia is characterized by dysmnesia. The memory impairment may be so slight that it resembles and, in fact, is explained by forgetfulness or absent-mindedness. The afflicted individual may compensate for his difficulties of absorbing and retaining information by keeping detailed appointment books and calendars or adhering to increasingly rigid daily routines. Family and friends may become aware of the deficits through their own irritations and annoyances when appointments, engagements and promises go unkept. At this point, the individual's memory deficits or rigidity can lead to interpersonal conflict. To compound the picture, the memory deficit and related complications appear inconsistently; he remembers some appointments and items while forgetting others. Often, such symptoms are virtually ignored or explained as nothing more serious than getting "old" or having "too much to worry about." Serious medical consultation is rarely sought, unless there is more dramatic pathophysiology, such as abdominal pains from gallbladder disease.

For a patient at this stage of dementia, a nursing process may look similiar to the following: heavy emphasis is placed on data collection and skilled observations (see Table 13-2: Nursing Process I).

As symptoms of dementia become more severe, the individual has difficulty remembering events of the recent past. The memory deficits are increasingly consistent. Subjects of conversation become increasingly historical, since recall of learning and events experienced prior to memory failure remains intact. Expressed thoughts are characterized by poverty and rigidity. Old, strongly held ideas are applied irrespective of the current circumstances.

As the individual's ability to compensate begins to break down despite increased rigidity and compulsiveness, his intellectual grasp weakens and thinking slows and becomes increasingly difficult and less effective. Attention is aroused and sustained only with great difficulty. He tires easily, especially when confronted with unaccustomed tasks (Slater and Roth, 1969). The individual may also be demonstrating the other symptoms of mild disorientation, especially an impaired sense of time and concrete thinking process. At this stage, professional or medical assistance may be sought. Incidences of work or social difficulties often occur prior to his seeking this assistance. He may also be brought by a family member who has become bewildered, angry or frustrated by the patient's seemingly irrational behavior.

Case Study

Mrs. L. is a white, Roman Catholic of Irish descent, 67-year-old female, who has lived alone since her husband died three years ago. Prior to her husband's retirement from the motel business six years ago, Mrs. L. kept the books for her husband's four motels. Since her husband's death, Mrs. L. had no major health problems, until she was hospitalized eight months ago with vague complaints of tran-

TABLE 13-2
Nursing Process I

Data	Interpretation	Problem	Nursing Actions
Forgets dentist appointment	Data characteristic of an individual showing signs of dementia—early stage:	Questionable impaired functioning secondary to mild dementia	Speak with family member (daughter) to assess recent changes in patient:
Daughter upset after mother did not come for supper as promised	1. More rigid daily routines
2. Reports of forgetfulness although inconsistent		1. Personal routines
2. Personality
—increased rigidity?
—increased obsessiveness?
—increased orderliness?
Requests that Public Health Nurse make her visit at 10:30— upset when nurse arrives late	3. Evidence of possible interpersonal conflict

Due to the vagueness of the data, other possibilities need to be considered: | | 3. Episodes of forgetting appointments
4. Evidence of bills not paid or other obligations not met |
| Adheres rigidly to meal times:
11:30 a.m.
5:30 p.m. | a. Obsessive/compulsive personality
b. Interpersonal or situational crisis | | Assess general state of health:
1. Observe for indications of recent illness including infections, flu |
| Remembers hair appointment every Wednesday at 10:30 a.m. | | | 2. Results of last physical: lab work, review of systems, borderline normals |
| Washes on Monday | | | |

(Continued)

TABLE 13-2 (Continued)

Data	Interpretation	Problem	Nursing Actions
Irons on Tuesday Errands on Wednesday Cleans on Thursday Visits on Friday			3. Current physical assessment with special attention to systems which have caused problems or have a change in status 4. Evidence of any change in a chronic physical or psychological health problem Recent events that may have produced an increased level of anxiety

sient dizziness, headaches and anxiety. Although there were no significant medical findings at that time, Mrs. L.'s daughter continues to talk about her mother being different. She states, "I have to check up on Mom, and I never had to before. Also, she seems so set in her ways."

Building on the previous nursing process as the patient's cerebral symptoms increase, identity of the problem areas becomes clearer and demands a more directive role on the part of the professional (see Table 13-3: Nursing Process II).

In the most severe incidences of dementia, the memory defects expand to include events prior to the onset of the illness. As the disease process expands, the memory deficits involve events further and further into the past, until the deficit is global. At this point, the individual neither understands the present nor remembers the past.

Disorientation

The symptom of disorientation is rarely detectable with appreciable memory impairment. First to be impaired is the sense of time. An individual is initially unable to recall when and, especially, in what order the current or previous day's events occurred. However, he may still be able to describe the events in some detail.

As the temporal disorientation increases in severity, the individual may be unable to tell the day of the month, month of the year, day of the week or year. At this point of deterioration, the individual begins to lose his orientation to place. Initially, he has difficulty identifying or locating unfamiliar places. As disorientation to place increases in severity, he has difficulty identifying familiar surroundings and, eventually, he is unable to remember his own address or present location.

As the individual becomes increasingly disorientated to place, he begins to experience difficulty identifying the people around him. Initially, he forgets their names then their relationships to him. Only after nearly all other intellectual function is impaired, does he have difficulty identifying himself or remembering his own name (Detre and Jarecki, 1971).

Concrete Attitude

Initial deficits in abstract thinking, like initial deficits in

TABLE 13-3
Nursing Process II

Data	Interpretation	Problem	Nursing Actions
Would not ride to grocery store with grandson because he had long hair	Behavior indicated symptoms consistent with a mild/moderate degree of dementia:	Dementia	Explain to the patient's family that her apparent intolerance of grandson's hair, lack of concentration and other changes in behavior are due to decreased cerebral efficiency
Went to hair appointment at 10:30 a.m. Wednesday even though beautician had called and changed appointment to 2:30 p.m. Thursday	1. Forgetting recent events and responsibilities 2. Preoccupation with past 3. Increasingly rigid routines	Lack of attention	Help family plan in order to avoid conflict:
Bank has called daughter in reference to overdrawn checking account	Intellectual deterioration:	Concrete thinking	1. Do not confront with grandson's long hair
Became angry with daughter when supper was delayed one and a half hours	1. Increased difficulty maintaining attention and decreased activities and poverty of conversation	Interpersonal conflict	2. Discuss with family the possibility of helping patient pay bills or setting up an automatic bill-paying account with the bank
Conversation topics often about childhood and young adult happenings	2. Concrete attitude, less flexibility of attitudes		

Less involvement in family discussion—seems to pay little attention or have little interest	Less aware of her impact on others and interpersonal conflict and deterioration in personal hygiene
Frequency of visits to Senior Citizens decreasing from 2-3 times a week to once every 1-2 weeks	
Dress often slightly soiled, hair combed less meticulously	
Family members voicing frustration and anger about apparent unthoughtfulness	

memory, are often mistakenly attributed to stress rather than to organic disease. To confuse the picture further, even when impairments are demonstrable or measurable—by asking the individual to bear several facts in mind simultaneously or to repeat five numbers in reverse order—he may appear lucid and remain competent in his performance of familiar tasks (Detre and Jarecki, 1971). If tasks or the individual's job depend on his ability to make decisions or deal with sensitive interpersonal situations, his impairments soon become apparent to those around him. Behavior and decisions appear inappropriate, as the individual overlooks obvious but vital factors, making his judgment become suspect and unreliable. The executive or professional could expect a greater degree of disability from the same degree of dementia than the factory assembly line worker.

As the dementia, disorientation and loss of intellectual abilities become progressive, more and more of his intrapersonal, interpersonal and social interactions are affected. His ability to meet basic hygiene needs, nutritional needs and financial obligations deteriorates, until he is totally unable to cope. At this point, if not before, a total or near total care setting is required to maintain life.

Emotional Reactions, Adaptive Efforts, Personality Changes

Emotional, adaptive and personality changes which are so characteristic of dementia generally mesh with the individual's intellectual deficits. At the onset, these aspects are particularly colored by the patient's premorbid personality, rate of deterioration, environmental demands, intrapersonal and interpersonal supports and general state of health. Initial changes are most likely an exaggeration and exacerbation of the existing characteristics and problems. Unlike the maturation process, which perfects and adds to the repertoire of adaptive skills, dementia causes the individual to rely on only those coping skills he knows best. Individuals whose pre-existing personalities were characterized by isolation, withdrawal, suspiciousness or social ineptness are particularly vulnerable to difficulties which arise out of decreased flexibility (Detre and Jarecki, 1971). The psychological defenses of sublimation, repression and denial are ultimately replaced by projection and a more paranoid attitude, which can result in a refusal to collaborate with the environment.

The individual may initially experience difficulty modulating his emotional responses. He is aroused or interested more slowly but, also, less able to suppress his reactions once aroused and, thus, appears to overreact (Detre and Jarecki, 1971). What initially appears as decreased vitality progresses toward constricted and shallow responses and decreased interest in the environment. At some point and often prior to readily observable intellectual impairments, the afflicted individual may develop irritability, depression, affective lability, euphoria and diffuse, unsubstantiated somatic complaints. Until the clinical picture of dementia becomes more dramatic, individuals experiencing such vague difficulties are often thought to be depressed, anxious, malingering or even psychotic.

The brain damaged individual's intellectual, emotional and biological reserves are so marginal, that most stressful events aggravate his symptoms, causing subclinical impairments to become evident. Events that decrease, overload or distort sensory imput are particularly stressful. Common events that cause aggravation of existing symptoms are electrical shock treatments, cataract surgery, barbiturates or many other psychotropic (CNS depressants) agents, physical illnesses, interference with sleep and placement in an unfamiliar environment, i.e., hospital, nursing home, even home of a relative (Detre and Jarecki, 1971).

This individual is also predisposed to a further decline in social functioning by factors only indirectly related to his intellectual deterioration. The following list of conditions can intertwine, placing those who are only minimally impaired in a life-threatening situation (Detre and Jarecki, 1971).

1. Impairment of vision and/or hearing; sensory imput may be so reduced or distorted that, in effect, there is no environmental feedback system to help determine the appropriateness of his behavior.
2. Nutritional deficiencies, if severe enough, cause an overlying delirium. These deficiencies, however, may be the result of living alone, inability to shop, inability to cook, insufficient funds, decreased appetite or inability to chew.
3. Inordinate demands on his time and energy result in impairing his ability to function and to care for himself. Common contributory conditions are physical problems, especially poor vision, missing teeth, constipation or arthritis.

4. Intrapersonal conflicts result in disturbed body image, decline in self-esteem or exaggerated fear of death.
5. Apathy, undesirable behaviors and withdrawal, which are symptoms associated with decreased intellectual functioning, can cause further decreases in the contacts with family and friends. Thus, sources of sensory and social stimulation are further decreased, compounding the original deficits.

Treatment-Nursing Actions

Medical and nursing interventions focus on identification and symptomatic management of the evident deterioration. Identification is especially important in those instances where treatment of underlying metabolic problems can reverse, or at least minimize, the resulting deficits. Even in those cases where a progressive deteriorating course is inevitable, early identification can save family associated frustration, prevent unnecessary alienation, help maximize the patient's remaining assets and allow for careful and realistic planning for a time when the patient can no longer meet his own basic needs. The following discussion is intended to assist the nurse in identifying the individual, who may be organically impaired, and provide some nursing observations and actions, which will assist in the diagnostic process and symptomatic management.

Assessment

Change is an important aspect of assessment, especially in the early stage or the diagnostic phase. In the assessment of change, someone who knows the patient well may be an important source of information. A familiar observer is more likely to know when and if change has taken place, and he is more able to provide a detailed description than the patient himself. In any case, it must be remembered that the changes may have taken place so slowly that they may not be immediately recognizable as changes. The following aspects should be considered:

1. Is there a decrease in intelligence?
    a) What is the individual's level of education? Is he functioning at a level consistent with his education?
    b) Has there been psychological testing? Results?

c) Has he had recent problems on his job? Describe
d) Has he had unanticipated or unusual difficulty learning a new skill or procedure? Has he become increasingly resistant to change, even insignificant change?
e) Does he enjoy jokes and/or wit less? Are his jokes increasingly off-color (sexual) or otherwise inappropriate?
f) Has his vocabulary decreased? Does he use words inaccurately?
g) Can he keep in mind several items at a time?

2. Is there a change in his personality?
    a) Depression . . . particularly if the individual has *no* previous history of depression or a depressive personality
    b) Irritability
    c) Unexplainable loss of interest in subjects and activities which were previously sources of pleasure. Withdrawal?
    d) Increase in interpersonal conflicts, especially with family members and close associates
    e) A less flexible attitude, even stubborness. More insistent on conducting affairs the "old" way. He may listen to new ideas but continues his old pattern, despite arguments for or benefits of adaptation
    f) Deterioration in personal appearance and/or habits. Change may be subtle and need not be unacceptable—only less acceptable by comparison with the individual's previous standards

3. Has there been a change in the individual's state of health?
    a) Head injury
    b) Metabolic disease - acute or chronic in nature
    c) Surgical intervention
    d) Initiation of or change in a medication regime
    e) Radical dietary change, i.e., vegetable or protein restriction, etc.
    f) Sensory deprivation

4. Is there an attempt to order the external environment in such a way as to avoid reference to or confrontation of his defects?
    a) Refusing to answer questions
    b) Feigning deafness
    c) Diverting discussion to a more acceptable physical symptom
    d) Answering questions other than the one asked
    e) Rationalizations for lack of appropriate or desired response

f) Confabulation
  g) Pretending the situation is social rather than medical. } Indication of more severe dementia
  h) Acting as if the interviewer were a guest - flattery; friendly conversation; flirtation; long, involved discussions of the past, especially about physical or sexual attributes, family social status or children's accomplishments
  i) Projection - accusing interviewer of trying to get him upset } Severe dementia

Management of dementia is most successful when the following principles are the basis for determining nursing observations and interventions:

1. Maximum independence and functioning can be facilitated by teaching the patient less complex ways of doing things, encouraging him and his family in their use of these techniques, and helping the individual and his family adapt to any remaining impairments.
2. If dementia is progressive and irreversible, help the patient avoid confronting his disabilities, but help the family confront them and make adequate, realistic provisions for the afflicted individual, as well as their own long-term well-being.
3. To maximize the remaining learning potential, the individual should be made comfortable (physically and emotionally), and initial tasks should be ones he is capable of performing. New material should be introduced simply and gradually, with attempts to insure maximum success at each step.
4. His living situation should be simple and well structured, with little opportunity for the individual to confront his incompetence.
5. There is the potential for more satisfaction from performing a simple job well than from unsuccessful attempts to return to a former occupation or activity or than from doing nothing at all.
6. As an individual deteriorates, meeting basic survival needs becomes more demanding of his energies and capabilities.
7. Sudden acceleration of deterioration (delirium) may indicate a superimposed treatable disease, i.e., infection, metabolic disorder.
8. An individual's disturbed perceptions are a fertile field for

development of delusional symptoms; the greater the deterioration of his intellectual functions, the greater likelihood of delusions.
9. More cohesive delusions reflect the patient's real life situation and everyday irritations, particularly his feelings of helplessness, loneliness and abandonment.

The following Tables provide outlines of the broad symptom categories associated with dementia and nursing actions and observations which might facilitate the management of the individual so impaired.

TABLE 13-4

Mild Organ Brain Syndromes—Dementia

Symptoms	Nursing Actions and Observations
Mild, transient, difficulty remembering	1. Share the observation with the patient that he seems to forget some appointments, instructions, etc. 2. Problem-solve—Inquire how patient has helped himself to recall obligations, etc., in the past. If suitable, apply to present difficulty.

Emotional reactions
  Diminished vitality
  Personality changes
  Depression
  Somatic complaints
  Hysteria
	3. Utilize past patterns of recall. Possible suggestions might be:
	  a. Appointment calendars and books
	  b. Tactful reminders from friends and associates just prior to the proposed activity.
	4. Give patient written instructions for such things as diet, care/treatment regime, medication, etc. in addition to verbal instructions.

Difficulty in abstract reasoning Decreased abstract reasoning	5. Attempt to adapt diet, care/treatment regimes to existing patterns and schedules (minimizing new learning necessary for compliance). 6. Encourage individual to establish daily routines, possibly converting it to a written schedule. 7. Respect individual's self-imposed schedules. 8. Minimize the complexity of new information and proposed medication and treatment regimes: focus on essentials, niceties and extras may be confusing—individual may remember to take medication once a day with his vitamin pill but may have difficulty taking medication at unfamiliar times. 9. Plan for additional time to accomplish new learning. 10. Utilize as many senses as possible—hearing, touching, smelling, seeing, tasting—to maximize sensory

(Continued)

TABLE 13-4 (Continued)

Symptoms	Nursing Actions and Observations
	input and, therefore, understanding of new information: a. Charts b. Verbal and written instruction c. Have patient taste, feel, smell as well as visualize new medication, etc. d. Encourage adaptation that enables successful performance, i.e., work, financial 11. Observe for indications that memory difficulties are becoming increasingly consistent: a. Appointment calendar, schedules, reminders no longer assist the individual to compensate for dysmnesia. b. Individual increasingly rigid and able to utilize only old, well-established coping skills with increasingly less success. c. Individual having greater difficulty with tasks of less complexity. d. Conversations and interests dominated by past; deals with the present in terms of the past—content of reminiscing about past incidents that reflect a current theme, such as loss, anger, joy, fun, etc. e. Individual more likely to incur feelings of frustration, anger or futility in family members, care givers or even acquaintances, especially when learning or remembering is involved.

TABLE 13-5

Organic Brain Syndromes of Moderate/Severe—Dementia

Symptoms	Nursing Actions and Observations
Immediate memory markedly impaired	1. Simplify and adapt new procedures and treatment regimes to previous habits and patterns.
Disorientation Time—recent Place—unfamiliar Person—recent—unfamiliar	2. Expect a lesser amount and more erratic compliance. 3. Authority—"The doctor ordered it; you have to take your pills," may be better understood than rationale, thus, more beneficial in obtaining compliance.
Difficulty in abstract reasoning	4. Although new content MAY still be taught, patient may not be able to transfer learning from one situa-

TABLE 13-5 (Continued)

Symptoms	Nursing Actions and Observations
Impaired judgment Unable to deal with complex Concrete attitude Deterioration in personal habits	tion to another; therefore, teaching needs to take place in the setting where the activity is going to be performed. Referral services of visiting nurse associations, home health care agencies, health departments, as well as supervision by families, may be necessary for an individual to perform satisfactorily those activities taught in the hospital in his home environment. Inter-agency communication needs to include detailed teaching plans, so that the individual is not unnecessarily confused with alternate ways of accomplishing the same goal. Hospital or institutional teaching should consider the realities of this individual's "home" environment.
Adaptive Limitation of coping mechanisms	5. Explain the deterioration of the patient's behavior, memory, capabilities, etc. to family members, thereby minimizing the possibility of alienation of the patient and maximizing these support systems in the management of this individual.

Intensification of premorbid personality	6. Realistically assess patient's memory and observe patient closely for indications of further memory loss:
	  a. Does not tell his stories in the same or similar manner; key factors such as who, when or where begin to vary.
	  b. Confabulation—especially to account for nighttime hours.
	  c. Content of conversation becomes increasingly historical.
	  d. Is content to reread the same magazines, work the same puzzles and is unable to identify television reruns.
	  e. Cannot participate appropriately in activities that require the taking of turns and/or building on another's responses, i.e., games, group participation.
	  f. Observe for indications of disruptions in other areas of cognitive functioning.

TABLE 13-6

Disorientation

Problem	Actions

Time—initial	1. Assist individual in ordering recent events according to time.
	2. Provide visual stimuli which continually orient the patient to time.
	   a. Large single-month/day calendars
	   b. Easily read, large clocks
	3. Provide verbal stimuli relating time to routine, e.g., "It is 5:00 p.m., supper should be along shortly," or to season, e.g., "Since it is winter, dusk will be about 4:30 p.m."
	4. Plan or assist the routines which help him orient himself to time.

Place	1. Provide for and/or encourage patient to seek accompaniment to unfamiliar places.
	2. Alert family that patient is likely to become lost in new environments.
	3. Provide for special orientation to new environments, e.g., hospital rooms, nursing homes, day care centers.
	4. Provide for sitters or family to stay with patient until he develops increased familiarity with environment, especially at night when sensory clues are decreased both by darkness and drowsiness.
	5. Provide for night lights to assist visual orientation.
	6. Observe for nighttime delusional thinking (sundowning), which is secondary to decreased sensory input and may compel the individual to wander or endanger himself by climbing out a window.
	
	   Provide for appropriate safety measures.
	   a. Non-opening or protected windows
	   b. Restraints
	      1) Physical
	      2) Chemical use of nonbarbiturate or Librium/Valium type drugs to control second-degree delirium. Low dosage phenothiazines provide sedation without second-degree delirium
	      3) Sitter
	      4) Frequent, regular nighttime observation of patient
	7. Facilitate highest level of functioning by attempting to maintain individual in his own home or familiar environment
	   a. Utilization of support measures and community services
	      1) Assistance with food shopping, personal hygiene, food preparation, financial guardianship, cleaning, etc.

TABLE 13-6 (Continued)

Problems	Actions
	2) Encourage family to maintain regular visits and arrange for outings to familiar locations such as church, favorite restaurant, concert, homes of close friends, etc. (Short regular visits are more beneficial than extended, infrequent visits.)
Person	1. Help family and friends understand that patient's severe OBS is the reason he does not immediately recognize them. 2. Suggest they facilitate patient's recall by immediately stating who they are and their relationship to the patient. 3. Care givers need continually to remind the patient of who they are and their role in respect to each visit or intervention. 4. Plan for consistency of professional and helping staff.

TABLE 13-7
Assessment of Individual's Ability to Maintain Independent Domicile

Problem	Evaluation
Meals	Evaluate critically the individual's ability to maintain independent domicile with external supports 1. Does he remember to eat? 2. Is the food of nutritional value? 3. Is the food prepared appropriately, e.g., pork fully cooked? 4. Is food stored appropriately—refrigeration? 5. Is food utilized, before it becomes spoiled? 6. Can he modify usual diet to meet restrictions in sodium, calories, potassium, etc?

Personal Habits	1. Personal cleanliness
	   a. Always wearing the same dress.
	   b. Clothes which are in poor repair, especially, if clothes are badly stained.
	   c. Neglect of hair, nails, beard, skin—dirt unexplained by recent activity or secondary skin irritations.
	   d. Odor of urine and/or feces.
	2. Inappropriate or careless smoking
	   a. Holes in clothing.
	   b. Ashes on floors and tables.
	   c. Used wrappers visible, crumpled and apparently forgotten.
	   d. Unemptied, overloaded ash trays.
	   e. Disregard for NO SMOKING signs or requests.

(Continued)

TABLE 13-7 (Continued)

Problem	Evaluation
	f. Use of inappropriate receptacles (paper cup) as ash trays. g. Indications patient may be smoking in bed. h. Inappropriate amusement with smoking accidents—fire in ash tray, ash drop in coffee.

Maintenance of the Domicile	1. Safety and appropriate use of appliances, especially electrical stove burners and oven left on—burned food.
	2. Evidence of grease fires.
	3. Coffee pot left plugged in.
	4. Electrical razors or hair dryers used while bathing.
	5. Use of flammable household or cleaning product near sources of heat—stove.
	6. Physical deterioration
	  a. Ever increasing clutter, some of which is obvious trash—empty cans, boxes, dirty dishes.
	  b. An increasing number of projects which never get finished, e.g., painting the kitchen, cleaning the closets, etc.—these often begin to add to the clutter.
	  c. Evergrowing number of excuses why physical conditions—dirt, clutter—accumulate.
	  d. Presence of exposed wires—phone cords stretched across halls, up stairs, etc.; stairways cluttered; inappropriate use of chairs and tables for climbing.
	  e. Physical deterioration due to unmade repairs; improper or inadequate cleaning, especially kitchen and bathroom.
	  f. Increasing evidence of pests, e.g., rats, roaches, ants; even an accumulation of stray dogs and cats.

Interpersonal Relationships	1. Evidence of increasing paranoia
	  a. Thinks "people" only want his money or some article of real or personal value.
	  b. Concerns about phone being tapped, house being broken into, or being followed.
	  c. Fearful for his own safety; strangers may be thought to be after him from the F.B.I., C.I.A. or Mafia.
	  d. Does not comprehend the nature of relationships, especially newly established ones.
	2. Increased conflict with those with whom he has had close relationships—family
	  a. Increased belligerence.
	  b. Use of harsh, crude language.
	  c. May be overtly combative.
	3. Appears insensitive to others' needs, wants, desires.

TABLE 13-8

Severe Organic Brain Syndromes—Dementia

Symptoms	Actions

Severe dysmnesia
  Remote past memory to global
 	
Disorientation
  Time—Does not know year, month, day or hour
  Place—Knows only most familiar or does not know where he is
  Person—Can't recall his own identify, name
 	
Difficulty with abstract reasoning
Unable to care for himself
 	
Emotional reactions
  No interest in the environment
 	
Adaptive: Projection
  Marked paranoia
  Negativism
  Limited to no collaboration with environment
	1. Do not ask or expect the patient to take responsibility for *any* aspect of meeting his own needs.
	2. Arrange for a total care living arrangement.
	3. Nutrition
	  a. Provide for complete nutrition.
	  b. Feed patient if unable or unwilling to feed himself.
	  c. Provide for tube feeding if unable to feed sufficiently.
	4. Cleanliness
	  a. Provide for daily showers and/or baths as dictated by physical limitations.
	  b. Wash those areas in need of special cleaning or attention.
	  c. Provide clean clothes and provide assistance with dressing.
	  d. Assist with toileting
	    1) Establish routine anticipatory pattern.
	    2) Take patient to the toilet if necessary.
	    3) Provide for condom drainage, diapers, etc.
	  e. Shave, wash hair, provide nail (finger and toe) care.
	  f. Exercise—walks in immediate environment—ROM exercises for those unable to walk.

DELIRIFORM SYNDROMES

The symptom complex of delirium is the hallmark of deliriform syndromes. These syndromes refer to a number of illnesses of organic origin, in which clouding of consciousness is the keynote symptom (Mathews and Miller, 1975; Slater and Roth, 1969). Associated symptoms of delirium include dysmnesia and disturbances of attention (Detre and Jarecki, 1971). These failures lead to the characteristic, secondary symptoms of disorientation and emotional disturbances. Neurological findings in deliriform syndromes include headache, dysarthria and EEG abnormalities—dominated by the development of slow waves, course, irregular tremors and sudden, non-rhythmic, non-patterned, gross muscle contractions in a resting person (Detre and Jarecki, 1971).

Delirium, per se, is not the primary pathology but a syndrome associated with a wide variety of infectious, metabolic and structural disorders. Although the primary disease or injury may be directly associated with the brain (cerebral tumor or head injury), more often the delirium is an expression of the systemic nature of such pathology as cardiac or respiratory disease, severe infections, hypoglycemia, liver failure, drug poisoning, uremia, thyroid disease and postoperative hypoxia.

At one time, the psychological symptoms of delirium were thought to be diagnostically significant to the practitioner of general medicine. Since Bonhoefler described the forms of delirium and demonstrated its universality and independence from the primary physical illness, these symptoms were viewed with less medical significance (Slater and Roth, 1969). If the symptoms are relatively mild, they are often ignored. Only when they intensify is the difficulty identified most often as a management rather than a medical problem. This attitude has, no doubt, suppressed systematic research into the phenomena of delirium, delaying our physiological understanding of the appreciation for this widely experienced syndrome.

Pathophysiology of Delirium

The degree of involvement of the nervous system and the severity of the symptoms are not always closely related. Depending on the nature of the underlying illness, different neuropathways for the production of neurological and psychological symptoms may be implicated. The following physiological occurrences are often associated with and used to provide explanations for the psychosis that accompanies infections (Slater and Roth, 1969):

1. Rise in body temperature
2. Vascular disturbances
3. Effects of bacterial toxins
4. Toxic, intermediate products of metabolism acting singularly and in combination.

However, these explanations seem to have some rather severe

limitations, and at best, they provide only the most rudimentary explanation for occurrence of delirium.

Although it has been generally recognized that mental symptoms frequently run parallel to fluctuations of fever in infections and subside when the temperature returns toward normal, psychological symptoms of delirium may precede a rise in temperature (typhoid fever) or occur after the temperature has returned to normal (post-febrile delirium). Secondly, it has not been demonstrated that experimentally induced febrile states result in significant mental changes; thus, it is unclear that fever is the causative factor in delirium associated with infections (Slater and Roth, 1969).

In infections and many systemic diseases, the regulation of capillary function is disturbed. If cerebral capillaries are involved, the cortical cells cannot receive adequate oxygen and, thus, express the psychological symptoms associated with delirium. Slater and Roth (1969) suggest that this theory of cerebral dysfunction is particularly applicable to psychosis accompanying cardiac decompensation and anemias.

Since many physically ill people show mental symptoms in the later and more severe stages of illness, exhaustion may well play a significant role in the development of delirium. This concept of exhaustion suggests that it is not the infection itself, but the resulting tiring or depletion of cerebral substances caused by the infection that precipitates the organic psychosis. However, the concept of "exhaustion" has yet to be adequately operationalized. One possible explanation is that depletion of nicotinic acid and other B vitamins interferes with cellular metabolism and, especially, carbohydrate metabolism of the central nervous system (Slater and Roth, 1969). However, further research may well demonstrate that numerous aspects, especially neurochemical substances, are involved in exhaustion. Depletion of any one or combination of these substances might result in psychological symptoms.

Toxic substances, particulary the toxins produced by microorganisms, have been implicated in the occurrence of delirium or organic psychosis. However, recent reexamination of this theory suggests that the role of these toxins is more complicated than originally thought (Slater and Roth, 1969). For instance, psychosis or delirium is an almost unknown complication of diphtheria or tetanus, despite the latter's reputation for exceptionally potent toxins and known effects on the peripheral nerves. If, in fact, delirium results from the action of bacterial toxins, then these toxins would seem to be highly specific in their action, yet produce a relatively nonspecific mental reaction, delirium (Slater and Roth, 1969).

Closely related to the concept of the action of bacterial toxins on cerebral function is the action of toxins, which are the immediate products of metabolism. This concept has long been utilized to explain the deliriums associated with uremia, diabetes (acidosis) and alcohol toxicity (Slater and Roth, 1969).

However, the role of vitamin deficiencies in Wernicke's encephalopathy, rather than liver dysfunction, is now generally accepted as a major causative factor of alcohol-related delirium. Thus, the symptom complex of delirium requires more explanation than is inherent in explanations based on organ malfunctions.

Other factors which appear to influence the development and course of delirium are the related factors of age and constitution. Although not clearly delineated, it is likely that some individuals are more prone to mental disturbances or delirium than others. Family or inherited tendencies are not clearly delineated; however, there are numerous clinical records of persons who become delirious every time they have an infection, although the infections are of significantly different natures (Slater and Roth, 1969).

> Intrinsic factors associated with age are known to affect the incidence of delirium. Delirious states complicating an infectious illness are more common in children than in adults; emotional disturbances following infectious illness are said to be particularly frequent in adolescents and young people, and the Korsakov syndrome occurs most frequently as a sequela of a symptomatic psychosis in the middle-aged and the elderly (Slater and Roth, 1969, p. 344).

By now, it is probably evident that delirium is produced by more than one and, probably, combinations of pathogenic mechanisms. Recent observations and knowledge point toward the reticular-activating system (see Figure 13-1 on p. 457) as the basis for evaluation unification of existing theories related to delirium, as well as the physiological focus for further research and understanding of this syndrome. The functions of the reticular-activating system are to regulate the tone of the cortex and to modulate its state (Luria, 1973). Thus, the functions of awareness and vigilance, therefore consciousness, are regulated by this system, which is comprised of structures of the midbrain, diencephalon and its diffuse connections with the cerebral cortex (Slater and Roth, 1969; Carpenter, 1972; Luria, 1973). Electroencephalographic abnormalities characteristic of delirious states commonly show bursts of rhythmic, slow activity. This slowed activity not only suggests interference with the reticular-activating system, but helps to explain why aged adults and children (age 10) are more vulnerable to delirium. Since these two groups, under normal metabolic circumstances, have slower EEG activity, they no doubt also have less tolerance for further slowing that occurs with various infections, metabolic diseases and syndromes.

Further evidence for interference with the reticular-activating system in the syndrome of delirium can be drawn from the nature of structural lesions, intracranial tumor, elevated intracranial pressure or cerebral vascular accident. Besides the resultant delirium, the common factor evident in these otherwise diverse conditions appears to be a basal lesion or indirect pressure causing at least partial occlusion of the arteries that supply the reticular formation from the circle of Willis (Slater and Roth, 1969).

If, in fact, slowing of EEG tracings is a necessary condition for the altered level of consciousness characteristic of delirium, then the fast EEG activity characteristic of both barbiturate intoxication and delirium tremens suggests a psychological syndrome other than delirium.

> Delirium tremens is now widely regarded as being a withdrawal phenomenon. Sudden withdrawal of drugs of addiction may precipitate epileptic attacks and, at times, status epilepticus. The EEG changes are of considerable interest in that bursts of spikes and wave complexes may be seen even in cases without convulsions. In place of a typical delirious state, the effect of withdrawal may be to precipitate an acute paranoid psychosis with little or no disturbance of consciousness (Slater and Roth, 1969, p. 345).

Differences between withdrawal syndromes and those producing alteration of consciousness with associated slowing of electrical activity are also suggested in the differences in their respective pharmacological treatment. Phenothiazines, in low dosages, are preferable in all but withdrawal syndromes (Detre and Jarecki, 1971). In fact, in cases of delirium associated with EEG slowing, CNS depressants often increase, rather than decrease, the patient's confusion and excitement and further decrease his level of consciousness. Even though alcohol and barbiturate withdrawal syndromes are classically considered to fall into the category of diseases and syndromes which produce a resultant delirium, further inquiries may clarify their pathophysiology and reassign them to another group of organic brain syndromes.

Clinical Manifestations of Delirium

The individual suffering from delirium may experience a variety of fluctuating symptoms. His disattention may range from distractibility to complete loss of contact with the environment. He may appear to pass from a state of wakefulness into the hypnagogic state of sleep, which is characterized by light sleep at dreaming and, finally, into deep sleep (Slater and Roth, 1969). In full-blown delirium, the patient also harbors illusions and experiences hallucinations (particularly visual) of a rapidly changing content (Detre and Jarecki, 1971). He may appear depressed and apathetic or excited and violent. It is this later behavior which usually draws attention to the patient and his delirium.

The mood of the delirious patient varies with his imagination but is most often characterized by fear and bewilderment. Since his perceptions of reality are confused and predominantly influenced by illusionary falsifications, his thinking is disconnected. His behaviors are reflective of his thoughts; thus, there are often repeated attempts to leave his bed, in order to flee or to fight his imaginary foes (Slater and Roth, 1969). In mild to severe delirium, the patient's behavior is characterized by irritability. The smallest inconvenience or provocation is capable of unleashing a tirade of criticism and verbal abuse. Some appear hysterical, over-acting to stimuli. Such an individual may call the police because her daughter is ten minutes overdue. Although there is some basis for the concern, the individual's actions are grossly out of proportion. The actions reflect the imaginative or delusional thinking, which is so characteristic of delirium. No matter what the configuration of symptoms, they are often exaggerated by darkness, when some degree of disorientation is within the range of normal experience.

Although there is some regularity in the symptom development and receding of delirium, no two cases develop exactly alike. General patterns of development include: (1) drowsiness which progresses toward stuporousness and even coma, (2) initial excitement which subsides to drowsiness only after the individual becomes exhausted, and (3) continual fluctuations—at one moment the individual is calm and lucid or only mildly perplexed, the next, excited and massively confused (Detre and Jarecki, 1971). Despite the clinical picture, shortly before recovery, many patients drift into a period of deep sleep known as "terminal sleep." This period of sleep ranges from 12 to 24 hours and usually marks the end of the psychosis (Detre and Jarecki, 1971; Slater and Roth, 1969). As a rule, recollection of the delirium is fogged or completely obliterated; however, some recall of isolated incidents may remain (Slater and Roth, 1969).

In instances of unfavorable outcome of delirium, the motor excitation subsides only with increasing exhaustion and weakness. As the patient's status deteriorates further, there remains only an ataxic fluttering of the hands and unintelligible muttering of the lips. Finally, the patient slips into a coma so deep that he does not react even to painful stimuli (Slater and Roth, 1969). Other less catastrophic complications of delirium include epileptic seizures, twilight states, residual delusions and residual paranoid attitudes. Also, there may be a resultant dementia, if there is permanent destruction of cortical tissue, either because of the primary injury or pathology or destruction secondary to effects of the underlying pathology.

Regardless of the characteristics or severity of the clinical picture, delirium, even in its mildest forms, must be considered a serious medical emergency. Detre and Jarecki (1971) identify three convincing reasons for considering delirium among the most serious of medical conditions:

1. The patient's behavior can become dangerously unmanageable.
2. The primary illness causing the symptoms of delirium can, if unchecked, lead to permanent brain damage and/or death.
3. Untreated delirium can progress to stupor, coma, convulsions or even status epilepticus.

Management

The treatment of deliriform syndromes is that of the underlying metabolic illness. Since delirium itself offers few clues to its cause, history and physical and laboratory findings—especially ventilatory status and acid-base balance—are of prime diagnostic significance. In the interim between successful diagnosis and control of the underlying disorder, supportive care becomes the focus of both medical and nursing management. The following provides an outline for this supportive care (Detre and Jarecki, 1971; Kyes and Hofling, 1974; Beland and Passos, 1975; Luckmann and Sorensen, 1974):

1. Maintain the patient's fluid and electrolyte balance
   a) Maintain and record accurate intake and output
   b) Observe for indications of dehydration
      (1) Increased thirst
      (2) Poor or deteriorating skin turgor
      (3) Dry, cracked mucous membrane
      (4) Decreased urinary output
          < 25ml per hr or 500ml per 24 hr
      (5) Increased specific gravity of the urine—above 1.030
      (6) Dry, cool, pale skin
      (7) Elevated temperature > 101°F
      (8) Increased blood viscosity
          Elevated hemoglobin
          Elevated hematocrit
      (9) Lowered blood pressure
      (10) Lowered venous pressure
      (11) Elevated serum Na^+ (above 145 mEq)
      (12) Muscle flacidity and/or tetany
   c) Check temperature every 2-4 hours
   d) Give adequate fluids per appropriate route (PO, IV, tube)
   e) Observe for indications of water or fluid intoxication
      (1) Absence of thirst
      (2) Polyuria—low specific gravity of the urine (normal kidney)
      (3) Twitching, hyperirritability, increased mental disturbances, convulsions, decreasing level of consciousness
      (4) Serum Na^+ below 130 mEq/L
      (5) Nausea, vomiting, weakness, muscle twitches
      (6) Development of dependent edema
      (7) Third space edema—ascities, pulmonary edema

2. Maintain the patient's nutritional balance
   a) Encourage high caloric, high protein, high vitamin intake meals
   b) Provide for supplementary feeding
   c) Administer tube feedings per physician's order
   d) Administer nutritional supplements per physician's order
   e) Administer vitamin (particularly vitamin B) supplements per physician's order
   f) Monitor weight
   g) Observe for indications of indigestion, constipation or diarrhea
   h) Observe for pre-existing nutritional deficiency—anemias, iron deficiency—low hemoglobin
3. Protect from complications
   a) Minimize risks of secondary infection
      (1) Limit visitors, especially those with any indication of viral or bacterial infection
      (2) Maintain strict asepsis and handwashing techniques in providing for care
      (3) Isolate from other patients who have or are suspected of having *any* infectious process
      (4) Observe for elevations in the WBC
      (5) Maintain the patient's personal hygiene
   b) Minimize the risks of cardiac embarrassment
      (1) Observe for and report the occurrence of
         (a) Heart rate above 100 or below 60
         (b) Rales or rhonchi in the lungs
         (c) Increased venous pressure (protrusion of the jugular vein, especially upon turning the head to the opposite side)
         (d) Bruits—pounding sound against the arterial wall
         (e) Absence or decreased peripheral pulses
         (f) Decrease in color and/or temperature of the extremities
         (g) Pupil dilatation
      (2) Avoid fluid and electrolyte imbalances
         (a) Observe for indications of K deficiency
         (b) Maintain fluid intake and output ratio
      (3) Prevent hyperthermia

- (a) Report elevations in temperature, especially those above 101° F
- (b) Administer antipyretic, as ordered, for elevated temperature
- (c) Institute measures to lower temperature, as ordered and/or indicated
  - (1) Alcohol sponge
  - (2) Cool bath
  - (3) Ice mattress
4. Control anxiety and agitation secondary to the confused state
   a) Simplify and structure the environment
      - (1) Night light
      - (2) Calendar—bold, large print, preferably single digit date, month, year
      - (3) Clock—bold-faced, with each hour numbered
      - (4) Familiar objects—own pajamas, family pictures, personal articles
      - (5) Remind the individual where he is, why, and what is expected of him
      - (6) Have someone sit quietly with him, especially at night
   b) Protect the patient from excessive stimulation
      - (1) Shade bright lights
      - (2) Avoid confusing stimuli, e.g., flashing lights, abstract pictures, difficult-to-identify sounds
      - (3) Provide for consistent care—limit the number of professionals interacting with the patient
      - (4) Limit visitors—maximum of one or two at a time, close family and friends
      - (5) Limit duration of visits to a 15- to 30-minute period and ask visitors to leave if patient shows indications of increasing restlessness or agitation
      - (6) When possible, avoid monotonous stimuli
   c) Report increasingly disoriented or agitated behavior
      - (1) Request and/or administer physical and/or chemical restraints, when delirious patient cannot be controlled by psychological measures
      - (2) Low dosages of phenothiazines preferable in all but CNS withdrawal syndromes or in instances of seizures—administered in dosages enough to diminish excitement

0.5-1.0 mg Prolixin fluphenazine
1.0-2.0 mg Trilifon perphenazine
10-20 mg Thorazine chlorpromazine
Administer at first indication of uncontrollable excitement or on a regularly scheduled basis (long-acting drug)
(3) CNS depressant drugs contraindicated—these drugs often escalate the patient's confusion and excitement as well as confuse the diagnostic picture
(4) Patients with cardiovascular or cerebral vascular illness receiving phenothiazines need special observations, because of secondary hypotension
   (a) Phenothiazines with little hypotensive effect preferable
   (b) Keep side rails up
   (c) Have patient move slowly and gradually from prone to upright position
   (d) Patient should be accompanied at all times when out of bed
   (e) Determine impact of hypotensive effects by comparing lying and standing blood pressures
(5) Patients may continue to receive phenothiazines in increased dosages after diagnosis and stabilization in order to diminish delusions
   (a) Administer as ordered
   (b) Observe for diminishing of delirium, especially delusional thinking
   (c) Observe for and report side effects of phenothiazine therapy

EPILEPTIFORM SYNDROMES

Seizure Disorders (Epilepsy)

Seizure disorder and epilepsy are often used interchangeably both in the medical literature and by laymen. Since most of our concept of seizure or epileptic phenomenon is based on observable clinical events and, as yet, poorly understood physiological phenomena, definitions of epilepsy are at best inadequate (Matthews and Miller, 1975). The symptom complex of seizure disorders or epilepsy, like those of other organic brain syndromes, is attributed to brain tissue dysfunction characterized by the origination and spread of abnormal electrical discharges (Detre and Jarecki, 1971). However, as Matthews and Miller (1975) point out, to define seizure disorders as a paroxysmal or episodic disorder of cerebral function would include a variety of transient cerebral ischemic attacks and seizure episodes secondary to reversible metabolic disorders. In addition, some individuals experience abnormal brain discharges consistent with epilepsy, yet appear to be entirely free of the related clinical symptoms. Although there is no completely satisfactory definition of epilepsy, the following characteristics are attributed to patients categorized as being epileptic:

1. The pattern of a seizure or fit depends not on the cause but on the site of the abnormal cerebral discharge (Matthews and Miller, 1975).
2. There is a paroxysmal and transitory disturbance of the function of the brain (Slater and Roth, 1969).
3. The disturbance tends to develop suddenly, cease spontaneously and recur (Slater and Roth, 1969).
4. In most instances, the abnormal discharge originates in and spreads to the same cerebral area, thus symptoms are similar with each occasion (Detre and Jarecki, 1971).

Incidence

Reported incidence of epilepsy ranges from 5 per 1000 population (Matthews and Miller, 1975) to 3.76 per 1000 (Slater and Roth, 1969) in the general population. When considering psychiatrically hospitalized populations, the incidence increases 3 to 10 percent of the total admissions (Slater and Roth, 1969).

About 40 percent of epileptics experience their first seizure prior to age 10, with an additional 30 percent experiencing first seizures by age 20 (Slater and Roth, 1969). According to Glaser (1975) more males than females are treated for epilepsy. Age seems to be only a factor in determining the type of disorder, not the actual presence of epilepsy.

Closely related, if not directly associated to the seizure activity, is a marked increase in psychiatric disorders. Approximately one-sixth to one-fourth of epileptics suffer identifiable psychiatric problems, and at least 10 percent are admitted to psychiatric hospitals for treatment (Slater and Roth, 1969). Especially at risk for epilepsy are males from the lower socio-economic class. However, it is unclear whether epilepsy contributes to social and psychological maladaption or may, in fact, arise from such hazards as malnutrition, infection, violence and poor obstetric care. According to Pond, Bidwell and Stein (Slater and Roth, 1969), this group of males is more impaired by the number and severity of their seizures plus intellectual and personality problems, making the finding and retaining of employment problematic.

Etiology

Secondary or Acquired—When a seizure appears secondary to an identifiable illness, it is referred to as symptomatic. Gross interference with brain function may occur during the course of such systemic illnesses as infections, intoxication (uremia and eclampsia) and severe or sudden cardiac decompensation. When seizure activity arises secondary to such systemic illnesses, the primary clinical concern is focused on the treatment and control of the underlying illness. The seizure activity, per se, is of limited importance.

Another, more significant cause of secondary seizure activity is that of local damage, which sets up a focus of abnormal discharge. Major causes of such foci are infections, such as meningitis, cerebral syphilis, local vascular damage, birth injuries (especially if combined with asphyxia), congenital malformations of the brain and/or skull, head injury (especially related to a period of unconsciousness) and cerebral tumors (Slater and Roth, 1969). Post traumatic epilepsy may develop within three years in upwards of 4 percent of open head injuries (Glaser, 1975). Physical factors, such as penetration of the dura (Slater and Roth, 1969), and severity and location of the wound (Glaser, 1975) interact with genetic and environmental factors in determining the occurrence of a seizure disorder of the magnitude of epilepsy.

Birth injuries, especially those associated with neonatal asphyxia, prematurity and breech delivery (Glaser, 1975), are probably an underestimated source of seizure foci. During the passage of the infant through the birth canal, a dramatic rise in intracranial pressure occurs. When this increase occurs, tissue in the hippocampal regions of the temporal lobes is at particular risk to infarct, resulting in temporal lobe seizures (Slater and Roth, 1969).

For 15-20 percent of individuals who suffer from brain tumors, a seizure is usually the first indication of pathology (Glaser, 1975). In 30-40 percent of the cases, seizures, especially of the focal nature, are subsequently experienced. According to Glaser (1975), when symptoms progress from focal seizures to hemiparesis and dementia, they are highly suggestive of a tumor. Likewise, when seizure onset occurs after 30 years of age with no history or evidence of a head injury, tumor is a likely cause (Detre and Jarecki, 1971).

Cerebral vascular disease is a cause of epilepsy, especially in those individuals who experience onset after 40 years (Detre and Jarecki, 1971; Glaser, 1975). Glaser (1975) reports that, although not always recognized, up to 25 percent of individuals with cerebral vascular disease experience seizures. Seizures associated with cerebral vascular disease are believed to be secondary to localized vascular insufficiency, ischemic hypoxia and lesions secondary to embolism, hemorrhage and thrombosis. Diffuse cerebral arteriosclerosis, cerebral degenerative diseases (Alzheimer, Pick) and demyelinating diseases (multiple sclerosis) also have a significant incidence of seizures.

Idiopathic—When a specific structural or biochemical cause cannot be found, the seizure disorder of epilepsy is said to be idiopathic; up to 75 percent of those with seizure disorders are so classified (Glaser, 1975). Petit mal epilepsy in childhood is regarded as the classical example of idiopathic epilepsy. However, as Slater and Roth (1969) point out, some think that fewer cases of seizures will be considered idiopathic, as the causal agents resulting in epilepsy become better known. In the meantime, this lack of understanding about the specific causative factors presents the patient, family and even the health care providers with a major problem in controlling and adapting to the related symptoms.

In either acquired or idiopathic epilepsy, the propensity for seizures is influenced by factors of heredity and psychological determinants, as well as the brain lesions and physiological disturbances discussed earlier. Individuals who develop a seizure disorder following post traumatic head injury report six times as many epiletics in their families as individuals suffering no seizures following a head injury (Detre and Jarecki, 1971). As Harvald (Slater and Roth, 1969) points out, the hereditary factor is probably multifactorial and additive. Although there may be a single gene which is determinant for seizures in some families, what is more likely is that there is an inherited predisposition to seizures. This lowered threshold or propensity for seizures (Detre and Jarecki, 1971) may be characterized by the increased tendency to produce cerebral paroxysmic discharges and the increased tendency for discharges to spread (Slater and Roth, 1969).

Stress of either physiological or psychological character is often an important factor in triggering seizures. In normal individuals, seizure activity develops only after major stress, such as electrical shock, severe electrolyte imbalance, hypoglycemia, hypocalcemia, hyperpyrexia or withdrawal from central nervous system depressant drugs (Detre and Jarecki, 1971). More susceptible individuals may have seizures provoked by less stressful events, such as sleeplessness, fatigue or psychological stress. While the nature of the triggering stimuli varies, it can be relatively innocuous, such as listening to music, reading, being touched without warning, seeing flickering lights or passing cars. The individual's dramatic response is, in part, determined by the emotional reaction to the participating event, as well as the event itself (Detre and Jarecki, 1971).

Clinical Manifestations

Categories of epilepsies are not mutually exclusive or even sharply defined. Several types of seizures may occur in a single individual; the patient with grand mal seizures may also demonstrate symptoms of focal seizures. In addition, those with petit mal seizures tend to develop other types of seizures as they approach adulthood. However, the traditional distinctions among grand mal, petit mal and focal seizures are useful in establishing an investigative plan, therapeutic program and prognostic formulation (Detre and Jarecki, 1971).

Although the EEG is an important diagnostic instrument in the diagnosis of epilepsy, the distinction among types of epilepsy cannot be based on the EEG alone. In fact, the diagnosis of epilepsy cannot be based solely on the EEG results. The instrument, sensitive to a wide variety of external factors, such as movement around the instrument and fluorescent lights, may indicate abnormalities when none exist. Other limitations to the ECG are as follows (Detre and Jarecki, 1971):

1. The EEG can only detect those abnormal discharges of sufficient voltage to be measured through the cranial bones and scalp.
2. The EEG is incapable of reproducing the original rhythms that originate in deeper areas of the brain.
3. Special EEG techniques are necessary to reveal occult cerebral dysrhythmia: (a) sleep EEG, (b) administration of drugs that activate epileptic foci, (c) use of special leads, and (d) repeated examinations and comparisons.

Generalized or Centrencephalic Epilepsy

Grand Mal Epilepsy

Grand mal seizures usually start with a prodromal phase, which may precede the attack by several hours and, on rare occasions, by several days. This phase may be characterized by mood changes, restlessness, headache, gastrointestinal symptoms and even skin eruptions (Slater and Roth, 1969). The prodromal phase often goes unidentified by the individual's family and associates. With the onset of the seizure, there is a brief sensory experience, indicative of the origin of the seizure and often regarded as an aura. Frequently experienced auras include a sense of fear or dread, upper gastric sensations, an unpleasant odor, hallucinations of a sensory, auditory or visual character, peculiar sensations in an arm or leg or localized movements in extremity or face (Glaser, 1975). Identification of an aura may distinguish between a seizure generalized from onset and one that becomes generalized after a focal onset.

The actual convulsion is often initiated with a sudden high-pitched scream ("epiletic cry"), loss of consciousness and tonic rigidity of the trunk and extremities. During a convulsion, arms are held close to the trunk, elbows are straight, wrists flexed, and fingers often dig into the palm with abducted thumbs (Slater and Roth, 1969). Lower extremities extend with inversion of the feet and flexion of the toes; these tonic movements are followed by clonic movements of impaired breathing with apnea, cyanosis and stertor

(Glaser, 1975). Incontinence of the bladder and bowel and biting of the tongue and cheeks occur during the clonic phase. The clonic phase movements are characterized by a series of jerks. After a brief partial relaxation of musculature, convulsive spasms recur with cyanosis increasing in proportion to the interval between spasms. The clonic stage concludes in a final violent jerk followed by flacidity and reestablishment of breathing and consciousness (Slater and Roth, 1969).

Within minutes of the conclusion of the clonic phase, the afflicted individual enters the postictal state; he may appear confused and fatigued and complain of a headache, then lapse into a deep sleep (Glaser, 1975). At times, residual neurological signs, such as an extensor plantar response, hemiparesis, sensory disturbances and dysphasia persist. As a rule, once the individual has awakened from the deep sleep, consciousness is recovered.

If the postictal sleep does not occur or is postponed, some degree of confusion is usually evident. The person may not be fully aware of his identity, be restless and demonstrate post-epileptic auromatisms and, occasionally, explosions of irritability (Slater and Roth, 1969). During such explosions of irritability, anger is evident, and the patient may pose a threat by aggressive attacks on others.

The individual, generally, is completely amnesic for the major events surrounding the seizure (with the possible exception of the prodromal phase and aura (Glaser, 1975). However, in differentiating between actual epileptic seizures and seizure-like states, the former is usually distinguished by an alteration of consciousness. Partial or complete retention of consciousness is more characteristic of focal attacks (Slater and Roth, 1969).

Petit Mal Epilepsy

Petit mal epilepsy, or "absences," is one form of a twilight state in which the mental state is near stupor. Brief lapses of consciousness typically last 5 to 10 seconds but, occasionally, as long as 30 seconds and may occur up to 100 times a day (Glaser, 1975). During these brief absences, the individual appears to stare, with only the slightest of motor manifestations, such as blinking of eyelids, a slight turning to one side and brief almost imperceptible movements of the lips and hands (Detre and Jarecki, 1971). After the seizure, the patient usually is able to resume his previous activity with mental clarity; however, it is possible for him to have a period of post-seizure confusion.

Petit mal seizures commonly arise in childhood between the ages of 3 to 10 years or, at the latest, early adolescence (Glaser, 1975; Detre and Jarecki, 1971). The cause is seldom known, and these seizures tend to diminish spontaneously by adulthood. However, the prognosis for the development of grand mal seizures or psychomotor seizures in adult years is significantly increased from that of individuals with no petit mal seizure history (Detre and Jarecki, 1971).

Petit mal seizures are often precipitated by flickering lights, such as sunlight or a television screen (Glaser, 1975). The phenomenon of self-induction of the seizure is related to the sensitivity to flickering lights. The individual can induce a seizure by staring at a light and then passing his hand in front of his eyes (Glazer, 1975). In such instances, there appears to be an accompanying pleasurable sensation.

As might be expected, petit mal attacks, especially if very brief and relatively infrequent, may go undetected or unappreciated for a period of time. However, as the seizures increase in frequency and/or last longer, the child may have difficulty in completing tasks and mastering complex learning skills (Glaser, 1975). As might be expected, the schoolroom is often the first place where these difficulties are identifiable. If the attacks reach status proportion, clouding of consciousness, confusion and disorientation occur:

> Instances of even more prolonged mental dullness with profound psychic disturbances, a change in personality, motor agitation, dreamy states, delusion and "dementing" syndrome have been found associated with this type of abnormality (Glaser, 1974, p. 320).

Closely related to petit mal seizures are akinetic seizures and myoclonic seizures. During akinetic seizures, the patient falls and briefly loses consciousness. These seizures are often associated with severe brain damage and intellectual retardation (Detre and Jarecki, 1971). Myoclonic seizures may be localized or general and, when severe, are associated with impaired consciousness. These can precede a generalized seizure or occur in association with petit mal seizures. Sensory influences such as lights or sounds, changes in posture, drowsiness or emotional upset can precipitate the sudden involuntary contractions of a single muscle or group of muscles (Glaser, 1975; Detre and Jarecki, 1971).

When a severe myoclonic seizure disorder appears in the first eighteen months of life along with dramatic cerebral deterioration, the disorder is called infantile massive spasms or jackknife seizures (Glaser, 1975). Although the cause is undetermined, jackknife seizures are seen in conjunction with phenylketonuria, Down's syndrome, bilateral subdural hematoma or hydrocephaly.

Focal Epilepsy

Focal seizures are characterized by those manifestations consistent with the specific region of the brain involved. When more generalized convulsions follow, these transient psychological, sensory or motor symptoms constitute the "aura"; but when the same symptoms occur in isolation, it constitutes a focal seizure (Slater and Roth, 1969). Motor phenomena with or without Jacksonian march, vocalizations, movement of the lips, tongue and mouth, adversion of the head and eyes, hallucinations, imposed and impulsive thoughts and recollection of special situations are among the possible manifestations of a focal seizure.

Psychomotor - Temporal Lobe—Although any region of the cortex or subcortex may develop seizure foci, certain regions are apparently more predisposed. By far the most common location of focal seizures are areas of the temporal lobe, including portions of the limbic system.

> The temporal lobe and its deeper nuclear masses, the amygdala and hippocampus and their associated limbic structures, as indicated previously, are particularly vulnerable to many pathological processes from the perinatal period onwards throughout life (Glaser, 1975, p. 325).

In the majority of cases, a definite structural lesion may be identified; these lesions are often secondary to trauma, encephalitis, ischemia, hypoxia or tumor (Glaser, 1975).

The psychomotor attack precipitates a disturbance of mental functioning resulting in alteration but not loss of consciousness. The seizures are of short duration and usually accompanied by complex mental states, motor automatisms, vegetative symptoms, disturbances of behavior and speech and hallucinatory experiences (Glaser, 1975; Slater and Roth, 1969).

Prior to the onset of the seizure, the individual may experience a wide range of auras. Some of the more common auras include a peculiar sensation in the epigastrium, which is felt to rise towards the throat, deja vu and deja vecu experiences, feelings of depersonalization or derealization, illusions, hallucinations and forced ideas. During the actual seizure, the individual arrests or suspends his activity. He then begins simple movements such as lip-smacking, chewing, sucking and purposeless motions of his extremities. Following these simple movements come stereotyped automatisms of varying complexity; these activities may be partially purposeful or inappropriate and bizarre. They are, however, often associated with environmental influences and can be related to unresolved psychological conflicts (Glaser, 1975). In children, psychomotor seizure symptoms tend to be more visceral in nature. The child is likely to complain of hunger, nausea, retching, vomiting and abdominal pain (Glaser, 1975).

During the post seizure or ictal stage, the individual's behavior may immediately return to normal, although he may experience affective disturbances of fear, anger or depression. Destructive or aggressive behavior has been reported postictally; however, the association with homicide remains problematic (Glaser, 1975; Pincus and Tucker, 1974). Occasionally, vague states last for extended times, during which the patient can wander some distance with no recall of his experience.

Psychomotor seizures may be misdiagnosed or ignored due to the complexity of the symptom complex. Further, the EEG is not always reliable, because of the deep cerebral origin of the seizure activity. Because the individual appears to remain in contact with his environment, the bizarre behavior is likely to become the focus of therapeutic intervention. Only after repeated hospitalizations and/or unsuccessful treatment is the behavior seen as a portion of a pattern induced by a seizure disorder. Detre and Jarecki (1971) pose five steps that assist in making the necessary distinction:

1. Aura
2. Stereotyped sequence of events
3. Presence of EEG abnormalities in the midst of a characteristic episode of the behavior in question
4. Concomitant motor manifestations, even if they are barely discernible
5. Previous history of seizures.

Focal Motor and Sensory Seizures—Other significant focal seizures include the focal motor seizure and focal sensory seizure. Focal motor seizures are produced by lesions in the motor cortex of the brain. The classical Jacksonian motor seizure is characterized by initiation of unilateral repetitive movement in the distal portion of a finger, toe or corner of the mouth. The clonic jerks spread up the extremity toward the trunk and may cease at any point or become generalized, spreading contralaterally. Only when the seizure spreads contralaterally is consciousness altered.

Focal sensory seizures may also be Jacksonian in character. These seizures originate in the sensory cortex and produce a unilateral march of sensations such as numbness, cold, pain and tingling. Focal seizures in the occipital lobes produce unformed visual hallucinations. If the visual hallucinations are more complex and identifiable, they have originated in the occipito-parietal region of the cortex. Auditory and olfactory experiences can be elicited by focal seizure activity in the related areas of the brain.

Psychological Considerations

Epilepsy, or a chronic seizure disorder, is an example of a symptom complex that, by its very nature, affects the individual physiologically as well as psychologically. Which symptoms predominate depends heavily on the focus and radiation of the paroxysmal discharges. In recent years, aggressive treatment, particularly with anti-convulsant drugs, has enabled better than 85 percent of affected individuals (Glaser, 1975) to maintain virtually normal, seizure-free lives. However, even the controlled epileptic experiences problems of living and adaptation, which reflect the interactions of all aspects of the individual's personality, physiological, intra-psychic, familial, interpersonal and reference group. Listed below are just a few of the more prominent areas of conflict:

1. Fear of losing control and dependence on medication to maintain control provide fertile pasture for intensification of dependency - independency conflicts
2. Lessened ability to trust one's emotions, sensations, thoughts or perceptions as being valid responses to a given situation
3. The individual's increased predisposition to a seizure when confronted with emotional or psychosocial stress, thus, exposing

him to accusations of using a seizure to avoid confrontation
4. Inability or compromised ability to maintain control over bodily functions and appearance
5. Family's perception of the individual's problem as a sign of weakness or inferiority
6. Society's restrictions on activities such as driving, marriage, entrance into some careers and trades, attendance at public schools, availability of insurance and workman's compensation and childbearing often put almost unmanageable strain on the individual's coping and adapting skills
7. Inappropriate, residually cultural reactions to the epileptic as being "possessed" or fears that the seizure is somehow contagious
8. Unrealistic fears that even the controlled epileptic is dangerous either to himself or others.

Management

Treatment of a patient with a seizure disorder must take into account all aspects of the patient (his family and life situation), as well as his particular disorder. For those whose seizures are secondary to such conditons as hypercalcemia, hypoglycemia or other clearly metabolic disorders, treatment of the underlying disorder can be expected to alleviate the seizures.

In the cases of cerebral tumors, seizures may subside if the tumor can be successfully removed. However, it is not unusual for the trauma of the surgical procedure itself to establish additional seizure foci. Thus, even though the tumor is removed, the individual may require anticonvulsant drug therapy.

Most cases of epilepsy are amenable neither to cure of the underlying disorder nor surgical removal. Patients with post-traumatic epilepsy, as well as idiopathic epilepsy, are often successfully treated with anticonvulsant drugs and a general psychosocial rehabilitative program (Glaser, 1975).

Anticonvulsant Drugs

Drugs are commonly utilized in the treatment of seizure disorders. Although there is no unanimity concerning the order and manner in which anticonvulsants are utilized, Detre and Jarecki

(1971) formulate some general guidelines consistent with the classical grouping of seizures.

Type of Seizure	Drug Classification
Grand Mal	Hydantoins and/or Barbiturates
Focal Motor Epilepsy	Barbiturates
Petit Mal	Succinimides, Oxazolidines
Psychomotor	Hydantoins and Barbiturates if effective
	Oxazolidines and Succinimides

Common representatives of each of the aforementioned categories of anticonvulsant drugs are listed below, along with common side effects and dosages (Glaser, 1975).

HYDANTOINS

Dilantin (diphenylhydantoin)
- Dose
  - Children 0.1 to 0.3 g.
  - Adults 0.3 to 0.6 g.
  - Effective blood level 10-20 μg/ml
- Symptoms — Grand mal, psychomotor, focal seizures
- Toxic effects — Rash, fever, gum hypertrophy, gastric distress, atoxia, hirsutism, drowsiness

Mesantoin (methylphenylethylhydantoin)
- Dose
  - Children 0.1-0.4 g.
  - Adults 0.4-0.8 g.
- Symptoms — Grand mal, psychomotor, focal seizures
- Toxic effects — Rash, fever, drowsiness, ataxia, agranulocytosis, aplastic anemia

Peganone (ethylphenylhydantoin)
- Dose
  - Children 0.5-1.5 g.
  - Adults 2.0-3.0 g.
- Symptoms — Grand mal, psychomotor, focal seizures
- Toxic effects — Similar to Dilantin but less severe; also generally less effective

BARBITURATES

Phenobarbital
Dose	Children 0.45-0.1 g. Adults 0.1-0.3 g.
Symptoms	All seizure states used in combination with Dilantin
Toxic effects	Drowsiness, dulling, rash, fever, irritability and hyperactivity in children

Mysoline (primidone) (a barbiturate congener)
Dose	Children 0.25-1.0 g. Adults 0.75-2.0 g. Effective blood level 5-15 μg/ml.
Symptoms	Grand mal, psychomotor, focal seizures; useful with Dilantin
Toxic effects	Drowsiness, ataxia, dizziness, rash, nausea, leukopenia

Mebaral (mephobarbital)
Dose	Children 0.06-0.3 g. Adults 0.3-0.6 g.
Symptoms	Grand mal, petit mal, psychomotor, focal seizures; useful in combination with hydantoins
Toxic effects	Drowsiness, irritability, rash

Gemonil (metharbital)
Dose	Children 0.1-0.3 g. Adults 0.3-0.6 g.
Symptoms	Myoclonic seizures, massive spasms, petit mal
Toxic effects	Drowsiness, rash

SUCCINIMIDES

Zarontin (ethosuximide)
Dose	Children 0.75-1.0 g. Adults 1.5 g.

Symptoms	Drug of choice for petit mal
Toxic effects	Blood dyscrasias, dermatitis anoxia, nausea, drowsiness, dizziness, euphoria

Milontin (phensuximide)
Dose	Children 0.25-1.5 g. Adults 2.0-4.0 g.
Symptoms	Petit mal, myoclonic, akinetic and occasionally psychomotor seizures
Toxic effects	Nausea, dizziness, rash, hematuria

Celontin (methsuximide)
Dose	Children 0.6 g. Adults up to 1.5 g.
Symptoms	Petit mal, psychomotor, myoclonic seizures
Toxic effects	Ataxia, drowsiness, blood dyscrasias, anorexia

OXAZOLIDINES

Tridione (trimethadione)
Dose	Children 0.3-1.8 g. Adults 1.2-2.4 g.
Symptoms	Petit mal, myoclonic, akinetic and occasionally psychomotor seizures
Toxic effects	Rash, gastric distress, visual symptoms, neutropenia, agranulocytosis

Other drugs that are commonly used as adjuncts to anticonvulsant treatment include the following (Detre and Jarecki, 1971):

Diamox (acetazolamide)
1. Petit mal epilepsy
2. Seizure disorders which increase in severity just before the menstrual period

Dexedrine (dextroamphetamine)
1. Seizures which are related to drowsiness
2. Anticonvulsant regimens that make the individual excessively drowsy

Valium (diazepam)

Librium (chlordiazepoxide)
1. Control of anxiety and tension experienced by some individuals with a seizure disorder

No anticonvulsant drug is capable of total seizure control in all patients. However, careful selection and utilization of anticonvulsant drugs, taking each individual and his special needs into consideration, usually provide optimal results. There is a certain amount of trial and error, as well as skilled observation and adjustment, necessary to reach optimal results. The cooperation of the patient and his family is essential in establishing the most satisfactory treatment regimen from the standpoint of seizure control, long-term compliance and personal life adjustment.

Nursing Care

Nursing Care During a Convulsion

A. Protect the patient from secondary injury
   1. Stay with the patient, send another person for additional assistance
   2. Observe for indications of aspiration and respiratory obstruction
   3. Provide safe environment
      a) Move obstructions away from patient
      b) Ease patient to the floor if he is standing or sitting
      c) Place small pillow, jacket, bathrobe or some cushion under the patient's head
      d) Do not attempt to restrain or move the patient during a seizure
      e) Do not attempt forcibly to open clenched jaws or force anything into the patient's mouth
      f) Make available a padded tongue blade for insertion into patient's mouth between the back teeth, prior to the clenching of the jaws, to prevent biting of tongue and mouth
      g) Accompany patient who is experiencing uncontrolled seizures
      h) Administer prescribed anticonvulsants

B. Maintain patent airway and adequate ventilation
   1. Loosen tight clothing
   2. Insert plastic airway, if possible, prior to clenching of jaws
   3. Without forcing, turn patient or his head to the side to facilitate drainage of secretions and prevent obstruction by the tongue
   4. Administer oxygen as indicated
C. Observe the patient during the seizure
   1. Describe behavior immediately prior to the onset of convulsion
      a) Position of head, body, extremities
      b) Activity - what the patient was doing
      c) Verbalizations - what was said - how it was said
      d) Mood
   2. Describe behavior that first indicated a convulsion was taking place
   3. Describe the convulsion
      a) Progression
      b) Type of activity
      c) Parts of the body involved
      d) Automatisms
      e) Neurological signs
         (1) Deviation of tongue or eyeballs
         (2) Change in pupils
         (3) Paralysis, hemiparesis
      f) Length or duration
   4. Describe the post convulsion behavior and activity
      a) Level of consciousness
      b) Any injury secondary to the seizure
      c) Disturbances of speech, coordination, thought processes, perceptual alterations, motor power, paresthesias
      d) Vital signs
      e) Presence and character of sleep post seizure
      f) Patients recall of any aspect of seizure and preceding feelings, behavior, etc. (Luckmann and Sorensen, 1974; Beland and Passos, 1975)

This same guideline may be used to facilitate a history of the patient's seizures from family and close associates. It must be remembered that the patient is usually amnesic for events surrounding a seizure, and that family members have accepted much of the patient's behavior without question. In addition, if the seizure is characterized by behavioral abberations, the seizure can be overlooked, since attempts are made to correct the unacceptable behavior.

Some additional questions that the nurse might ask are as follows:
1. Were there any known complications related to the pregnancy and delivery of the patient?
2. What serious illnesses or injuries has this patient experienced? Particularly:
    a) Illness involving the central nervous system or associated with high fevers—above 105°F
    b) Injuries to the head, especially those that resulted in even brief unconsciousness
3. Is there *any* family history of seizures?
4. Has this patient ever been thought to have had a seizure—even febrile?
5. Have there been times when the patient's behavior suddenly changed or he did not seem to respond appropriately (e.g., to the call of his name)?
6. Has this patient ever been thought to have emotional problems or behavioral problems, including sexual deviations and aggressive outbursts?
    a) Arrests
    b) Mental hospitalizations
7. Does the patient seem to have undue difficulty concentrating or completing even routine tasks?

Special Nursing Care Considerations During Status Epilepticus

In the special instances of status epilepticus, the major focus is on the immediate control of the intractable seizures. The following drugs are commonly used in the emergency treatment (Glaser, 1975):

Sodium phenobarbital 0.25—0.50 IV
Sodium amytal 0.25—0.50 IV
Valium (diazepam) 10 mg. IV
Dilantin sodium 0.25 g. IV or IM

In addition to administering and recording the ordered medications, the nursing care focuses on the maintenance of vital system functions and the safety and protection of the patient. Related nursing goals would include:

1. Continual assessment and maintenance of fluid and electrolyte balance
2. Maintenance of the airway
3. Temperature control
4. Assessment for changes in cardiac and renal function
5. Provisions for a safe environment to prevent self-injury during the seizures.

Nursing Care Related to the Long-term Management of Epilepsy

For the individual who has epilepsy, establishing diagnosis and initial control of the seizures is only the beginning, since epilepsy is a life-long proposition. Thus, the afflicted individual not only has to make the initial intrapsychic and psychosocial adjustments but readjusts continually as he grows, develops and assumes different roles and responsibilities. How great a factor the seizure disorder is or should be in an individual's life is often left to chance, which may actually encourage two extremes in adaptation: denial, seen in discontinuing medication or choice of an extremely risky and dangerous occupation; or a life of unnecessary restriction, even invalidism. Assisting the individual and his family to make these readjustments is an important, if not vital, nursing function. Listed below are those factors that need to be considered repeatedly with the patient and his family:

1. Control of seizures is not a cure. Thus, following some treatment regime is a long-term, if not life-long, endeavor.
2. Due to the continual change in an individual's physiology and living pattern, the original treatment regime may not remain indefinitely successful or even tolerable. Thus, the treatment regime needs to be reevaluated at scheduled intervals.
    a) Anticipating stress inherent in particular developmental phases, e.g., adolescence.
    b) Continued reassessment for toxicity to the anticonvulsant drugs.

    c) Reevaluation of the regime in light of changes in individual, family and social circumstances.
    d) Reevaluation of the treatment in relation to changes in pertinent medical, drug and treatment knowledge.
    e) The first indications of exacerbation of seizures may be an unexpected overt seizure but may also be a personality change such as irritable, inappropriate behavior or lability of mood.
3. Realistic consideration of activities which are contraindicated or restricted by the individual's seizure disorder.
    a) Most children can and should attend public school and take part in related activities, including sports.
    b) After a two-year, seizure-free period, driving a car need not be restricted.
    c) Career choices need not be unduly restricted. Special consideration may need to be given to those jobs that require climbing to extreme heights, using heavy power equipment or dangerous chemical substances.
    d) Marriage and childbearing are *not* contraindicated.
    e) For most, a special protective environment is not required or desirable.
    f) The individual can and should be expected to function normally within his family, school and social setting.
4. Consideration should be given to the present social stigmas and legal restrictions which affect people with epilepsy.
    a) The patient and/or his family need factual information about state and local laws and their enforcement that apply to individuals with seizure disorders.
    b) Myths and social stigma about epilepsy need to be openly discussed, including how to avoid or deal with them.

Two other conditions closely related to epilepsy are narcolepsy and somnambulism. Although these conditions are not epileptic, they share the commonality of paroxysmal occurrence of symptoms (Detre and Jarecki, 1971).

Narcolepsy

Narcolepsy is a syndrome of unknown origin, although some disturbance in the alerting mechanisms of the reticular formation is suggested. It is characterized by an irresistible urge to sleep (Matthews and Miller, 1975). The attacks may last for a few hours, but the majority subside within 10 to 15 minutes (Detre and Jarecki, 1971). Initially, the attacks occur during a period of rest or relaxation, when some drowsiness can be regarded as normal.

> Falling asleep in public transport, in the cinema, or even on the hard benches of the outpatient department can be described as little more than an exaggeration of normal behavior. . . . (Matthew and Miller, 1975, p. 309).

If the condition worsens, the individual may be overcome by sleep during a meal or even while standing upright. He can be easily aroused, but, if left undisturbed, will sleep for minutes or hours.

Other characteristic disturbances of attention are often found in conjunction with narcolepsy. Among the more common accompanying disturbances are the following (Detre and Jarecki, 1971):

1. Cataplexy—attacks of becoming akinetic and falling down without falling asleep
2. Hypnagogic hallucinations—during the period just before falling asleep or awaking, the individual sees and/or hears things that seem real but are not
3. Sleep paralysis—just before falling asleep or awakening, he feels as though he is fully awake but unable to move.

The individual who suffers from narcolepsy is likely to have difficulties in addition to falling asleep. Since much of his energy is taken up attempting to remain awake, he is likely to appear anxious, fatigued and even hypochondriacal (Detre and Jarecki, 1971). Other difficulties which appear more frequently in these patients include severe obesity, development of a passive-aggressive character disorder and even psychosis (Detre and Jarecki, 1971).

Diagnosis of narcolepsy is based on the following criteria (Detre and Jarecki, 1971):

1. Brief, recurrent sleep attacks followed by feelings of alertness
2. One or more of the associated disturbances—cataplexy, hypnagogic hallucinations, sleep paralysis
3. History beginning in adolescence
4. Family history of similar disorders
5. No identifiable causative factors.

Treatment is symptomatic. Amphetamines, often in large doses, can provide some relief without disturbing nocturnal sleep. Cataplexy responds well to imipramine (Matthews and Miller, 1975).

Somnambulism

More commonly known as sleep walking, somnambulism is the opposite of narcolepsy. The wakeful state or alert state intrudes into the nocturnal sleep pattern (Detre and Jarecki, 1971). During such an episode, the individual has his eyes open, initially, and activities are repetitive, but as he becomes increasingly oriented, behavior may become quite complex and purposeful. He will briefly answer questions, but it is difficult to maintain his attention or waken him (Detre and Jarecki, 1971). The individual has little, if any, recollection of his night activities upon normal wakening in the morning.

Associated, possibly related, symptoms to somnambulism are enuresis nocturna and pavor nocturnus (night terrors). These three symptoms are often seen together, especially in children (Detre and Jarecki, 1971). Various forms of treatment, psychotherapy and drugs have been tried to control somnambulism but, to date, there is no generally prescribed management.

Organic Brain Syndrome / 457

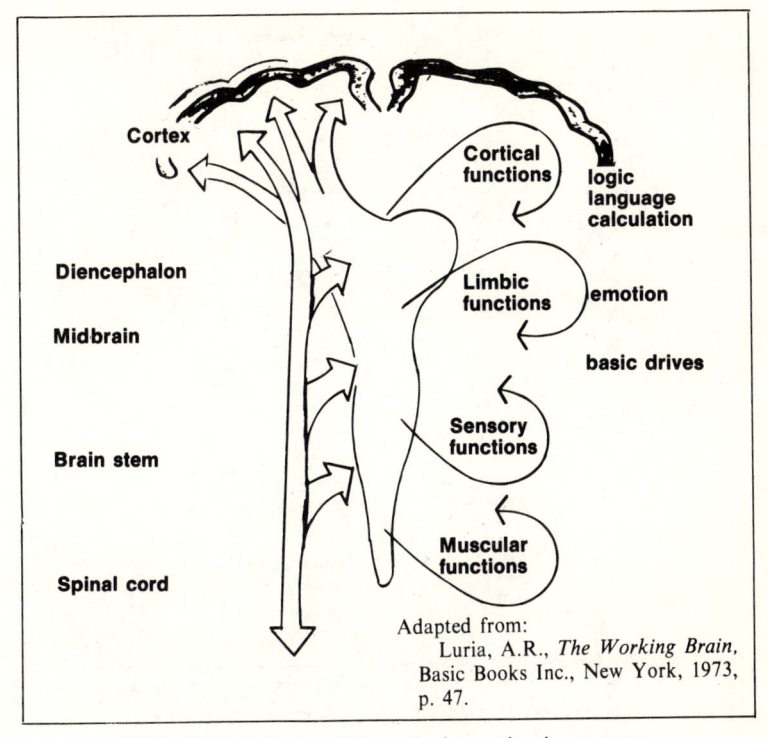

Figure 13-1: Scheme of the reticular-activating system.

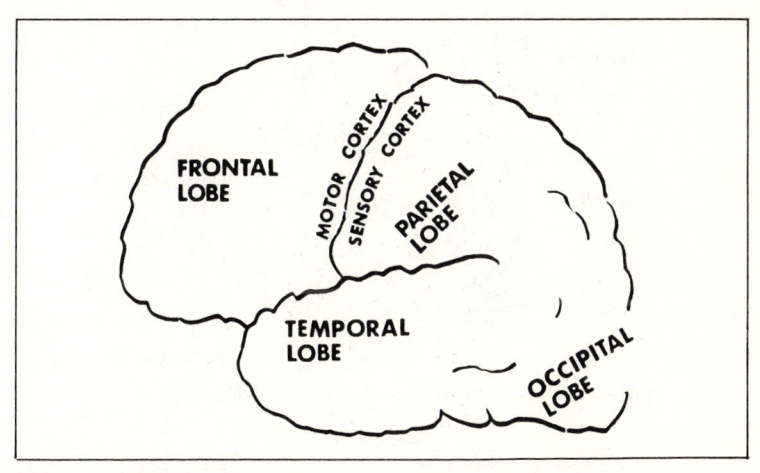

Figure 13-2: Lateral view of left cerebral hemisphere.

458 / ADULT PSYCHIATRIC NURSING

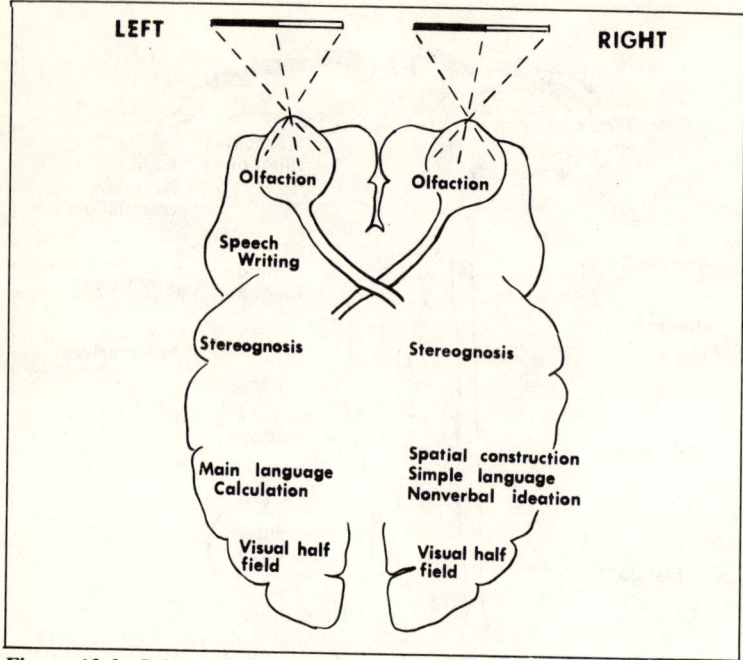

Figure 13-3: Schematic diagram of visual fields, optic tracts and associated brain areas, showing left and right lateralization in man.

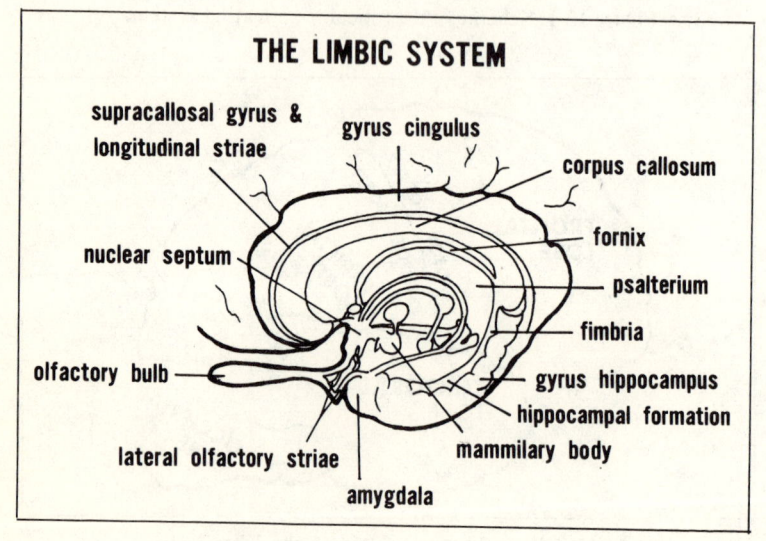

Figure 13-4: The limbic system.

BIBLIOGRAPHY

Beland, Irene, and Passos, Joyce. *Clinical Nursing: Pathophysiological and Psychosocial Approach.* 3d ed. New York: The Macmillan Publishing Co., 1975.

Carpenter, Malcolm B. *Core Text of Neuroanatomy.* Baltimore: Williams & Wilkins Co., 1972.

Detre, Thomas, and Jarecki, Henry. *Modern Psychiatric Treatment.* Philadelphia: J. B. Lippincott Co., 1971.

Glaser, Gilbert H. "Epilepsy: Neuropsychological Aspects," in *American Handbook of Psychiatry.* Vol. IV. 2d ed. Edited by M.F. Reiser. New York: Basic Books Inc., 1975, pp. 314-355.

Greenberg, Owen. Classnotes. Yale University, 1966.

Heller, Stanley S., and Kornfeld, Donald S. "Delirium and Related Problems," in *American Handbook of Psychiatry.* Vol. IV. 2d ed. Edited by M. F. Reiser. New York: Basic Books Inc., 1975, pp. 43-66.

Kyes, Joan, and Hofling, Charles. *Basic Psychiatric Concepts in Nursing.* 3d ed. Philadelphia: J. B. Lippincott Co., 1974.

Luria, A. R. *The Working Brain. An Introduction to Neuropsychology.* New York: Basic Books Inc., 1973.

Lezak, Muriel D. *Neuropsychological Assessment.* New York: Oxford University Press, 1976.

Luckmann, Joan, and Sorensen, Karen. *Medical-Surgical Nursing: A Psychophysiologic Approach.* Philadelphia: W. B. Saunders Co., 1974.

Matthews, W. B., and Miller, Henry. *Diseases of the Nervous System.* 2d ed. Oxford: Blackwell Scientific Publications, 1975.

Pincus, J. H., and Tucker, G. J. *Behavioral Neurology.* New York: Oxford University Press, 1974.

Slater, Eliot, and Roth, Martin. In *Clinical Psychiatry.* 3d ed. Baltimore: The Williams & Wilkins Co., 1969.

PART IV: Treatment Approaches

CHAPTER 14

Somatic Therapy

David P. Colvin, M.S., D.O.

INTRODUCTION

Somatic therapy consists of treating the body or *soma* of the patient by a variety of biochemical or physical means. As it relates to the treatment of mental disease, somatic therapy is designed to effect structural, as well as biochemical changes with the goal of modifying symptoms and symptomatic behavior (Eaton, 1976). Some of the more traditional methods of the somatic therapies used in the treatment of mental disorders include pharmacotherapy, electroconvulsive therapy (ECT), insulin shock, psychosurgery and various forms of narcosis.

This approach has its place in the arsenal of psychiatric interventions for several reasons. The somatic therapy approach is used to treat purely psychiatric disorders such as schizophrenia, as well as those disease processes known to have an organic origin. This approach is not used to treat directly the primary mental disorder but, rather, to facilitate the treatment process by improving the patient's physical and psychological well-being.

In any case, nurses must not only be aware of their collaborative role in the management of mental disease using somatic therapies but must also know the possible side effects and dangers of these interventions. Standard VI of the ANA Standards of Psychiatric-Mental Health Nursing Practice serves as a guideline to those involved in delivering somatic therapy to patients (Congress for Nursing Practice, 1973).

STANDARD VI

Knowledge of somatic therapies and related clinical skills is utilized in working with clients.

Rationale

Various treatment modalities may be needed by clients during the course of illness. Pertinent clinical observations and judgments are made concerning the effects of drugs and other treatments used in the therapeutic program.

Assessment of Function

1. Pertinent reactions to somatic therapies are observed and interpreted in terms of the underlying principles of each therapy.
2. A patient's responses are observed and reported.
3. The effectiveness of somatic therapies is judged and subsequent recommendations for changes in the treatment plan are made.
4. The safety and emotional support of clients receiving therapies are provided.
5. Opportunities are provided for clients and families to discuss, question and explore their feelings and concerns about past, current or projected use of somatic therapies (Congress for Nursing Practice, 1973).

SOMATIC INTERVENTIONS

Psychopharmacology

Since the introduction of reserpine and chlorpromazine in the early 1950s, the use of psychotropic drugs has become widely accepted. Their widespread use has led to more humanistic treatment of the mentally ill. For example, there has been a dramatic decrease in the incidence of isolation and restraint of hospitalized patients. Also, hyperactive patients can be sedated, so that they do not harm themselves or others while undergoing psychiatric treatment.

ANTIPSYCHOTIC DRUGS

The antipsychotic drugs consist of four major drug classifications: the phenothiazines, thioxanthenes, butyrophenones and Rauwolfia alkaloids (Eaton, 1976). The properties and side effects of the four classes are so similar that the phenothiazines are commonly considered as the prototype class (Goodman and Gilman, 1975). It is well established that the antipsychotic drugs produce a specific improvement in the mood and behavior of psychotic patients without excessive sedation and have low addictive properties. When the antipsychotic agents reach therapeutic levels, the destructive, antisocial behavior decreases, thus enabling the patient to enter into psychotherapy and supportive therapy.

The following common antipsychotics are currently in use:

Drug	Brand Name	Daily Dosage Mg.
1. *Phenothiazine*		
Butaperazine	Repoise	15-30
Chlorpromazine	Thorazine	50-100
Fluphenazine	Prolixin	1-45
Perphenazine	Trilafon	8-64
Prochlorperazine	Compazine	5-150
Promazine	Sparine	25-300
Thioridazine	Mellaril	50-800
Trifluoperazine	Stelazine	4-40
Triflupromazine	Vesprin	100-150
2. *Butyrophenone*		
Haloperidol	Haldol	2-15
3. *Thioxanthene*		
Chlorprothixene	Taractan	30-600
Thiothixene	Navane	6-10
4. *Rauwolfia Alkaloids*		
Ceserpidine	Hormonyl	0.1
Veserpine	Serpasil	.5-5

Phenothiazines

The phenothiazines are used effectively in the treatment of the functional psychoses and the behavioral disorders resulting from organic brain disease. The antipsychotic effects of the various phenothiazines are similar. The specific drug is chosen in order to minimize a particular side effect. Specific side effects are dealt with later in this section.

Butyrophenones

The therapeutic effects of this class are similar to the phenothiazines. Empirical evidence suggests, however, that they are less likely to produce orthostatic hypotension or weight gain when compared to the phenothiazines (Goodman and Gilman, 1975).

Thioxanthenes

The thioxanthenes are chemically related to the phenothiazines and have similar pharmacologic effects (Goodman and Gilman, 1975).

Rauwolfia Alkaloids

These agents are derived from the juices of the snakeroot plant. Still widely used in many branches of medicine, they are now less utilized as psychotropic agents, because the phenothiazines and butyrophenones are considered to be more effective (Goodman and Gilman, 1975).

Drug Action

The properties of the phenothiazines, butyrophenones, and thioxanthenes are so similar, that the phenothiazines are classically presented as the prototype drug in the study of the pharmacologic action of the antipsychotic medications. In this discussion, emphasis is placed primarily on chlorpromazine, a phenothiazine, as the model drug.

Chlorpromazine exerts important effects at all levels in the nervous system. Central nervous system centers primarily affected are the cerebral cortex, basal ganglia, hypothalamus, limbic system and brainstem. The peripheral nervous system sites primarily affected are the autonomic ganglia (Goodman and Gilman, 1975). Clinically, chlorpromazine relieves or significantly reduces free-floating anxiety; thus, it may be used in reduced doses to treat neuroses and personality disorders, when overt symptoms of anxiety are present. In the psychotic patient, chlorpromazine and related antipsychotic drugs improve thought disorder, improve the blunted effect, improve withdrawal and autistic behavior and relieve or significantly reduce hallucinations, hostility and aggressiveness (Eaton, 1976).

The Rauwolfia alkaloids are also effective in treating free-floating anxiety. With an increase in dosage, they are also effective in the treatment of schizophrenia. The major disadvantage in using the Rauwolfia derivatives resides in the fact that they sometimes precipitate severe depression, thus increasing the potential for suicide in some patients (Eaton, 1976).

Contraindications

Because of potential side effects of the drugs, several medical conditions serve as relative contraindications to the use of antipsychotic agents. Severe cardiovascular disease is a contraindication, due to the physiological embarrassment of the autonomic nervous system by these medications. Since the liver metabolizes these drugs, extreme caution is warranted in the face of serious liver disease. Also, as is the case with most drugs, the use of antipsychotic agents in early pregnancy involves a calculated risk (Goodman and Gilman, 1975).

Side Effects

The four major classes of antipsychotic drugs have similar side effects and will be considered in this discussion as one unit (Goth, 1974).

Subjective Discomfort

Drowsiness is the most common subjective complaint. This sedative effect rapidly develops and usually dissipates at the end of the first week of therapy. Other subjective complaints, including dry mouth, nasal congestion and blurred vision are related to their antihistaminic properties.

Convulsions

Antipsychotics, especially the phenothiazines, reduce the convulsive threshold and may produce convulsions in susceptible patients. Convulsions may also occur if there is rapid withdrawal of an anticonvulsant medication followed by phenothiazine medication.

Depression

Frequently, an apparent depression develops as the psychotic symptoms improve with medication. There are two reasons for this: (1) feelings of despair are common complications of psychoses; (2) the depressive phenomenon reflects the patient's growing awareness of the seriousness of his illness, as his psychotic thinking is cleared.

The Rauwolfia derivatives may cause a paradoxic depression, generally thought to be due to depletion of norepinephrine, a neurotransmittor. The use of antidepressant medications is generally discouraged, because tricyclic antidepressants may worsen schizophrenic symptomatology.

Metabolic

Of the possible metabolic problems, weight gain is the most frequently encountered. The best approach to the management of this problem is through rigid dietary management. Other metabolic derangements to be watched for include galactorrhea, amenorrhea and gynecomastia.

Dermatologic Changes

Urticaria (hives), contact dermatitis and photosensitivity may all appear. These symptoms usually reflect hypersensitivity to the drug, and withdrawal is usually indicated.

Liver

Jaundice (of the obstructive type) is a possible side effect that requires discontinuance of the drug being used.

Cardiovascular

Arrhythmias may occur. Syncope is not uncommon and is related to the hypotensive effects of the drugs. Many patients develop tolerance to this side effect fairly rapidly, whereas others must have their drug dosages reduced.

Blood Dyscrasias

Leukocytosis, leukopenia, and eosinophilia are all common side effects. Agranulocytosis occurs rarely. When present, it usually becomes evident after 4-10 weeks of therapy. Complaints of sore throats, fevers and other symptoms of infection should be investigated, for they may be related to leukopenia or agranulocytosis.

Extrapyramidal Signs

Extrapyramidal signs are a frequent side effect of antipsychotic drug therapy. They are more common in the elderly and in individuals with central nervous system disease.

There are five neurological sequelae which can develop in patients taking antipsychotic drugs. They are akinesia, akathisia, acute dystonia, pseudoparkinsonism and tardive dyskinesia.

Akinesia—(weakness and muscle fatigue) the most common disorder. Patient complaints include generalized muscle weakness, lethargy and easy fatiguability.

Akathisia—(motor restlessness) occurs in 20 percent of patients and is twice as common in women. It most frequently involves the lower limbs and takes the form of regular rhythmical motor movements.

Acute Dystonic Reaction—(inappropriate muscle tonicity) very dramatic in appearance. It affects men twice as often as women and is more common in adolescents and children. The patient appears frozen in position with torticollis, and the eyes may be opened and rolled back in their sockets (oculogyric crisis). This early complication is often misdiagnosed as the the opisthotonos of tetanus or the catatonic stupor of schizophrenia.

Pseudoparkinsonism—occurs in about 17 percent of patients taking antipsychotic drugs and usually occurs within the first three months of therapy (Goth, 1974).

Tardive Dyskinesia—(a late occurring impairment of voluntary movement) one of the more serious side effects associated with antipsychotic agents. This is a persistent disorder of rhythmical involuntary movements of the face, mouth, jaw and tongue. It is particularly prevalent in elderly patients, and there is no established treatment for it. It is sometimes associated with rapid discontinuance of antipsychotic medication, particularly after prolonged use.

GUIDELINES FOR NURSING INTERVENTION

The nurse's role in somatic therapy assumes greater proportions once the appropriate drug and effective dosage are determined. It is then the nurse's responsibility to establish and maintain the drug regimen. This entails securing the cooperation of patients in the taking of their medication. Patient compliance may have to be earned by recognizing the blocks to taking medications and overcoming them by careful listening and counseling. Before administering medication to a patient, the nurse should be aware of the expected reactions and possible side effects. Also, errors can be minimized, if the nurse is familiar with usual drug dosages. Observations should be reported to the physician so that the proper drug level can be ascertained.

More specifically, the nurse should develop the following procedures as part of routine care of patients undergoing drug therapy for mental disorders.

After a comprehensive drug history has been obtained and before instituting therapy with any psychotropic drugs, baseline blood pressures should be recorded in both the standing and reclining positions.

Parenteral routes of medication are generally used during early phases of hospitalization, when patient cooperation is often low. The nurse should administer the injection deep into the muscle to prevent local tissue necrosis from some of the more irritating drugs. At least 20 percent of hospitalized, emotionally disturbed patients do not take their oral medication. It is the nurse's responsibility to observe closely for tell-tale signs of poor patient compliance, such as persistent symptoms of hostility, anxiety or other signs that should be responding to the drug therapy.

Following the first few I.M. injections, the patient should be instructed to lie down and remain quiet for about an hour, because of possible fainting spells due to a rapid lowering of the blood pressure.

Because of the tendency to gain weight rapidly, the nurse should assist the patient in obtaining weekly weights, and, if indicated, the patient's weight gain can be controlled by diet, rather than by the use of appetite suppressants.

With Thorazine, there is also an increased sensitivity to the sun. Nurses should see that patients are protected from direct exposure to the sun or make use of sun-blocking creams to prevent severe sunburn during outings.

Subjective side effects, such as nasal congestion, blurring of vision, depression and allergic pruritus are often distressing to patients, and their anxiety may be allayed by reassurance from the nursing staff.

As drug levels are increased, each patient reaches his point of tolerance and extrapyramidal symptoms, such as involuntary tremors, convulsions and motor retardation should be carefully observed for.

ANTIDEPRESSANT DRUGS

According to a recent National Institute of Mental Health survey, some eight million people per year suffer from a depression severe enough to warrant treatment. Expressed in terms of having the illness in an individual's life, about 8 percent of men and 16 percent of women can expect to have one of the depressive syndromes during their lifetime. Thus, the somatic treatment of depressive illnesses is an area about which the nurse should be well informed (Eaton, 1976, p. 378; Goth, 1974, p. 235-239).

There are three main groups of antidepressant medications:

	Brand Name	Daily Dose Mg.
1. *Tricyclic Antidepressants*		
Amitriptyline	Elavil	150

	Brand Name	Daily Dose Mg.
Desipramine	Norpramin	150
Doxepin	Sinequan	150
Imipramine	Tofranil	150
Nortriptyline	Aventyl	50

2. *Psychomotor Stimulants*

Dextroamphetamine	Dexedrine	5-15
Methamphetamine	Methedrine	5-15
Methylphenidate	Ritalin	10-30
Phenmetrazine	Preludin	25-75
Racemic Amphetamine	Benzedrine	5-15

3. *Monoamine Oxidase Inhibitors*

Isocarboxazid	Marplan	10-30
Pargyline	Eutonyl	10-30
Phenelzine	Nardil	10-75
Tranylcypromine	Parnate	10-30

Tricyclic Antidepressants

The tricyclic antidepressants are considered the most useful antidepressants. They are slower acting than the amphetamines, and therapeutic results are observed only after 10-14 days of therapy. They are chemically related to the phenothiazines and are considered to be safer than the monoamine oxidase inhibitors. The tricyclic antidepressants are indicated for the treatment of involutional melancholia, neurotic depressions, psychotic depressive reaction and other psychiatric syndromes where depression is the central clinical feature (Goth, 1974; Goodman and Gilman, 1975).

Side Effects

Many somatic complaints associated with antidepressant medications are also associated with depression. Thus, one must constantly evaluate the patient's complaints in terms of their being associated with the drug or with the illness.

Central Nervous System Effects—The tricyclics may cause involuntary muscle tremors of the upper extremities similar to the extrapyramidal signs of the phenothiazines. Rarely, tremors, convulsions, paresthesia and ataxia may occur. Occasionally the tricyclics bring about angry states, as well as manic and excited schizophrenic episodes. This has been called the "manic shift." Some researchers attribute this shift to a missed diagnosis (schizophrenia is made worse by tricyclics), while others believe the drug causes the patient with bipolar manic-depressive illness to shift from the depressed to the manic state.

Autonomic Nervous System Effects—The autonomic nervous system side effects range from slight subjective complaints of dry mouth, palpitations, tachycardia, visual blurring and dizziness to more unpleasant episodes such as vomiting, profuse sweating, urinary bladder dysfunction and constipation.

Those patients with certain types of glaucoma may notice exacerbation of this disease.

Cardiovascular Effects—Cardiovascular status is occasionally compromised, resulting in postural hypotension, especially in the elderly.

Hypersensitivity Effects—Photosensitivity and jaundice are rarely seen. Also seen rarely are the blood dyscrasias including agranulocytosis. The same precautions should be taken with the side effects of this class of drugs as with the antipsychotic agents.

Withdrawal Effects—In patients receiving long term therapy in excess of 150 mg. daily, a sudden withdrawal of the drug may cause nausea, vomiting, headache, dizziness, abdominal cramps, diarrhea, anxiety and irritability.

Monoamine Oxidase Inhibitors

Monoamine oxidase (MAO) inhibitors are of lesser clinical importance than the tricyclic antidepressants. These inhibitors of MAO stimulate the central nervous system in a manner similar to those of the amphetamines and related stimulants. Clinical evidence indicates that some patients who do not respond to tricyclics may respond to MAO inhibitors, so that a trial on MAO inhibitors may be useful (Goodman and Gilman, 1975).

Side Effects

The MAO inhibitors have frequent and rather serious side effects. Some of these drugs have been withdrawn from the market because of side effects.

Psychological Effects—These drugs can convert a retarded depression into an agitated one and may, occasionally, cause hypomania or precipitate an acute schizophrenic psychosis.

Acute confusional episodes with disorientation and clouded mentation may also occur.

Central Nervous System Effects—Slurring of speech, increased muscle tone, dizziness or generalized weakness may be precipitated by these drugs.

Autonomic Nervous System Effects—The autonomic side effects are similar to those described for the tricyclic antidepressants. The most serious side effect is related to the hypertensive crises seen as several related syndromes. The concomitant administration of tricyclic antidepressants or sympathomimetics with the MAO inhibitors may produce such crises and may be fatal. The MAO inhibitors are also incompatible with food-stuffs high in tyramine content. Because of this incompatibility, patients on MAO inhibitors should be educated regarding the potential danger of consuming cheese, chianti wines and other foods containing tyramine.

Symptoms of this hypertensive syndrome include chest pains, headache, high blood pressure, palpitations and profuse sweating.

Psychomotor Stimulants

The psychomotor stimulants are rapidly acting stimulants which act directly on the central nervous system. Their stimulating effect increases alertness and elevates mood. Their antidepressant effect is rarely strong enough to be therapeutic in severe depressions. They are helpful in the mild psychic depressions characteristic of the cyclothymic personality. These drugs cause increased motor activity and an upsurge of energy. Unfortunately, these feelings are quickly dissipated as the drug effect wears off. This short span of action creates a "letdown" with concomitant increase in depressive symtoms and an occasional increase in suicide risk. This is seen especially in the treatment of neurotic depressions (Goth, 1974; Eaton, 1976).

Side Effects

Common side effects include hyperactivity, high blood pressure, increased pulse rate, sweating, difficulty in concentration, insomnia and anorexia. Because of their euphoric effects, there is a tendency of abuse of these agents, which may lead to impaired judgment and hypomanic behavior.

LITHIUM CARBONATE TREATMENT OF ACUTE MANIA

The efficacy of lithium carbonate for the treatment of acute mania has been well established. Its action is anti-manic, without the sedation that is seen when using the antipsychotic agents. The onset of therapeutic effects are seven to ten days, as opposed to the antipsychotic agents which begin working immediately. Lithium also serves to prevent the manic and depressive phase of the manic-depressive disorder (Goth, 1974; Goodman and Gilman, 1975).

Side Effects

Most patients treated with lithium develop side effects. They usually occur during the first two weeks of therapy and rarely necessitate discontinuance of the drug.

Early side effects include:

1. gastrointestinal complaints such as diarrhea, nausea and vomiting
2. CNS symptoms such as dizziness and drowsiness
3. neuromuscular effects such as tremors, fatigue and muscular weakness
4. renal complaints of urinary frequency and excessive thirst.

Symptoms of severe toxicity are seen as an increase in the amplitude of the above symptoms but, principally, an increase in the CNS side effects.

ANTI-ANXIETY DRUGS

The anti-anxiety agents, also known as minor tranquilizers, are widely used for the symptomatic treatment of anxiety and tension in non-psychotic patients. These drugs help to control mild to moderate degrees of emotional distress in neurotic patients and in normal individuals undergoing unusual stress. Some have muscle relaxant properties. These drugs are prone to abuse and are physically addicting.

Anti-anxiety agents can be divided into two general groups (Goodman and Gilman, 1975, p. 187-193):

	Brand Name	Daily Dosage Mg.
1. *Benzodiazepines*		
Chlordiazepoxide	Librium	10-100
Diazepam	Valium	4-40
Oxazepam	Serax	30-120
2. *Non-Benzodiazepines*		
Diphenhydramine	Benadryl	25-400
Hydroxyzine	Atarax, Vistaril	75-400
Meprobamate	Equanil	600-1200

Side Effects

The anti-anxiety drugs are relatively safe as long as they are taken as prescribed and are not used along with other drugs which potentiate their effects.

A very common side effect is sedation. This property is potentiated by alcohol and other CNS depressants. Patients should be warned against the slightest use of alcohol or other sedative agents while on these medications. Other CNS side effects include double vision, fine muscle tremors, slurred speech and hypotension.

Paradoxical hyperexcited states are sometimes seen with symptoms of angry outbursts or depersonalizations.

These drugs are potentially addicting, and the patient should be warned to take them only as prescribed. The withdrawal syndrome from these medications may not appear for up to two weeks after the last dose and can lead to convulsions and death.

SEDATIVE-HYPNOTIC DRUGS

These drugs have a very limited place in psychiatry today and are mentioned here for the sake of completeness. These drugs are frequently abused and have withdrawal effects when abruptly stopped. When severe sleep disturbances are refractive to phenothiazine sedation, either chloral hydrate or paraldehyde is recommended because of their lower abuse potential (Goodman and Gilman, 1975, p. 102-134).

Chemically, these drugs are divided into the barbiturates and non-barbiturates:

	Trade Name
1. *Barbiturates*	
Amobarbital	Amytal
Pentobarbital	Nembutal
Phenobarbital	Luminal
Secobarbital	Seconal
2. *Non-Barbiturates*	
Ethchlorvynol	Placidyl
Glutethimide	Doriden
Chloral hydrate	Noctec

Side Effects

These drugs can progressively cause ataxia, general anesthesia, medullary depression and, ultimately, death, if taken in overdose quantity. Repeated administration is habituating, and physical dependence becomes a problem.

ELECTROCONVULSIVE THERAPY

Electroconvulsive therapy, introduced in 1937 by Cerletti and Bini, is the most widely used of the older somatic therapies. Until the advent of the antidepressant drugs, it was the treatment of choice for depressive illness. It consists of electrically inducing a generalized grand mal convulsion via electrodes placed on the head. It is indicated in the treatment of serious depressions, refractory to drug therapy, or where rapid results are necessary (Kalinowsky, 1975, p. 1970-1976).

Prior to therapy, the patient must remain NPO at least 4 hours. Thirty minutes prior to therapy, the patient's vital signs are taken, and he is instructed to empty his bladder. Items such as dentures or contact lenses are removed. At this time, a small dose of a sedative may be given to reduce anxiety. Atropine is also given to decrease tracheobronchial secretions to obviate aspiration. The patient is placed on a padded table, and a quick-acting anesthetic, such as sodium pentothal, is given. A muscle relaxant, such as Anectine, is then given to decrease the severity of the clonic seizures. If spontaneous respirations are decreased as a result of Anectine, then positive pressure oxygen therapy is administered, until the patient resumes breathing on his own. A tongue depressor is placed in the mouth to prevent swallowing or biting the tongue. Then a shock is delivered through electrodes placed on the skull. The limbs are restrained to prevent fractures. The patient usually sleeps 20-30 minutes after treatment and frequently evidences some confusion and memory loss upon awakening. During recovery, the vital signs are taken again. The nurse then stays with the patient until the senses are cleared and he can care for himself.

The nurse is an important source of emotional support during the course of therapy. Most patients have fears or other feelings about ECT and find a sense of relief in being able to discusss them with their nurse.

Electric current can be administered in such a way as to produce loss of consciousness with a minimum, though sustained, muscle contraction. The typical grand mal seizure threshold is not reached. This type of treatment usually lasts from 3-5 minutes and is called electronarcosis.

Contraindications to ECT are rare. Cardiac patients are poor candidates for this procedure. Patients with known brain tumors should definitely not receive ECT.

Side effects are commonly confined to memory disturbances and rare skeletal complications, such as fractures or vertebral compressions.

INSULIN SHOCK THERAPY

The treatment of pychosis by insulin shock was developed in 1933 by Sakel. It was first used to treat schizophrenia in 1940. Due to the increased knowledge and use of psychotherapy, psychotropic drugs and ECT, insulin shock has lost much of its practical importance (Kalinowsky, 1975).

Its purpose is to induce a coma by the administration of increasing doses of insulin to a fasting patient and requires a skilled clinical team to monitor constantly the patient's treatment. The attending nurse needs to be completely familiar with the signs and symptoms of hypoglycemic coma in order to know at what stage of insulin shock the patient is in at all times. Usually, patients go into a true coma about the third hour after the insulin dose has been given. Therapy is then terminated by glucagon injection, which should enable the patient to wake in 10-20 minutes.

The nurse in attendance should guard against a possible second hypoglycemic coma several hours after therapy by giving the patient sugar and encouraging him to stay awake and active in group activities.

INDOKLON THERAPY

This recent addition to the convulsive therapies utilizes the inhalant gas, hexafluorodiethyl ether (Indoklon), which induces rapid loss of consciousness, tremors and clonic seizures. Nursing interventions in this procedure are similar to those in the other convulsive therapies (Kalinowsky, 1975).

PSYCHOSURGERY

All operations performed on the central nervous system, primarily designed to affect the patient's psychological state, are called psychosurgery. The concept has been around since ancient times, but the modern method, known as the prefrontal lobotomy, was developed by Moniz in 1936. Since his pioneering work, many similar procedures have been devised (Kalinowsky, 1975).

Simply stated, the lobotomy consists of the surgical separation of the nerve tracts of the frontal lobe cortex from the subcortex and basal ganglia, which is considered the seat of the emotions.

A variation of this procedure is known as the transorbital lobotomy. The transorbital approach is probably the most popular method of recent years, because it is simpler to perform and tends to have fewer post-operation complications.

Although the lobotomy has lost its widespread clinical use, there is some resurgence in this therapy, using newer techniques. Details of these techniques, and the nursing problems inherent in them, are for those planning to work in the few research centers still employing this method and are beyond the scope of this chapter.

PHYSIOTHERAPY

The application of some types of physical therapy to the treatment of the psychiatric patient consists mainly of hydrotherapy and massages. As with some other somatic therapies, these physical techniques are used less, since the advent of the psychotropic drugs. However, these measures have certain characteristics that still make them a viable part of psychiatric patient care. They have prompt and short-lasting therapeutic effects and little or no side effects. Also, they may be used with little fear of interfering with the diagnostic process.

THE NURSE'S ROLE IN SOMATIC THERAPY

The nurse plays a very important role in the somatic therapy of psychiatric patients. Whatever the somatic intervention happens to be, it is the nurse who serves as its humanizing element. Routine administration of therapy has its interpersonal setting. It is the nurse who sets the tone of this setting—be it showing personal interest or showing unconcern. Hopefully, the professional nurse will recognize this dimension to somatic therapy and use it as an opportunity to listen and give reassurance when needed. Simply stated, it is the nurse who makes "routine care" less "routine" and more "personal."

BIBLIOGRAPHY

Congress for Nursing Practice. *Standards of Psychiatric-Mental Health Nursing Practice.* Kansas City, Mo.: American Nurses' Association, 1973.

Eaton, Merrill T., et al. "Somatic Therapy," in *Psychiatry*. 3d ed. Garden City, N.Y.: Medical Examination Publishing Co., 1976, pp. 364-387.
Goodman, Louis S., and Gilman, Alfred. *The Pharmacological Basic of Therapeutics*. 5th ed. New York: The Macmillan Publishing Co., 1975.
Goth, Andres. *Medical Pharmacology*. St. Louis: C.V. Mosby Co., 1974.
Kalinowksy, Lothar. "Organic Therapies," in *Comprehensive Textbook of Psychiatry*. Vol. II. 2d ed. Edited by Alfred M. Freedman, Harold I. Kaplan, and Benjamin J. Sadock. Baltimore: Williams & Wilkins Co., 1975, pp. 1921-1990.

CHAPTER 15

Treatment Modalities in Psychiatric Nursing

Linda Colvin, R.N., M.S. and
Jeanette Lancaster, R.N., Ph.D.

INTRODUCTION

Various professionals—social workers, ministers, nurses, physicians, psychologists—work with clients in a psythotherapeutic manner. In-depth study and numerous hours of supervised clinical experiences are prerequisite to the practice of psychotherapy or counseling. The American Nurses' Association speaks to the requirement needed for the practice of psychotherapy:

STANDARD X

The practice of individual, group, or family psychotherapy requires appropriate preparation and recognition of accountability for the practice.

Rationale: Acceptance of the role of therapist entails primary responsibility for the treatment of clients and entrance into a contractual agreement. This contract includes a commitment to see a client through the problem he presents or, if this becomes impossible, to assist him in finding other appropriate assistance. It also includes an explicit definition of the relationship, the respective roles of each person in the relationship, and what can realistically be expected of each person.

Assessment Factors

1. The potential of the nurse to function as a primary therapist is evaluated.
2. The accountability for practicing psychotherapy is recognized and accepted.
3. Knowledge of growth and development, psychopathology, psychosocial systems and small group and family dynamics is utilized in the therapeutic process.
4. The terms of the contract between the nurse and the client, including the structure of time, place, fees, etc., that may be involved, are made explicitly clear.
5. Supervision or consultation is sought whenever indicated and other learning opportunities are used to further develop knowledge and skills.
6. The effectiveness of the work with an individual, family or group is routinely assessed (Congress for Nursing Practice, 1973).

Nurses, as team members, find it necessary to have a basic idea of the various forms of treatment, including those beyond their primary responsibility. The common types of treatment are presented, beginning with psychoanalysis, the classic method of psychotherapy.

PSYCHOANALYSIS

Sigmund Freud, a Viennese neurologist, neurophysiologist and psychiatrist, is described as the father of psychoanalysis. The theories of Freud and his followers comprise the core of American psychiatry. Although often criticized, psychoanalysis provides the basis of various contemporary psychiatric therapies.

In psychoanalysis, the sessions typically last 50 minutes, four to six times a week for at least two years and often more than five years. Generally, the psychiatrist sits in a chair at the head of the couch, upon which the patient is lying. While the therapist is able to watch the patient, the patient cannot see the therapist. The treatment is expensive, intense and takes a great deal of time.

In the United States, the psychoanalyst has medical, psychiatric and additional training at a psychoanalytic institute, including a thorough personal analysis. He also does course work in psychoanalytic theory, undergoes supervision in psychoanalytic treatment and must attain a satisfactory score on an examination (Kyes, 1974).

In the process of psychoanalysis, the unconscious factors influencing the patient's behavior are thoroughly explored. Different techniques used to obtain the desired exploration of unconscious factors and childhood memories include free association, dream analysis and transference. Free association, the unobstructed flow of thoughts, is encouraged. By not consciously controlling thoughts, the patient evidences a flow of words that represent his spontaneous thoughts, allowing unconscious forces in the personality to reveal themselves. The analyst does not guide the patient, nor does he advise or counsel. Rather, the analyst's role is to listen carefully, occasionally ask a question and make timely interpretations concerning the meaning of the person's associations. In order for analysis to be effective, the patient must be completely candid about everything that comes to mind, thereby revealing information not consciously known to the patient. Dreams and "slips of the tongue" are also explored, as they are seen as expressions of unconscious. A further construct of psychoanalysis is transference. Transference, an unconscious process, is evidenced in a variety of therapeutic relationships. In transference, one person reacts to and holds attitudes toward another person in the present, which are influenced by a prior relationship. For some reason, the patient retains unresolved feelings toward the past relationship and confuses them with the feelings toward the person in the present situation. In psychoanalysis, the transference is toward the analyst.

The goal of psychoanalysis is to elicit repressed material and go over memories previously unavailable to consciousness, so as to integrate this content into the total personality. The process of psychoanalysis is slow and tedious. Psychoanalysis is needed by some patients; however, there are many cases in which other types of therapy are the treatment of choice. Such forms of therapy include psychoanalytic psychotherapy, which is based on analytic concepts short of classical psychoanalysis (Stewart, 1975).

PSYCHOANALYTIC PSYCHOTHERAPY

In psychoanalytic psychotherapy, the patient sits in a comfortable chair, and the therapist and patient are in full view of each other. The psychiatrist interacts with the patient and is seen as a real person. The sessions generally last 50 minutes and are at least once a week. Like psychoanalysis, the therapy is intense and expensive.

The focus of therapy is on the patient's interactional patterns, which are leading to difficulty in everyday life. The relationship is one in which the patient is expected to develop maturation. This is accomplished through the mechanism of the therapy. As a first step, the patient must feel accepted by the therapist. One of the benefits of this acceptance is a lessening of the guilt that the patient feels concerning his inadequacy. Another step is the development of an ability to touch his inner world, the unconscious. As with psychoanalysis, transference is an important part of the treatment. Psychoanalytic psychotherapy falls into three major types: insight therapy, supportive therapy and relationship therapy.

Other forms of therapy are, frequently, the treatment of choice for a variety of patients.

BEHAVIOR THERAPY

Behavior therapy, begun in the late 1800s and early 1900s, has its roots in the animal learning laboratories of Bekhterev, Pavlov and Thorndike. In this type of therapy, the observable and measurable behavior of the patient and the way the behavior affects the environment are of utmost importance.

Systematic desensitization, a basic technique of behavior therapists, was originated by Joseph Wolpe. This technique is applicable to a wide range of behavioral disorders and phobias. The patient is taught to reach a psychophysiological state that inhibits anxiety, such as deep muscular relaxation. After this relaxation training, the patient identifies the stimulus causing anxiety. A hierarchy of ten to twelve scenes is developed according to the degree of anxiety that visualizing each scene causes the patient. Following the learning of deep relaxation and the listing of the scenes in the order of increasing anxiety, the desensitization begins. The patient, in a deeply relaxed state, imagines each scene on the hierarchy beginning with the least anxiety-producing scene and progresses, over a period of time, to the most anxiety-producing scene. The scene that produces the least anxiety is imagined by the patient and discussed until it is no longer anxiety-producing. The patient begins to associate the relaxed and pleasant state with the previously upsetting situation. This process is continued, and each scene is dealt with until it is no longer anxiety-producing. Then when the imagined situation occurs in a life situation, the patient no longer experiences the previously felt fear or anxiety.

Another technique of behavior therapy is positive reinforcement. The basic belief behind positive reinforcement and extinction is that behavior is affected by the outcome or results of the behavior. When a behavioral action is followed by a good or rewarding event, it is encouraged and will occur more often; when followed by a disliked or aversive event or by no response, it will occur less often.

As with most therapies, behavior therapy sessions last about 50 minutes once a week. The importance of acceptance by the therapist is once again emphasized. It differs from many other types of treatment in that learning theories and scientific investigation play a major part in the theoretical framework.

HYPNOSIS

Hypnosis is helpful in that it accelerates the impact of therapy. Although the word hypnosis is from the Greek word hypos, meaning sleep, it actually is a process of heightened concentration. In both sleep and hypnosis, peripheral awareness is reduced, but focal awareness is decreased in sleep and increased in hypnosis.

Hypnosis was first mentioned as a therapeutic tool in the eighteenth century by Mesmer. The medical use of hypnosis, pioneered by M. H. Erickson, has been accepted in the United States since the 1930s.

Different methods are used to lead the patient into this state of deep concentration on areas of concern or unresolved problems.

"Hypnosis can be described as an altered state of intense and sensitive interpersonal relatedness between hypnotist and patient characterized by the patient's nonrational submission and relative abandonment of executive control to a more or less regressed dissociated state" (Spiegel, 1975). Basically, the value lies in the fact that unconscious material may be revealed and that as the patient concentrates intensively on an area, he may find clarification in that area.

GROUP PSYCHOTHERAPY

Group psychotherapy, a rapidly growing field of psychiatry, "is a form of treatment in which carefully selected emotionally ill persons are placed in a group, guided by a trained therapist, for the purpose of helping one another effect personality change. By means of a variety of technical maneuvers and theoretical constructs, the leader uses the group members' interactions to bring about change" (Sadock, 1975).

In 1907, an internist, Joseph Pratt, organized a group in a Massachusetts tuberculosis sanatorium. He is given credit as the originator of group therapy in this country. Other men in the early history of group therapy include Marsh, Lazell, Burrow, Wender, Schilder, Slavson, Wolf, Moreno, Freud, Adler and Lewin.

Group therapy employs almost as many technical maneuvers and theoretical constructs as do practitioners. There are many ways in which groups can be categorized and labelled. Commonly used group categories include:

1. population making up the group
2. group process or mechanisms that are emphasized
3. leadership styles
4. theoretical framework
5. types of interactions
6. specific goals sought.

Therapists, naturally, have different backgrounds and frames of reference (Freudian, neo-Freudian, transactional, behavioral, client-centered, etc.); therefore, looking at and describing group therapy, in general, can be confusing and complex. Generally, the group has between four and twelve patients with one or two therapists. When there are two therapists leading the group, this is referred to as co-leading. Groups generally meet once or twice a week for 45 to 90 minutes.

Nurses frequently find themselves in groups of patients. These times of dining, exercising, doing handcrafts and watching television can be times of group work if the nurse makes the situation a therapeutic one. Also, the nurse who specializes in psychiatric mental-health nursing will frequently be the primary or co-leader of organized group therapy sessions. The nurse, being one member of the team, will find that working with other professionals in the group therapy sessions is often essential.

FAMILY THERAPY

The exact origin of family therapy, a relatively new and exciting treatment approach, is unknown; however, it emerged in literature around the mid-1950s. Several persons working independently are considered as the founders of the basic tenets of family therapy.

An important concept identified by Bateson, Jackson, et al., was the "double bind" (Satir, et al., 1977, p. 24). They pointed out that a child who received conflicting messages from someone in the family, usually the mother, was placed in a "double bind"—he could not do the right thing regardless of his actions. Take the case of John: he was criticized for mowing the lawn one week, because he might have hurt himself and ended up causing the family trouble by going to the hospital and running up a medical bill; the next week, when he did not mow, his mother, who had criticized him the week before for mowing, now criticized him for being lazy and not helping out by mowing the lawn. He could not win; whatever he did was the wrong thing. A child might also receive incongruent messages. John received an incongruent message when his mother's covert and overt messages did not match. She said, with a frown on her face and through clenched teeth, "John, how I love you." The identification of this "double bind" concept has helped in the development of family therapy.

Another concept which helped lay the foundation for family therapy, developed by Wynne, et al., described the rigid family system where individual growth or moving from an established role was not permitted (Wynne, 1958). In this rigid family system, the family would wear a mask of harmony and well-being, labeled "pseudomutuality." The main goal of the family was to present an appearance of harmony and the absence of family problems. In this same time period, Ackerman (1966), Bowen (1960), Satir (1964) and Bell (1961) were discussing and developing ideas about the family and family therapy. These and others led to the ever-changing area of psychiatry known as family therapy.

Because family therapy was started by various people who were not working together, there is no consensus as to exactly what family therapy is. Some describe it as each family member having his own therapist; some see it as one therapist seeing each member of the family separately; some say it is seeing the parents together;

others describe it as occasionally seeing members of the family for the patient's interest; and still others say family therapy is seeing the whole family together. Nathan Ackerman states:

> Family treatment, although relatively new, offers promise. It gives an expanded understanding of the relations between inner and outer experience. It lends explicit emphasis to the principle of emotional contagion in family process, the transmission of pathogenic conflict and coping from one generation to the next. . . . It is the therapy of a natural living unit; the sphere of therapeutic intervention is not a single individual but the whole family. . . . Family psychotherapy absorbs selected features of each (of the older traditional methods of psychotherapy) but extends beyond them to evolve a new form of therapy, one that utilizes a natural group rather than the isolated individual or a contrived collection of individuals (Ackerman, 1966).

Although controversy exists as to the exact nature of family therapy, the family is considered a unit or a system. The whole family is the patient, although most families request help initially for one member. The family member chosen, the identified patient, may not be the sickest person in the family. Because the family is a system, with each member a subsystem, a change in one family member affects the other family members. This makes the family an ever-changing system that must work to maintain a balance. The family's methods of keeping the balance may not be healthy, and, in such cases, one of the goals of therapy will be to help the family system develop healthy ways in which to maintain a balance, as the members change.

The family therapist uses various techniques and methods of treatment to help the family work out individual and family problems. The type of therapy used when treating families varies between therapists; they have in common the belief that working with the family unit is more beneficial to everyone involved than treating individuals alone.

OTHER APPROACHES TO PSYCHOTHERAPY

Due to an ever-increasing number of psychotherapeutic systems and techniques, a few of the representative modalities are summarized. In order that the student might read more about any of the treatment types, a reading list is included on p. 493.

Client-centered Psychotherapy

Carl Rogers (1961) noted in the period 1938 to 1950, that the highly diagnostic, probing and interpretative methods he saw used in psychotherapy were not effective. His observations and beliefs about therapy led to the development of a "client-centered approach."

Rogers presents the idea that the relationship between the organism (the locus of experience) and the self is either one of "congruence" or "incongruence." Incongruence, the less healthy state, can be changed to a state of congruence by placing the person in a non-threatening situation, in which he examines his feelings in the presence of a therapist who is warm, real, caring, deeply sensitive, non-judgmental and accepting. Rogers indicates that the client-centered approach is a way of being with people to facilitate growth and change.

As with some other current therapies, in the client-centered approach a diagnostic label is not considered important. Rather, emphasis is placed on the process of the relationship, not the cure of particular symptoms. The role of the therapist is to help the person see his own ability to develop. The attitude of the therapist creates an atmosphere which facilitates the growth of the client. The inner experiences of the client direct and set the pace of the therapeutic process.

Rogers lists ten questions, as criteria, which the person hoping to enter a helping relationship could ask himself (Rogers, 1961):

1. Can I *be* in some way which will be perceived by the other person as dependable or consistent in some deep sense?
2. Can I be expressive enough as a person, that what I am will be communicated unambiguously?
3. Can I let myself experience positive attitudes toward this other person—attitudes of warmth, caring, liking, interest, respect?
4. Can I be strong enough as a person to be separate from the other? Can I be a sturdy respector of my own feelings, my own needs, as well as his? Can I own, and if need be, express my own feelings? Am I strong enough in my own separateness that I will not be downcast by his depression, frightened by his fear, nor engulfed by his dependency? Is my inner self hardy enough to realize that I am not destroyed by his anger, taken over by

his need for dependence, nor enslaved by his love, but that I exist separate from him with feelings and rights of my own?
5. Am I secure enough within myself to permit him his separateness? Can I permit him to be what he is—honest or deceitful, infantile or adult, despairing or over-confident? Can I give him freedom to be? Do I feel that he should follow my advice, or remain somewhat dependent on me, or mold himself after me?
6. Can I let myself enter fully into the world of his feelings and personal meanings and see these as he does? Can I step into his private world so completely, that I lose all desire to evaluate or judge it? Can I enter it so sensitively that I can move about in it freely, without trampling on meanings which are precious to him? Can I sense it so accurately, that I can catch not only the meanings of his experience which are obvious to him, but those meanings which are only implicit, which he sees only dimly or as confusion? Can I extend this understanding without limit?
7. Can I be acceptant of each facet of this other person which he presents to me? Can I receive him as he is? Can I communicate this attitude? Or can I only receive him conditionally, acceptant of some aspects of his feelings, and silently or openly disapproving of other aspects?
8. Can I act with sufficient sensitivity in the relationship, that my behavior will not be perceived as a threat?
9. Can I free him from the threat of external evaluation?
10. Can I meet this other individual as a person who is *in process of becoming*, or will I be bound by his past and my past?

Gestalt Therapy

Frederick Perls (1969), a man trained in the psychoanalytic tradition, is credited with the evolution of a Gastalt therapy in the mid-1950s. Gestalt theory suggests that if a need is met and emotions expressed, the need is dissipated, thereby allowing other needs to come into focus. This person is in proper biological and psychological adjustment with his environment. On the other hand, a person who has a consistent inability to recognize feelings, like anger, develops psychopathology, just as the failure to recognize hunger leads to an empty stomach and death. Repression of needs and actually hiding the needs is considered the major problem of the neurotic person. For example, the person who is hurt and angry but smilingly says,

"Oh, how nice," is denying his true feelings; thus, the need is unmet, and he cannot move on to another need. Since this repression is not alleviated with intellectual knowledge of the process, therapy stresses sensorimotor awareness and acting out of repressed desires. Gestalt techniques include various sensorimotor and psychological "exercises" to help the patient become aware of his repressed needs. The concern is only with the here and now. The therapist actively encourages the patient to encounter and deal with feelings and other stimuli in the environment that he is blocking out. The patient is asked not to rationalize or explain his behavior but to take responsibility for his actions.

One technique used in Gestalt therapy is the exaggeration of a feeling, word or symptom. The following example shows how a feeling of nervousness was recognized, allowed to come to full awareness by overexaggeration of the symptom, and consequently subsided:

Linda was going for a job interview and felt her hands trembling. Instead of trying to hide the trembling, she focused on the feeling of anxiety and her shaky hands. Remembering the technique of exaggeration of the feeling, she allowed herself to feel the tension and shook her hands vigorously until she was tired from the exaggerated movement. She then realized that the anxiety was greatly reduced, and her hands were no longer trembling.

Other techniques include role reversal, hot seat, empty chair dialogue and many more with the common aim of increased awareness of one's feelings and needs.

Logotherapy

Logotherapy, a humanistic or existential psychotherapy, was developed by Victor Frankl (1969), a psychiatrist with psychoanalytic training. He seems to have been influenced by existential philosophers such as Heidegger, Scheler, Jaspers, Binswanger and Sartre.

Frankl's premise is that a patient's discomfort is directly related to his inability to find meaning in life. One symptom of this existential vacuum is boredom. Logotherapy stresses the spiritual part of existence, and the focus of therapy is the individual's search for meaning.

Each patient is responsible for filling his life with meaning. Suffering is accepted as part of life and regarded as a challenge. Love and creative work are of utmost importance and value. Frankl uses the term "paradoxical intention " when the person brings about that which he fears and then sees that his anxiety is unrealistic, since that which he feared would happen did not come about.

Another technique in logotherapy, "dereflection," is the process of changing the person's focus from himself onto some external goal. Thus, as his attention is directed onto the outside world, he is less preoccupied with himself and has less anxiety.

Primal Therapy

Arthur Janov (1972) developed the theory and techniques of primal therapy around 1970. He asserted that when parents deny the infant's basic needs, the child feels psychological and physiological pain. The defense against such pain leads to a separation of feeling from consciousness. All of these needs that are not met have pain that is saved or accumulated, and this is what Janov calls the "Primal Pool." Because the pain is repressed, it is not conscious and manifests itself as tension.

The aim of therapy is to help the patient experience and integrate the "Primal Pain," alleviating the tension. In primal therapy, following a complete physical examination and a written life history, the patient follows a set of instructions, including spending 48 hours prior to the initial interview isolated in a hotel room. After this period of softening up and weakening of the person's defenses, the patient undergoes three weeks of intense individual therapy. Each session continues, until the exhausted patient requests a halt. In the therapy sessions, the patient lies on a couch with his arms and legs spread out from his body to increase the feeling of defenselessness. The room is usually quiet and darkened. As the therapist identifies the patient's defense mechanisms, he tells the patient not to use them. The patient is ordered to let strong feelings overtake him. Experiences of early childhood are considered very important, and scenes may be reenacted. The therapy is painful, since forgotten memories are dealt with. "The primal is a totally engulfing experience, in which the patient may assume the fetal position, use baby talk, and even cut teeth!" (Strupp and Blackwood, 1975).

After this individual therapy, the patient joins a group as an outpatient. In group therapy, the individuals deal with their own primals, and the session ends as they discuss their feelings during the primal and think about how the feelings lead to their tensions or neurotic behavior. Primals become less frequent, and neurotic behavior begins to disappear as the patient becomes more satisfied with himself and decreasingly ruled by unconscious needs.

Reality Therapy

William Glasser, the founder of reality therapy, puts emphasis on the individual's responsibility. His basic premise is that persons in need of psychotherapeutic help deny reality and are unable to fulfill essential needs. He identifies the basic needs as the need to love and be loved and the need to be worthwhile to self and others. Responsibility refers to the ability to fulfill one's own needs without interfering with another's fulfillment of his. Mental patients either never learned or forgot how to be responsible. "Responsible" is equated by Glasser with mental health, and "irresponsible" is synonymous with mental illness. Glasser says, "therapy is a special kind of teaching or training which attempts to accomplish in a relatively short, intense period what should have been established during normal growing up" (Glasser, 1965).

The first step in therapy is for the therapist to become "involved" with the patient. "Involvement" may take a day, or it may take several weeks to develop. Following the development of involvement, the patient can be helped to become responsible. The patient is directed to look at his actions and decide if they are good or bad. This value judgment is an important step in therapy, as the identification of the problem and the plan is the patient's responsibility. The therapist helps the person look at his life and aids him in making decisions about the irresponsible areas. With the help of the therapist, a plan is developed. The therapist, who is responsible himself, cares about the patient and helps him work with the problems of life in a responsible way.

The following is an example of reality therapy: Bill came in to see the therapist and requested medications for his nerves. The reality therapist avoided this request for medications and began a process of involvement. They talked about various topics, and a sense of trust developed. The therapist asked Bill to tell about what he did the day before. Bill said that nothing special happened and did not seem to know where to begin. The therapist told him to begin with getting up in the morning and not to leave out one single little thing for the rest of the day. This detail of the day brought out that Bill, who was married, had called a girl friend during the course of the day. After discussing this relationship, the therapist directed Bill to look at it and decide if it was good or bad. Was the girl friend helping his wife or children? Bill decided that to have the girl friend was wrong and not the responsible thing to do. As he felt more responsible, his sense of self-worth increased, and his nervousness decreased.

Transactional Analysis

Transactional analysis, usually called TA, was originated in the 1960s by Eric Berne, a psychiatrist with psychoanalytic background. A basic concept in TA is that people have three "ego states"—the Parent, Adult and Child. Each behavioral response or statement of a person indicates the ego state in control of the personality at that moment. The ego state's development includes both intellect and emotion. The Child ego state, which develops first, is considered the spontaneous and feeling part of the personality. Next, the Parent ego state, which contains introjected parental values, rules and commands, evolves. Lastly, the Adult ego state develops, as the child puts two and two together and gets four. The Adult ego state is sometimes referred to as a computer that can give facts and evaluate objectively.

With the groundwork of ego states laid, communication and interactions between people can be examined. In TA, communication between individuals is labeled as "transactions." Transactions which give "payoffs" are called "games." A long list of identified games that individuals participate in is described by Berne (1964).

In therapy, emphasis is placed on analysis of the person's "life script," which Berne states was fixed in the Child ego state, when the person was between 3 and 7 years old. Life scripts are discussed with clients, and they are helped to see how decisions made about themselves at very early ages are affecting them now. Clients are taught the principles of TA, including "life scripts," "ego states" and "games." The therapist points out the client's games as they become apparent and refuses to become involved in playing the games with the client. An educational process takes place, as the client becomes aware of the ego states and recognizes the ability to control them.

To obtain a full presentation of the therapeutic approaches summarized here, the following suggested readings will be helpful. In reading about the therapies described, the complexity of the theoretical foundations is evident. The following readings are listed alphabetically, rather than by importance.

SUGGESTED READINGS

Client-Centered Approach
Rogers, Carl R. *On Becoming a Person*. Boston: Houghton Mifflin Co., 1961.

Gestalt Therapy
Perls, Frederick S. *Gestalt Therapy Verbatim*. Lafayette, Cal.: Real People Press, 1969.

Logotherapy
Frankl, Viktor E. *The Will to Meaning: Foundations and Applications of Logotherapy*. New York: World Publishing Co., 1969.

Primal Therapy
Janov, Arthur. *The Anatomy of Mental Illness: The Scientific Basic of Primal Therapy*. New York: G.P. Putnam's Sons, 1970.

Reality Therapy
Glasser, William. *Mental Health or Mental Illness? Psychiatry for Practical Action*. New York: Harper & Row Publishers, 1970.

Transactional Analysis
Berne, Eric. *Games People Play: The Psychology of Human Relationships*. New York: Grove Press, 1964.

ACTIVITY GROUP THERAPY

Activity group therapy, similar in scope to remotivation therapy, refers to a group situation in which interaction is stimulated by the use of simple tasks, such as drawing pictures, reading and/or listening to music. In activity groups, members are encouraged to direct their attention to a group goal outside themselves. Psychiatric patients tend to be preoccupied with themselves, therefore, the "externalization" needed to heed a group goal may, in itself, be advantageous.

Activity therapy is discussed in regard to four specific types of programs. Traditionally, three of the categories are primarily guided by members of the health care team other than nurses. Activity programs may be in the form of occupational therapy, recreational therapy, psychoeducational therapy and activity therapy groups led by nurses.

In a nurse-led activity group, the goal is to utilize an activity for facilitating interaction, rather than for the activity to serve as the group focus. Patients, especially those anxious or withdrawn, often have difficulty relating to traditional group therapy. The goal of activity group therapy encourages patients to relate to some object outside themselves and, by so doing, practice ways of interacting with group members. Further, group members are provided with opportunities for problem-solving similar to situations anticipated outside the hospital.

An initial activity is to provide the ingredients for coffee and tea. Preparing tea or coffee may seem trivial, yet, for some psychiatric patients, this amount of initiative and self-responsibility is a step forward.

As members work together, they receive cues from others as to the impact of their actions and communications. Patients frequently provide astute feedback to one another regarding each one's behavior. Often, patients listen more carefully to comments and observations from one another than to those from the staff.

Reading, drawing and listening to music serve as beginning activities for a group. In each activity, the patient is allowed a choice in what he draws or reads. Poetry serves as a beneficial tool in activity groups, in that the rhythm and linkage of words, different from those of normal speech, tend to capture the patient's attention and interest. Similarly, a patient may respond to a request to read aloud, before he would speak spontaneously, as reading does not involve stating one's personal knowledge or opinions.

Drawing clearly sets forth a patient's perceptions. Any perceptual distortions are pointed out to the patient. For example, if one object in the drawing is not in proportion to the others, this is pointed out, so the patient can see the objects as they really exist. Not pointing out obvious distortions reinforces disordered thinking.

Activity group therapy is especially beneficial for patients who have difficulty in interpersonal relationships, such as schizophrenia. Schizophrenic patients frequently perceive their problems as major catastrophies for which no solutions are available. The group situation provides an opportunity for patients to realize that others experience similar feelings and problems.

Although the group situation has been found useful for helping patients learn to interact with each other, some schizophrenic patients have difficulties verbalizing in a group. Jones (1966) notes that, frequently, interactions seem to be easier for patients when they are participating in some activity. The activity may serve as a stimulus for the conversation.

Schizophrenic patients tend toward passivity, as well as self-centeredness. Activity group therapy enables the members to do things for themselves and for one another. They learn how to cooperate to carry out a group goal which, in turn, helps in decreasing the passivity and directs the patients' attention away from themselves. The group members are provided with opportunities in which they can learn to cope with some aspects of living which may arise following discharge. Members are further assisted in trying new ways to modify the environment, rather than responding with frustration and withdrawal. For example, the leader might secure the supplies for the members to make coffee during the meetings. If the members are to benefit from the presence of the coffee, they must take the initiative to prepare it and, further, must add sugar and cream to meet their individual needs.

Activity group therapy meetings frequently include from ten to twelve members. They usually meet for one hour a week for a duration of twelve weeks. The initial step in conducting an activity group therapy meeting is to establish rapport among the members. The leader may introduce himself first and then ask each member to do likewise. It is important for the leader to address each of the members by his surname, as this helps to preserve dignity and self-esteem.

After the patients are introduced to each other, the next step is for the leader to assist the members in focusing their attention upon the world of reality. The leader may use one of many techniques to get the group members to think about a selected topic having content which may be of interest to the group.

Following the period which is devoted to an activity, the next step is to engage the members in discussions. The various visual aids utilized in the beginning of the meeting serve as stimuli for discussion.

PSYCHODRAMA

Psychodrama, initially introduced by J. L. Moreno, is a method of psychotherapy which explores past, present and potential experiences through the medium of drama. Moreno observed that drama seemed to have a marked impact on both the actors and the audience. Identification with roles and characters indicates strong empathetic attachment, and, in some cases, catharsis or the release into awareness of repressed material from the unconscious. In psychodrama, the individual is encouraged to recapture the emotional tone of significant past experiences (Moreno, 1959).

Psychodrama is a form of group therapy in which individuals express their problem in words, gestures or facial expressions, as they recreate an experience through acting it out. The setting, designed to approximate closely the problem-situation, facilitates a corrective emotional experience as the actors relive past traumas and events in an attempt to work toward new avenues for coping. The support and suggestions of others provide opportunities for relearning. In the psychodrama, the actor is provided with a medium for identifying his feelings, as well as maladaptive behaviors, and for considering and practicing new adaptive behaviors.

The major goals of psychodrama are to assist the group members develop spontaneity and a more realistic self-view and to identify and practice more facilitative interactional tools.

Structure

A psychodrama session generally consists of the three distinct phases of warm-ups, presentation and group discussion. The warm-up phase seeks to create a relaxed, supportive climate with spontaneous participant interaction. Secondly, warm-up leads to clarification, as members focus on a real-life episode or concern. The format for the warm-up phase may be informal or carefully structured. In either case, it is important that this period lead to a supportive, spontaneous climate with a specific focus.

The presentation phase is the spontaneous dramatic reenactment of the situation under scrutiny. The purpose is to solve "here and now" problems by reenacting past fears, conflicts and situations. During group discussion, opportunities are provided to summarize impressions gleaned from the psychodrama, as well as to validate these impressions with others.

Instruments

Psychodrama uses five primary instruments: the stage, protagonist, director, auxiliaries and audience. The stage, possibly little more than a designated area of a room, provides a setting to recreate a situation with protection from the reality consequences.

The protagonist or leading figure in the psychodrama performs as himself, rather than assuming the identity of another. Essentially, it is his story and perceptions which comprise the plot.

The director, serving as producer, director and therapist, stages the scene, casts parts, insures clarity and dramatic rapport with the audience and facilitates dramatic enactment of the plot. He is instrumental in setting the dramatic tempo. Choosing avenues for plot development and assisting in the choice of a problem to be reenacted are within the realm of the director's responsibility. He also assures that problems presented are handled to the satisfaction of all participants. That is, he avoids allowing a psychodrama to end in the middle, thus leaving participants feeling anxious and unsettled. He also leads a discussion of the presentation, attempting to "tie" loose ends together.

The fourth instrument, the auxiliary ego or therapeutic actor, is both an extension of the director, clarifying and facilitative, as well as an extension of the protaganist portraying the actual or imagined personae of his life drama. By persona is meant a personality mask or facade an individual presents to the outside world. The auxiliary ego participates in scenes in a variety of ways, ranging from playing roles and serving as doubles to commenting on and assessing the action.

The fifth instrument, the audience, may help the protagonist or be helped by him. In helping the protagonist, the audience, serving as a sounding board for public opinions, responds much like the patient. After a scene, the audience may comment and analyze the interaction.

Techniques

A variety of techniques is used in psychodrama to replicate problem situations. Techniques are generally used spontaneously, in response to expressed content for the psychodrama, in contrast to being carefully planned in advance. The following are frequently used techniques:

1. *Role-playing* forms the basis for most psychodrama sessions, with the protagonist playing himself in a situation important to him. Auxiliaries and other group members assume the roles of other characters in the situation. Participants are not necessarily assigned to roles which resemble them; a person may profit more from identifying with a role quite different from his actual manner. Assuming a diverse role provides the person an opportunity to explore new avenues of interacting, as well as to increase flexibility. The aim of role-playing is to simulate the real situation as accurately as possible, so that participants can assess the situation and practice new ways of reacting. Role-playing allows participants to risk behaving in ways they hesitate to try in reality, as well as to express emotions in a protective, non-threatening atmosphere. Role-playing can be spontaneously used in a variety of nurse-patient situations; it is not confined to the domain of psychodrama. Instances in which a nurse and a patient can role-play in advance of the patient confronting the reality situation include:
   a) Employment interview, which is particularly effective if the patient is struggling with whether or not to tell the employer of his psychiatric history.
   b) Reentry into the community, such as ways to meet friends, relatives and co-workers.
   c) Explaining to children where the patient has been and what kind of illnes he had.
   d) Expressing one's actual feelings after many years of glossing over them and, subsequently, internalizing feelings. (An example would be the person who wants to tell a co-worker that some aspect of his behavior upsets her.)
2. *Role-reversal* occurs when the participants exchange roles, thus enabling the protagonist to play the "relevant other " so that he might learn to identify and understand the other person's feelings and reactions. This technique further provides an opportu-

nity for the protagonist to see himself and his behaviors as others see them. Rapid switching of roles and behaviors increases the spontaneity and flexibility of the actors. Role-reversal, like role-playing, can be utilized in a variety of nurse-patient situations. It provides an ideal continuum for the role-playing examples described in the preceding section.
3. *Doubling* can be used in combination with other psychodramatic techniques. The double, an auxiliary or other group member, expresses the unspoken feelings and thoughts which the player is hesitant to present. He may also intensify feelings, such as fear, anger, sadness or love which the actor presents in a mild, "toned-down fashion." Further, the double often provides cues to the action to enlighten the situation. The double, a supportive role, conveys to the actor that he is not alone in the situation, and that at least one other person understands him and cares enough to stand with him.
4. *Mirroring* refers to a technique in which an auxiliary portrays the protagonist, in his presence, to provide instant feedback as to the way he is being perceived. The protagonist is encouraged to comment on or react to the way the auxiliary is presenting him. This technique often proves helpful for confronting a person who resists examining his maladaptive behavior. It also provides a framework in which the protagonist can examine the effect he has on others.
5. *Soliloquy* is a technique in which the protagonist paces back and forth across the stage, speaking his thoughts aloud. A double may pace with the protagonist, verbalizing what seems to be implied, yet left unsaid. This format provides an opportunity for the protagonist to express himself in an uninterrupted fashion (Moreno, 1959).

These psychodrama techniques can be used spontaneously or in planned sessions. Each can be used singly or in a variety of combinations. The technique often facilitates free expression for patients who may experience difficulty speaking in a more formal setting. Patients may be able to free themselves from defensive shields in psychodrama and express real feelings.

THERAPEUTIC COMMUNITY

Plato's *Republic* was an early attempt to set forth the belief that man is a product of the environment and the more perfect the environment, the more perfect man will be (Denber, 1960). In accordance with the theme of the therapeutic community, that the hospital environment provides a decisive factor in the patient's recovery, Pinel's "Moral Treatment" offers an example of an early therapeutic hospital community in which kindness, patience, avoidance of force and restraint and the use of occupational and recreational activities were encouraged.

A twentieth century therapeutic community, the Borstal, in England, had a marked impact on the evolution of the concept in American hospitals. The Borstal, begun in 1902 for correction of youths who had committed crimes, was characterized by:

1. Team work of staff.
2. Emphasis on productive occupations.
3. Preparation of the inmates for subsequent return to the community.
4. Review with the prisoner of all events pertaining to him (Denber, 1960).

Many of the characteristics of the Borstal were direct predecessors of the therapeutic community concept, as introduced in America by Maxwell Jones. Bringing a conceptual framework from England, Jones began a therapeutic community at the Belmont Hospital Unit which was distinguished by three characteristics:

1. Patients were included in practically all information sharing processes on the ward.
2. Patients' opinions were included in decisions about other patients' readiness for such things as passes out of the hospital and discharge.
3. Patient inclusion in the democratic community process was considered an essential, if not major, treatment component.

Consistent with the three characteristics, a primary focus in the therapeutic community is upon group meetings. The patient-staff group becomes a primary interactional unit, with decisions made by the group, rather than allowing one person to dominate. The interaction taking place in group meetings is considered therapy, in that patients and staff jointly consider problems and arrive at possible approaches and solutions.

Group meetings vary in format. The community meeting, a daily meeting attended by unit residents and staff, varies in format from one agency to another. Common purposes include making decisions relating to the entire group, such as deciding on community rules, planning activities and discussing community problems. Some therapeutic communities subdivide the total community into smaller groups to meet daily for group therapy. These group meetings generally focus on psychopathology and interactional problems of group members. In group discussions, patients learn to consider others, observe their impact on others and identify ways in which they differ or resemble others. The traditional, one-to-one relationship between patient and therapist is supplanted by a complex network of relationships with staff and other patients. The purpose of multiple relationships is that each person can have an impact on the well-being of another. This focus takes the magical healing component away from the one-to-one relationship by implying that persons other than staff can facilitate treatment.

Each patient is expected to participate responsibly and actively, not only in his own treatment but in that of fellow patients. The emphasis in the therapeutic community is upon the here and now. Current behavior is focused on, so that staff and patients alike can confirm for one another how they seem at the moment. Efforts are consistently made to help patients recognize, understand and assume responsibility for their behavior and, ultimately, examine other action alternatives. Reality is pointed out, and any distortions or use of defense mechanisms are interrupted.

The value placed on communication implies a change in the status of patients from traditional settings. When patients are encouraged to collaborate with staff, they become active participants in their therapy, as well as that of other patients. This collaborative aspect differs markedly from the traditional passive, recipient patient role. In an attempt to improve the quality as well as quantity of communication, a democratic community atmosphere is created with reduced social distance between patients and staff. Each community member, patient or staff person, is expected to be responsible for the successful functioning of the milieu by attending meetings and, particularly, by decision-making, sharing impressions and feelings and validating reality constraints.

The delicate blurring of roles in the therapeutic community to foster the democratic process is often frightening to both patients and staff. Patients frequently search for some authority figure who will tell them what to do and, at the same time, assume part of the responsibility for their behavior. Staff may be frightened by loss of traditional power assigned to various levels of the hospital hierarchy and may undermine the premise of democratic functioning by giving "lip service" to the conceptual framework of the therapeutic community, while behaving in an altogether different manner. When staff are able to cope with decentralized authority and allow patients to be responsible for their behavior, they provide growth opportunities for patients.

VALUES CLARIFICATION

Values refer to one's set of beliefs, attitudes and opinions about the worth and significance of a thought, object or behavior (Rath, Harmin and Simon, 1966). Values clarification is a process originally introduced as an educational tool for helping children and young people make more effective decisions. Values clarification does not teach a particular set of values; rather, it is a technique designed to help individuals sort out, talk about and think through their own value systems. The emphasis in values clarification is on the process in which a person defines his value system and makes constructive and responsible decisions.

Since individuals experiencing psychological disequilibrium frequently are beset with difficulties in making decisions, the process of values clarification readily translates from the educational to the health care area. Dependency and reluctance to assume responsibility for one's actions often characterize individuals seeking psychiatric treatment. Nurses can easily integrate values clarification techniques or strategies into the problem-solving format of the nursing process. As mentioned in Chapter 6, the nursing process demands patient involvement. Nursing care is not done *to* the patient, but care is mutually planned and implemented. Thus, the need for self-awareness cannot be underestimated: patients must know what they think, feel and choose to do, if the nursing process is to facilitate a state of psychological equilibrium or growth.

Being a process, values clarification is action-oriented, although the action may refer to either physical movement or a public statement. The theoretical framework of values clarification is consistent with that of both psychodrama and therapeutic milieu. The difference between values clarification and psychodrama is that psychodrama moves past the awareness techniques of a values clarification exercise to focus on new ways of handling similar situations. Values clarification is consistent with the tenets of a therapeutic milieu which recognizes that thoughts, feelings, personal responsibility for one's self and group interaction facilitate more effective human functioning.

Values clarification theory states that for any belief, attitude, or feeling to be called a value, it must meet seven criteria:

Choosing: 1. A value must be freely chosen and not forced on the person.
2. The value must be chosen from alternatives, in contrast to being the only possible choice.
3. Values are chosen after giving careful consideration to the consequences which are likely to occur.

Prizing: 4. Values are prized and cherished; values flow from choices each one is glad to make.
5. One's values are publicly known, as others observe one's actions and words.

Acting: 6. Values become a part of each one's behavior.
7. Action upon the value is done repeatedly, not just once or occasionally.

Valuing is the process by which values are determined (Uustal, 1977). It is a process aimed at enabling a person to become aware of his needs and wishes, as well as to explore alternatives and the implicit consequences of them. The valuing process assumes that a person's awareness and life circumstances can change. The process is applicable to a variety of settings, as long as the one utilizing and guiding the session has tried the technique himself.

Four steps are identified in the process of values clarification:

1. *Open up; get information out:*
Stimulate the person to think about a value, to talk about his beliefs.

2. *Acceptance:*
Accept the other person's thoughts and beliefs without judging them. This step tells him it is safe to be honest with both you and himself.

3. *Push for clarification:*
   a) Stimulate the person to do some additional thinking. A clarifying response is a question or comment that invites another person to look at his situation and reflect upon his alternatives and their possible consequences. The response seeks to avoid moralizing, criticizing or advising.
   b) Accept the individual's response.
   c) Clarifying keeps in mind that the individual retains responsibility to look at each behavior but may elect not to change.
   d) Clarifying avoids asking "why" questions, as they often challenge the motives and sincerity of the other person.
   e) Clarification attempts to identify specific and concrete illustrations of behavior as compared to abstract generalizations.
   f) In clarifying, ask questions that enable the person to focus and weigh his alternatives and consequences.
4. *Acceptance:*
   Accept the other person's response.

Clarifying responses useful in implementing the valuing process:
1. Choosing freely
   a) How long have you felt that way?
   b) Where do you suppose you first got that idea?
   c) What do others (parents, spouse) want you to do?
2. Choosing from alternatives
   a) What else did you consider before you decided to do——?
   b) Was it a hard decision?
   c) Did you consider another alternative?
3. Choosing thoughtfully and reflectively
   a) What do you see as the primary consequence of each of your alternatives?
   b) Is this what you are saying?
   c) Now if you do this, what do you think will happen?
4. Prizing and cherishing
   a) Are you glad you feel this way?
   b) How long have you wanted it?

c) In what way would life be different without it?
5. Affirming
   a) Would you tell the group the way you feel?
   b) Are you saying you believe (repeat idea)?
   c) Are you willing to stand up for that belief?
6. Acting upon choices
   a) What is your first step?
   b) Are you saying you believe (repeat idea)?
   c) Are you willing to stand up for that belief?
7. Repeating
   a) Have you felt this way for some time?
   b) Have you done anything about——yet?
   c) Where will this lead you?

A spectrum of strategies is described to apply values clarification theory. The strategy, a structured approach for facilitating interaction, enables individuals to interact under controlled and specified conditions. Some beginning strategies include:
1. Take a sheet of paper and make a name tag, writing your name in the center. In one corner, write the names of four people, other than relatives, who have had a significant impact on your life; in another corner, the names of four geographical locations where you underwent change. In a third corner go three years:
   a) A year in which you were deliciously happy for at least five consecutive days.
   b) The year of your most intense love affair.
   c) The year you did the most good for another person.

In the fourth corner goes a rank order; you are given three abilities and asked to rank them in accordance with your desire for personal improvement. Examples of items to rank order include:
1. to have my anger the same on the outside as on the inside and to be able to use my anger as a disciplined tool
2. to always be able to admit when I'm wrong
3. to be able to ask boldly for affection.

Lastly, write on the paper at least six self-descriptive words ending with "able" (likeable, capable, impressionable). Now pin the name tag on and, without talking, mill around the room and find a partner. Read the data on your partner's card and try to communicate nonverbally. At one-minute intervals, move to a new partner.

Afterwards, break into groups of three persons who do not know one another well. This is called focusing, where each participant takes a turn at being the focus of the other two in his group for five minutes. The focus person talks about any of the four people on his name tag and how that person influenced him.

After the first focus session, the leader provides three rules:

1. *Focus.* Members of the group maintain eye contact with the focus person. They may ask him only those questions that do not shift the focus away from him.
2. *Accept.* Listeners are warmly interested and understanding, and their facial expressions and postures reflect this.
3. *Draw out.* Listeners try to understand the focus person's position, beliefs and feelings, and avoid questions that reveal negative feelings. The rules are followed to the letter in round two, talking about what happened in one of the years on the focus person's name tag.

Focusing can be a useful part of almost any activity that includes small-group discussion. A topic recommended to introduce students to focusing is: "I feel best (and then worst) when I am in a group of people who. . . ." Participants may want to volunteer "I learned" statements based on the focusing exercise.

SUMMARY

A variety of treatment modalities in psychiatric care are identified, ranging from psychoanalysis to values clarification. Each therapeutic approach has implications for nursing practice. While psychiatric nurses may use a selected approach in nurse-client interactions, an understanding of the tenets of widely used treatment techniques and their respective theoretical foundations is essential.

To some extent, the practice setting of the nurse determines the predominant approach to intervention. The skill and educational background of the nurse also influence the framework for practice.

PRINCIPLES

1. Unknown, untried or new situations or roles lead to increased anxiety.
2. The need to defend implies perception of attack or threat.
3. Clarification leads to increased communications.
4. Feelings are often expressed more clearly in actions than in words.
5. There is both a covert and an overt aspect to every behavioral response.
6. Activity tends to decrease anxiety.
7. One's actions are directly influenced by one's values.
8. The provision for the satisfaction of the individual's existing needs allows for the emergence of more mature needs.
9. The individual in the American culture satisfies most of his needs through relationships with others or with groups.
10. Reflection of feelings leads to increased communication.

BIBLIOGRAPHY

Ackerman, N.W. "Interlocking Pathology in Family Relationships," in *Changing Concepts of Psychoanalytic Medicine*. Edited by S. Rado and G. Daniels. New York: Grune & Stratton, Inc., 1956, pp. 135-150.

———. "Family Therapy," in *American Handbook of Psychiatry*. Vol. III. Edited by Silvano Arieti. New York: Basic Books, Inc., 1966, p. 209.

Bell, J. "Family Group Therapy," *U.S. Public Health Monograph*. No. 64. Washington, D.C.: U.S. Government Printing Office, 1961.

Berne, Eric. *Games People Play: The Psychology of Human Relationships*. New York: Grove Press, 1964.

———. *What Do You Say After You Say Hello?* New York: Grove Press, 1972.

Bowen, M. "A Family Concept of Schizophrenia," in *The Etiology of Schizophrenia*. Edited by D.D. Jackson. New York: Basic Books, Inc., 1960, pp. 346-372.

Congress for Nursing Practice. *Standards of Psychiatric-Mental Health Nursing Practice*. Kansas City, Mo.: American Nurses' Association, 1973.

Denber, H.C. *Therapeutic Community*. Springfield, Ill.: Charles C Thomas, Publisher, 1960.

Glasser, William. *Reality Therapy*. New York: Harper and Row. Publishers, 1965, p. 24.

Janov, Arthur. *The Primal Revolution: Toward a Real World*. New York: Simon & Schuster, Inc., 1972.

Jones, M. "Group Work in Mental Hospitals," *British Journal of Psychiatry,* CXII, No. 12 (October, 1966), 1007-1011.

Kyes, J., and Hofling, C. *Basic Psychiatric Concepts in Nursing.* 3d ed. Philadelphia: J.B. Lippincott Co., 1974, p. 480.

Moreno, J.L. "Psychodrama," in *American Handbook of Psychiatry.* Vol. II. Edited by Silvano Arieti. New York: Basic Books, Inc., 1959, pp. 1375-1395.

Perls, Frederick. *Gestalt Therapy Verbatim.* Lafayette, Cal.: Real People Press, 1969.

Rath, Louis, Merrill, Harmin, and Sidney, Simon. *Values and Teaching: Working with Values in the Classroom.* Columbus, Ohio: Charles E. Merrill Publishing Co., 1966.

Rogers, Carl R. *On Becoming a Person.* Boston: Houghton Mifflin Co., 1961, pp. 50-57.

Sadock, Benjamin. "Group Psychotherapy," in *Comprehensive Textbook of Psychiatry.* 2d ed. Edited by A. Freedman, H. Kaplan, and B. Sadock. Baltimore: Williams & Wilkins Co., 1975, p. 1850.

Satir, V.M., Stachowiak, and Taschman. *Helping Families to Change.* 3d ed. New York: Jason Aronson Inc., 1977.

———. *Conjoint Family Therapy.* Palo Alto, Cal.: Science and Behavior Books, Inc., 1964.

Spiegel, H. "Hypnosis: An Adjunct to Psychotherapy," in *Comprehensive Textbook of Psychiatry.* 2d ed. Edited by A. Freedman, H. Kaplan and B. Sadock. Baltimore: Williams & Wilkins Co., 1975, p. 1844.

Stewart, R. "Psychoanalysis and Psychoanalytic Psychotherapy," in *Comprehensive Textbook of Psychiatry.* 2d ed. Edited by A. Freedman, H. Kaplan, and B. Sadock. Baltimore: Williams & Wilkins Co., 1975, pp. 1797-1817.

Strupp, H. and Blackwood, G. "Recent Methods of Psychotherapy," in *Comprehensive Textbook of Psychiatry.* 2d ed. Edited by A. Freedman, H. Kaplan, and B. Sadock. Baltimore: Williams & Wilkins Co., 1975, pp. 1911-1912.

Uustal, Diane. "Searching for Values," *Image,* IX, No. 1 (February, 1977), 15-17.

Wynne, L.C., et al. "Pseudomutuality in Family Relationships of Schizophrenia," *Psychiatry,* XXI (May,1958), 205-220.

CHAPTER 16

Psychiatric Nursing in the Community

Jeanette Lancaster, R.N., Ph.D.

HISTORY AND DEVELOPMENT OF COMMUNITY MENTAL HEALTH NURSING

Rapid advances are being made in psychiatry as in most other medical specialties. The 1970s are witnessing the third revolution in the treatment of the mentally ill since the beginning of the century. To appreciate the scope of community mental health nursing, the historical evolution of mental healing must be considered.

Origins

The origins of mental healing date back to ancient and prehistoric times. Primitive man viewed disease as an evil spirit that took possession of the body as a punishment for an offense against the spirit world. The primitive art of mental healing was the art of driving hostile spirits away. This view of illness was believed to be in effect around 250 B.C. and was dominated by fear and superstition. Treatment in this era was either by restraint or actual physical rejection.

The fifteenth–seventeenth centuries were characterized by more drastic handling of mentally ill individuals, in that they were legally prosecuted and burned as witches. Their treatment was determined by the underlying belief that they were a threat to the community.

The next mode of mental healing, custodial care, dates to Greek and Roman times. Care at this time included sedation with opiates, music therapy, good physical hygiene and humane management of the patient's daily activities. This concept of care was abandoned when the Roman Empire deteriorated, and the supernatural concept was resumed.

The first and, perhaps, most significant impact on the treatment of the mentally ill began at the end of the eighteenth century. Humanitarian reform of mental hospitals received its great impetus in France, with the work of Philippe Pinel. In 1793, Pinel received reluctant approval from the French officials to remove the chains from some of the hospital inmates at La Bicetre Hospital in Paris, so that he might test his belief that mentally ill individuals should be treated as sick individuals, rather than as criminals housed in filthy dungeons. Chains were removed; rooms were cleaned and aired. Peace and quiet replaced the chaos and noise of the recent past, leading to astounding treatment results.

In England, concurrent with the work of Pinel in France, William Tuke established the "York Retreat," a pleasant country house where mental patients lived in a quiet atmosphere. The success of Pinel and Tuke influenced treatment of the mentally ill throughout the civilized world (Coleman, 1972).

Humanitarian methods in psychiatry were first seen in America in the work of Benjamin Rush, who has since been called "the father of American psychiatry." Rush is considered a transitional figure in American psychiatry, in that he encouraged more humane treatment, yet continued to use remedies like bloodletting, purgatives and a torturelike device called "the tranquilizer" (Coleman, 1972).

During the nineteenth century, all mentally ill individuals were collected in one spot with a paid attendant to watch them. Since mental illness at this time was considered irreversible, these deranged individuals were put in institutions as a societal protection. This era saw the development of a custodial state hospital system offering no treatment.

An energetic New England schoolteacher, Dorothea Dix, carried on the beginning humanitarian work of Rush. In 1841, Miss Dix appointed herself inspector of institutions for the mentally ill and began crusading for humane treatment of the mentally ill (Deloughery, 1971). She is credited with the establishment of thirty-two mental hospitals in the United States. Due to the work of

Dorothea Dix, the "asylum" became a familiar American landmark in the last half of the nineteenth century.

During the custodial era of psychiatric care, the primary responsibility of the nurse was to guard the patients. Mental illness was viewed as a disease process, and the "treatment" goal was to keep the patients in a safe place. During the custodial care era, psychiatric nursing began to evolve, with the first psychiatric training school for nurses in the United States begun in 1882 at the McLean Hospital in Belmont, Massachusetts (Sills, 1973). Numerous obstacles were encountered in the development of psychiatric nursing in the United States. The greatest of these related to the lack of demand for the "asylum-trained" nurses. As late as 1916, one-half of the United States mental hospitals operated schools for their nurses; hospitals without schools preferred to employ attendants at a low wage to "care" for patients. The tendency to educate nurses in psychiatric care at a school within a psychiatric institution was due to the belief that if a nurse needed to know about mental illness, the knowledge and experience should be acquired in a psychiatric hospital. This approach later led to the development in nursing education of affiliations. During an "affiliation," the nursing students went as a group to live for six weeks to three months in a dormitory at a large state hospital. This approach furthered the dichotomy between illness of the mind and the body, because the total patient system was not presented.

Public interest in mental health was noted at the close of the nineteenth century. In 1908, the first Mental Hygiene Committee was established, largely due to the publication of Clifford Beers' autobiography, *A Mind That Found Itself*. Beers, a distinguished businessman, described his mental collapse and subsequent treatment in the mental hospital so vividly, that the mental hygiene movement was launched (Freedman, 1967).

The development of the scientific method also furthered the work of psychiatry. This method gave a foundation for viewing behavior. The rigid separation of "mind and body," and the notion that all mental illness was caused by organic disease were successfully challenged. The work of Adolf Meyer in the early 1900s greatly influenced psychiatric education. Meyer promoted the study of a patient's total life experiences, in search of causation of illness and in planning psychotherapy. The work of Freud and other behavior scientists had an impact on psychiatric treatment (Gregg, 1965).

Twentieth-Century Psychiatric Revolutions

The first psychiatric revolution of the twentieth century was the emergence of psychoanalysis, due to the work of Sigmund Freud. Initially, psychoanalysis, viewed as a means of understanding mental functioning, was the treatment of choice for the neuroses. In recent years, due to waning interest in psychoanalysis, regional areas such as the Eastern Coast constitute centers for this form of treatment, with varied modes of treatment used extensively in other areas of the United States.

The second twentieth-century revolution began with the advent and widespread use of psychotropic drugs. Enthusiasm for drug usage in psychiatric treatment began in the early 1960s, with somatic or drug treatment viewed as a panacea for all psychiatric ills. To date, psychotropic drugs have greatly altered the course of treatment for many patients due to shorter hospitalizations and diminished severity of symptoms, with a simultaneous increase in the rate of hospital readmissions.

The Federal Government first entered the health field in 1935 with the passage of the Social Security Act. During the Depression, the view developed that if a local community could not provide care for its sick, the government should do so. Additionally, the changing tax structure of the country during the 1930s and 1940s provided greater Federal government income and lesser income to state and local communities (Freedman, 1967). At this point in American history, health care came to be viewed as a right of all, rather than as a privilege of a few (Deloughery, 1971). World War II had a significant impact on the community mental health movement, when 1,767,000 draftees were rejected from military service on the basis of mental or neurological grounds. Following World War II, the clearest evidence of Federal assumption of responsibility was seen in 1946, when the National Mental Health Act created the National Institute for Mental Health. Initially, the function of the National Institute for Mental Health was research of the origins of mental illness and development of treatment methods. The Institute's other area of responsibility was in the distribution of training and other grants by providing Federal funds to improve, expand and initiate training programs in the mental health fields. Further advances in the field of mental health were slow in coming, with the next major thrust beginning in the early 1950s.

In 1953, at the Fifth Mental Hospital Institute in Little Rock, Arkansas, American Psychiatric Association president, Kenneth Appel, called the nation's attention to the need for greater public support for the care and treatment of the mentally ill, and for training, research and prevention (Talkington, 1973). Following this report, Appel and other leaders in the psychiatric area evolved the idea of a committee sponsored by organizations serving the mentally disabled. The purpose of this committee was to examine the nation's resources and make recommendations for better ways to serve the mentally ill in the United States.

In 1958, Irving Goffman presented the view of mental illness as a social process rather than a disease process. He emphatically described the effect of institutionalization and hospitals designed for the management of staff rather than the care of patients (Goffman, 1961). Simultaneously, the therapeutic community concept, originating in England, was introduced to the United States (Jones, 1953). The therapeutic milieu (or community) concept emphasized open and direct communication between patients and staff, with patient participation in planning decisions. At this juncture, psychiatric nurses became actively involved in patient care and began defining the role of the nurse in the therapeutic community (Holmes, 1966). Basically, until the mid-1960s, psychiatric nursing was primarily oriented toward treatment of the hospitalized patient.

In 1961, the Joint Commission on Mental Illness and Health published *Action for Mental Health*. Following this report, President Kennedy appointed a Cabinet-level committee to review the report. The committee report influenced the President to submit to Congress in 1963 the first Presidential message on behalf of the mentally disturbed. He called for a "bold new approach" to bring psychiatry "back into the mainstream of medicine and community life" (Rubins, 1971). As a result of the President's report to Cogress, the Community Mental Health Center Act was passed, which provided support for construction of mental health centers. The advent of community mental health centers called forth the third twentieth-century revolution in psychiatry by moving the treatment area from the confines of hospital walls to the community domain.

The intent of the Community Mental Health Center Act was to provide comprehensive mental health services to meet the needs of all persons living in the specific area being served. The initial goal was to establish 500 comprehensive mental health centers by 1970, with each center serving a population of between 7,500 and 200,000 individuals, depending on the population density (Rubins, 1971). Although the original legislation made money available for construction of mental health centers, no funds were provided for program development. Moreover, in order to receive funding, each institution had to commit itself to operate a program for a minimum of twenty years (Marwalk, 1971).

The Federal legislation proposed that local communities develop methods of delivery of care designed for their unique needs, but these same regulations required five essential services. These services included:

1. inpatient care for patients requiring short-term hospitalization
2. partial hospitalization which includes day hospital for those patients who could return to their own homes at night, and night hospital for patients who were able to work but needed some care each day
3. outpatient treatment which allows patients to live at home and go to the center at regular intervals
4. emergency care with services available around the clock
5. consultation and education to members of the community (Coleman, 1972).

Essentially, the mental health program was designed to serve the people in close proximity to their local communities through a variety of programs for prevention, treatment and rehabilitation.

The work environment of the psychiatric nurse moved from the confines of the institutions' walls to the horizons of the community with the third psychiatric revolution. As the environment changed, so did the title of the care-giver. Titles now include: psychiatric nurse, community psychiatric nurse, community mental health nurse and psychiatric-mental health nurse. Osborne (1973) emphasizes that the first two terms refer to nurses working in traditional psychiatric hospital settings, providing care for patients defined as mentally ill. The term "community mental health nurse" describes the nurse whose role is that of strengthening health in the population and preventing mental illness (Osborne, 1973). "Psychiatric-mental health nurse" describes the nurse who functions both in the treatment and prevention of mental illness. The latter two terms are considered synonymous in the text with the community, representing the entirety of man's environments including the hospital environment. The nurse's role can be defined, using Gerald Caplan's concepts of intervention. The ultimate goal in community mental health nursing is that of primary prevention, referring to the processes involved in reducing the risk that people in the community will fall ill with mental disorders (Caplan, 1964). Secondary prevention is the early identification of emotional disorders by efficient case-finding, early diagnosis and effective treatment. The last category of prevention, tertiary prevention, attempts to reduce the residual effects of mental illness by early rehabilitation efforts (Caplan, 1964).

Each aspect of intervention can occur in either the hospital or the community. Primary prevention frequently occurs in the community, whereas secondary prevention may or may not involve some degree of hospital stay. Tertiary prevention is likely to begin in the hospital and continue when the patient returns to the community. Community mental health nurses are prepared to assume significant roles at each intervention level. Nursing is grounded in both the biological and social sciences, providing practitioners an ideal vantage point to assess a client's problems and to intervene or refer the client, as necessary. The psychiatric-mental health nurse must view the "whole" patient, no matter where he is found. There can be no dichotomy between "mind and body." Interaction between the patient and his environment must be considered in each interaction and each alternative mode of behaving.

As the practice and scope of nursing expands, previous models for providing care no longer seem relevant. Past models for dealing with health and illness are not suitable and comprehensive enough for the current complex health problems.

HUMAN ECOLOGICAL APPROACH TO COMMUNITY MENTAL HEALTH NURSING

The systems or human ecological approach provides a framework for community mental health nursing which takes into account each force impinging on the nurse-patient/client interaction. This approach or model is founded on the belief that man's health status results from the dynamic interaction between his internal environment and the external multi-environments in which he exists. The human ecological or systems approach is utilized in community mental health nursing to provide a holistic view of man as he relates to his environment.

Man's environment encompasses the physical and biotic realms, as well as the sociocultural realm; man relates both to an intrinsic as well as an extrinsic environment. His relationships to his multi-environments are never static but, rather, are dynamic and constantly being altered. Each of a person's responses comprises a unique attempt to maintain homeostasis. The complexity of his adaptive efforts are accentuated by recognizing that the human organism responds to the total environment. One cannot sort out those environmental components which seem most tolerable, but, rather, each responds in one way or another to the total environmental impact. This elementary concept is basic to the knowledge base of the nurse working in community mental health. One has only to make a limited number of home visits to appreciate fully the scope of an individual's response to the total environment.

Human ecology seeks to understand man and his problems by studying the effects of physical, biological and cultural environments upon man, and his influence upon the environment. According to Hinkle (1965), man is viewed as an open-ended system constantly interacting with the environment to maintain life and effective functioning.

The assumption is made in human ecology that "everything affects everything else" (Bruhn, 1970, p. 40). The belief is held that a human population is an aggregate of individuals, and each individual must have access to an environment which provides sustenance.

It is at this juncture in the scope of human ecology that systems theory offers a sound foundation.

According to Odum (1972), the center of professional ecology is the ecosystem concept. The term "ecosystem," first proposed by the British ecologist, A.C. Tansley in 1935, can be applied to a single cell, as well as to tissues, organs, organisms or populations at increasingly complex organizational levels. Each level can be viewed as an ecosystem, if the total environment is included as part of the environment (Bruhn, 1970).

Man and his multi-person systems are natural systems, in that they do not owe their existence to conscious human planning and execution. A perspective of man's hierarchy of systems includes: "We are natural systems first, living things second, human beings third, members of a society and culture fourth and particular individuals fifth" (Laszlo, 1972, pp. 23-25). Certain characteristics of natural systems apply to man and must be given serious consideration by the community mental health nurse. Basic system principles or characteristics include:

1. The whole is equal to more than the sum of its parts. The constancy of the whole remains the same, or essentially unchanged, even though components may undergo change. (This principle is readily applied to the family, in that the family maintains a considerable portion of its previous structure when one member leaves or behaves in a dysfunctional manner.)
2. Systems are arranged in hierarchies or levels. Each component of the suprasystem can be considered as a separate system. (Each person can be described as a system, with his bodily parts and functioning comprising his subsystems and his family or significant others comprising the suprasystem. Similarly, the family can be viewed as the system, with each member a subsystem and the group, the suprasystem.)
3. All living systems are open systems which continuously exchange information with the environment. Exchanges refer to matter, energy and information. These exchanges take the form of inputs (information taken into the system) and outputs (energy or information expelled by the system as a result of its operations). The process by which inputs are taken in, processed and expelled is known as the system transaction. (In each person or family, certain information is taken in, processed according to the person's perception, needs, intelligence and psychological functioning, and discharged as an output.) It is important to recognize that no two persons hearing the same message perceive it exactly alike. The input is different for each one. This principle is particularly important for the community mental health nurse, in that the client or patient perceives each communication and event in keeping with his needs and psychological state at the time.

4. Each system strives to arrive at a steady state or homeostasis; symptoms are signals of system distress. Each one strives to reach his highest plateau of physical or mental health. Rene Dubos (1969) aptly describes health as a goal, "a mirage." He says that health is a state each man continually strives for but cannot reach, because his environments change more rapidly than he can make advances.

The ecological or systems perspective provides one way of looking at man's journey toward health. Ecology's primary contribution to the field of health is the way in which it views the man-environment system. Ecology looks at the total organism, not just at the mind or body as isolated, unrelated parts.

The health status (physical and/or mental) of a community is determined by the dynamic interrelationships among three ecological components:

1. The agent of disease
2. The host which is affected
3. The environment which contains both

The role of the community mental health nurse necessitates an understanding of these ecological components as an integral aspect of assessment. When working in the community, the nurse must broaden her scope beyond the individual patient or client and examine the suprasystem (community), in which the individual strives to attain homeostasis.

In order to prevent illness, it is necessary to assign causal factors to the illness and then seek to eradicate the cause. Thorough assessment is implicit in determining causal factors of illness. Basic to identifying the causal factors in mental illness is the necessity to define mental health. Mental health is "that state in the interrelationships of the individual and his environment in which the personality structure is relatively stable, and the environmental stresses are within its absorptive capacity" (Marmor, 1950, p. 30). Mental health is defined by Mary Liston (1958) as a broad continuum of:

1. promotion and maintenance of optimal mental health
2. prevention of mental disorders
3. provision for and assistance with remedial and curative care
4. promotion of and provision for reeducation and rehabilitation (Liston, 1958).

The American Nurses' Association describes the nurse-patient relationship as including care, cure and coordination (Ujhely, 1965). The care component means that community mental health nurses must care enough not only to care for those who come into the hospital, but also to go out into the community and, using primary prevention, promote mental health and prevent mental disorders. In community psychiatry, this may mean to focus, initially, on basic material or physiological needs. Are the community residents fed, warm and protected? If basic needs are met, the focus can center on psychological needs. What is the emotional climate of the community? Are the residents lonely, aggressive or apathetic? The care component may take the nurse into the schools to talk with children about life stresses before these stresses accumulate, or it may mean talking formally or informally with small groups of new mothers regarding their new roles, expectations and apprehensions. The systems approach stresses that interrelationships maintain or defeat the organism in his environment. In applying the systems approach to the care component of nursing, the multitude of inputs would have relevance, as would the effects of these inputs on the transactions and outputs of each individual.

The cure component is consistent with secondary prevention. For example, when working with a family who has a mentally disturbed adolescent, the curative function would not be to consider the adolescent as a separate organism, but, rather, as one component of a family system. In families, the whole is greater than the sum of the parts, in that the family interaction constitutes a new aspect of a system—indeed, forms a new system composed of the members, who alone are individual systems, but, now, who become subsystems in the new larger system.

The coordinating function is consistent with tertiary prevention. An important recognition at this point is that each professional brings to the relationship a unique set of skills, needs and, possibly, goals. If the patient is viewed from an ecological perspective, it makes it clearer for the helpers to focus on the patient's needs and to share responsibility for the well-being of the patient.

The role of the nurse in community mental health cannot be implemented in isolation; collaboration and interdisciplinary planning comprise essential components of the work role for the nurse. Standard XI of the ANA Standards of Psychiatric-Mental Health

Nursing Practice describes the collaborative role of the nurse (Congress for Nursing Practice, 1973).

STANDARD XI

Nursing participates with other members of the community in planning and implementing mental health services that include the broad continuum of promotion of mental health, prevention of mental illness, treatment and rehabilitation.

Rationale

In our contemporary society, the high incidence of mental illness and mental retardation requires increased effort to devise more effective treatment and prevention programs. There is a need for nursing to participate in programs that strengthen the existing health potential of all members of society. In this effort, cooperation and collaboration by all community agencies becomes imperative. Such concepts as early intervention and continuity of care are essential in planning to meet the mental health needs of the community. The nurse uses organizational, advisory or consultative skills to facilitate the development and implementation of mental health services.

Assessment Factors

1. Knowledge of community and group dynamics is used to understand the structure and function of the community system.
2. Current social issues that influence the nature of mental health problems in the community are recognized.
3. High risk population groups in the community are delineated, and gaps in community services are identified.
4. Community members are encouraged to become active in assessing community mental health needs and planning programs to meet these needs.
5. The strength and capacities of individuals, families and the community are assessed, in order to promote and increase the health potential of all.
6. Consultative skills are used to facilitate the development and implementation of mental health services.

7. The needs of the community are brought to the attention of appropriate individuals and groups, including legislative bodies and regional and state planning groups.
8. The mental health services of the agency are interpreted to others in the community. There is collaboration with the staff of other agencies to insure continuity of service for patients and families.
9. Community resources are used appropriately.
10. Nursing participates with other professional and nonprofessional members of the community in the planning, implementation and evaluation of mental health services.

Dorothy Ozimek of the National League for Nursing (1974), in describing what society expects of the baccalaureate graduate, reaffirms the collaborative nature of nursing. She notes:

> The health needs of the majority of people are not of a critical nature, but are clearly needs for maintaining health and dealing with long-term disabling health problems. It is evident, then, that primary community health care must be a role of the nurse. The nurse must deliver health care, coordinate health services, deliver humanistic care and engage in health assessment and health maintenance. Nurses must practice in areas of primary, acute, and long-term care (Ozimek, 1974, p. 4).

In order to meet societal expectations, the nurse must continually upgrade her nursing practice and keep abreast of new concepts, developments and research in nursing practice. Continuing education is an essential component of professionalism. Standard XIII of the ANA Standards of Psychiatric-Mental Health Nursing Practice describes the need for ongoing, continuing education and professional development (Congress for Nursing Practice, 1973). The area of psychiatric nursing is filled with opportunities for further development, with workshops, symposia and group experiences providing innumerable growth opportunities.

STANDARD XIII

Responsibility is assumed for continuing educational and professional development, and contributions are made to the professional growth of others.

Rationale

The scientific, cultural and social changes characterizing our contemporary society require the nurse to be committed to the ongoing pursuit of knowledge which will enhance professional growth.

Assessment Factors

1. There is evidence of study of one's nursing practice to increase both understanding and skill.
2. There is evidence of participation in inservice meetings and educational programs, either as an attendee or as a teacher.
3. There is evidence of attendance at conventions, institutes, workshops, symposia and other professionally oriented meetings and/or other ways to increase formal education.
4. There is evidence of systematic efforts to increase understanding of psychodynamics, psychopathology and avenues of psychotherapeutic intervention.
5. There is evidence of cognizance of developments in relevant fields and utilization of this knowledge.
6. There is evidence of assisting others to identify areas of educational needs.
7. There is evidence of sharing appropriate clinical observations and interpretations with professionals and other groups.

As community mental health nursing moves away from the hospital and diversifies its practice, the independent nursing role assumes greater magnitude. Psychiatric nurses have made considerable noteworthy inroads in the area of reimbursement for services. Indeed, psychiatric nurses have been pacesetters in independent practice. Concurrent with the advances in independent practice has been the recognition of the need for certification of psychiatric nurses. Certification is based on an assessment of each applicant's knowledge, demonstration of ongoing, supervised clinical practice and recognition and endorsement by colleagues. Certification provides recognition and acknowledgment of professional achievement and clinical expertise in one area of nursing practice.

Implicit in the role of the psychiatric nurse is the responsibility for management and supervision of other health team members. Frequently, the nurse is responsible for 24-hour supervision of patient care. This supervision may be provided by three shifts of nursing coverage, or one nurse may supervise nonprofessional personnel during the evening and night shifts on an "on-call" basis.

The nurse is responsible not only for her personal development but, also, for persons working under her supervision. Standard XII speaks to the role of the nurse in providing learning opportunities and supervision for other nursing care personnel.

STANDARD XII

Learning experiences are provided for other nursing care personnel through leadership, supervision and teaching.

Rationale

As leader of the nursing team, the nurse is responsible for the team's activities and must be able to teach, supervise and evaluate the performance of nursing care personnel. The focus is on the continuing development of each member of the team.

Assessment Factors

1. Leadership roles and responsibilities are accepted.
2. Team members are encouraged to identify strengths and abilities. A climate is provided for the continuing self-development of each member.
3. A role model in giving direct nursing care is provided for the team.
4. The supervisory role is used as a tool for improving nursing care.
5. The client's needs, as well as the abilities of each member of the nursing team, are evaluated and assignments are based on these evaluations.

Psychiatric nurses must engage in research activities to advance theory development and test out new clinical approaches. While it is unreasonable to imply that each nurse will be continuously involved personally in research, each can keep abreast of research developments made by other practitioners. Standard XIV describes the nursing role in regard to research.

STANDARD XIV

Contributions to nursing and the mental health field are made through innovations in theory and practice and participation in research.

Rationale

Each professional has responsibility for the continuing development and refinement of knowledge in the mental health field through research and experimentation with new and creative approaches to practice.

Assessment Factors

1. Studies are developed, implemented and evaluated.
2. Responsible standards of research are used in investigative endeavors.
3. Nursing practice is approached with an inquiring and open mind.
4. The pertinent and responsible research of others is supported.
5. Expert consultation and/or supervision is sought, as required.
6. The ability to discriminate those findings which are pertinent to the advancement of nursing practice is demonstrated.
7. Innovations in theory, practice and research findings are made available through presentations and/or publications.

SUMMARY

The twentieth century has witnessed tremendous advances in the treatment modalities for psychiatric patients. Custodial care has greatly decreased as a treatment method, to be replaced by action-oriented approaches designed to assist patients to function more effectively in the community. Until recent years, secondary and tertiary prevention comprised the vast majority of treatment approaches to the mentally ill person. Attention is now paid to the benefits of primary prevention, so as to provide persons with coping skills in advance of psychological dysfunction.

The community mental health nurse, whose practice is based on principles from both the biological and social sciences, is ideally suited to provide care for patients in all three preventive areas: primary, secondary and tertiary. Implicit in implementing the nursing role is the need for a conceptual framework for practice. The human ecological approach, essentially a systems approach, provides a framework for dealing with the whole patient.

BIBLIOGRAPHY

Bruhn, John. "Human Ecology in Medicine," *Environmental Research,* III (January, 1970), 37-53.

Caplan, Gerald. *Principles of Preventive Psychiatry.* New York: Basic Books, Inc., 1964.

Coleman, James. *Abnormal Psychology.* 4th ed. Glenview, Ill.: Scott Foresman & Co., 1972.

Congress for Nursing Practice. *Standards of Psychiatric-Mental Health Nursing Practice.* Kansas City, Mo.: American Nurses' Association, 1973.

Deloughery, Grace, Gebbie, Kristine, and Neuman, Betty. *Consultation and Community Organization in Community Mental Health Nursing.* Baltimore: Williams & Wilkins Co., 1971.

Dubos, Rene. "Human Ecology," *WHO Chronicle,* XXIII (November, 1969), 499-501.

Freedman, Alfred. "Historical and Political Roots of the Community Mental Health Centers Act," *American Journal of Orthopsychiatry,* XXXVII (April, 1967), 487-494.

Goffman, Erving. *Asylums.* New York: Doubleday and Co., 1961.

Gregg, Dorothy. "The Role of Post-baccalaureate Nurse Specialists: Psychiatric Nursing." A position paper prepared for the Sterring Community, San Francisco, Cal., April 30-May 1, 1965.

Hinkle, Lawrence. "Studies of Human Ecology in Relation to Health and Behavior," *Bio Science,* XV (August, 1965), 517-520.

Holmes, Marguerite, and Werner, Jean. *Psychiatric Nursing in a Therapeutic Community.* New York: The Macmillan Co., 1966.

Jones, Maxwell. *The Therapeutic Community: A New Treatment Method in Psychiatry.* New York: Basic Books, Inc., 1953.

Laszlo, Ervin. *The Systems View of the World.* New York: George Braziller, Inc., 1972.

Liston, Mary. "Selection of Learning Experience in Psychiatric Nursing in the Basic Program," in *Teaching and Implementation of Psychiatric-Mental Health Nursing.* Edited by Mary Redmond and Margery Drake. Washington: Catholic University of America Press, 1958, pp. 71-80.

Marmor, Judd and Pumpian-Mindlin, Eugene. "Toward an Integrated

Conception of Mental Disorders." *Journal of Nervous and Mental Disease,* III, No. 1 (January, 1950), 19-29.

Marwalk, Meyer. "An Indictment of the Community Mental Health Centers Act," *Hospital and Community Psychiatry,* XXII (March, 1971), 79-81.

Odum, Eugene. "Ecosystem Theory in Relation to Man," in *Ecosystem Structure and Function.* Edited by John Wiens. Corvallis, Ore.: Oregon State University Press, 1972, pp. 7-21.

Osborne, Oliver. "Anthropological Issues in Mental Health Nursing," *Contemporary Issues in Mental Health Nursing.* Edited by M. Leininger. Boston: Little, Brown & Co., 1973, pp. 39-61.

Ozimek, Dorothy. "The Baccalaureate Graduate in Nursing: What Does Society Expect?" New York: National League for Nursing, 1974.

Rubins, Jack. "The Community Mental Health Movement in the United States Circa 1970," *American Journal of Psychoanalysis.* XXXI (January, 1971), pp. 68-79.

Sills, Grace. "Historical Development and Issues in Psychiatric-Mental Health Nursing," in *Contemporary Issues in Mental Health Nursing.* Edited by M. Leininger. Boston: Little, Brown & Co., 1973, pp. 125-136.

Talkington, Perry. "Critical Issues in Psychiatry: A Call for the Reassessment of Our Nation's Mental Health Care," *Hospital and Community Psychiatry,* XXIV (January, 1973), 17.

Ujhely, Gertrud. "The Nurse in Community Psychiatry," *American Journal of Nursing,* LXIX, No. 8 (August, 1965), 517-520.

CHAPTER 17

Crisis Intervention

Brenda Riley, R.N., M.S.

Crisis intervention is a significant aspect of nursing; it is a short-term, relatively inexpensive therapy that enables many people to receive help. Nurses frequently encounter crisis situations within the health care setting. Crises often involve the client's family, friends and/or neighbors. As crisis intervention deals with socially dynamic phenomena extending beyond the medical milieu in which the nurse is involved, it is important for the nursing professional to appreciate the broader social context, as well as to have a detailed understanding of the nursing role in crisis intervention.

So that the reader may gain insight into the application of crisis intervention as a technique, the following example of a crisis is offered. Thereafter, the definition, types of crises, stages of crises and operational steps are discussed and applied to the example. In addition, the nursing process is presented in the form of the problem-oriented record system.

CASE STUDY

Jane was one of the most promising nursing students at her university. Approximately midway into the first semester of her senior year, she and her husband divorced. The emotional strain surrounding the divorce, as well as the acutely felt sense of responsibility for her 1-year-old daughter, distracted Jane from her studies to the degree that her usually excellent grades dropped. Warnings from her instructors only added to her anxieties. Subsequently, as the first semester ended, Jane's grades deteriorated to the point that she was called to the dean's office and notified that she had failed her course work, thus making her ineligible for continuance in the program, whereupon she began crying uncontrollably.

After a few minutes, she said she knew she had failed and did not know what she was going to do about it. Then she began sobbing and appeared to be in despair. This continued for some time, with occasional utterances of, "I don't know what I'm going to do." The dean made an appointment and directed Jane to the counseling center.

Jane entered sobbing, staring at her hands, and fidgeting with a facial tissue. The nurse therapist asked Jane to tell her what had happened. Jane said she had just flunked out of school, had recently gotten divorced, had a child to take care of and had financial problems. The nurse therapist decided to concentrate on the first and most recent problem which Jane mentioned.

Jane told her that until this year, she had been a good student. Because of numerous problems, she was unable to spend as much time studying as required; when she did have study time, she was unable to concentrate. Jane indicated that her whole life depended on her graduation and ability to support herself and her child. Again, she said she did not know what she was going to do.

Although she received alimony, she discovered that it was not enough for living expenses, school supplies and tuition. It was too late to apply for a loan through the school, so she obtained an education loan from a local bank. She was to begin repayment of the loan two months after graduation. "What will I do?" she asked.

The nurse therapist at the counseling center asked her to explore the possibilities. She had stopped crying by now and began listing the possibilities, hesitantly, and with the therapist's help. She could go home and live with her parents, but she did not want to do that because she did not want to be a burden on them. She could get a job and stay in her present home, but it would have to be in unskilled labor and that was not appealing; but it was better than living with her parents, she thought.

The therapist asked about her desire to be a nurse, but there was no hope for that now. She had flunked out, and the loan was due soon after her previously scheduled graduation. The therapist asked if she were interested in exploring the possibility that she might still become a nurse. She agreed but did not see any way. She would have to have special permission to be readmitted, and she would have to wait until summer session to repeat the course if she had permission. "And what would I do about the loan?" she asked.

Jane and the nurse therapist discussed the idea of seeking readmission to the college of nursing. Even though she had negative feelings about school because of her failure, she really wanted to become a nurse. Finishing school as soon as possible was also important, in order for her to earn an independent income. With the nurse therapist's encouragement, Jane decided to make an appointment with the dean to seek permission to take the course in the summer. In the event the visit with the dean was positive, Jane was to talk with the loan officer at the bank and see if arrangements could be made to postpone the time the loan would be due. Also she was advised to return to the center in a week or less to report the results of her efforts. The nurse therapist verified with Jane that she had fewer negative feelings about her life. Knowing that people in crisis often have self-destructive tendencies, she questioned Jane to be sure that she had no thoughts of harming herself or anyone else. Jane, appearing more calm and in better control, said she had no suicidal or homicidal intentions.

Over the course of three more visits to the counseling center, Jane made specific plans for continuing in the nursing program and for taking care of her financial problems. She discussed her divorce and what that had meant to her, as well as the problems of being a single parent.

Definition of Crisis

According to most definitions of crisis, Jane experienced a crisis. A crisis is any situation 1) that causes a sudden alteration in the individual's expectations of himself, 2) that has a duration of at least several days (usually four-six weeks) and 3) that cannot be handled by the individual with usual patterns of coping (Mishel, 1965; Rapoport, 1965).

Jane's perceived failure caused a sudden change of expectations of herself with respect to others. She was doubtful that she would ever be able to support herself and her child, and she knew her failure would be disappointing to her parents. Also, she wondered what her classmates would think of her. She was embarrassed and hurt.

The second part of the definition indicated that a crisis lasts several days, usually four-six weeks. Jane's situation lasted approximately three weeks.

Finally, the definition states that the crisis situation cannot be handled by the individual with his usual pattern of coping. Jane repeatedly said she did not know what she was going to do. She finally asked the nurse therapist for help. In the past, she had been able to rely upon her husband, but he was gone now. She had no one close who could be supportive of her.

The example discusses Jane as an individual in crisis. Families experience crises also. The whole family may have acute emotional reactions based upon inability to cope with destruction of all their possessions by fire, flood or storm; death of a family member; sudden financial problems and the like.

Loss and Crisis

A crisis usually results from a threatened or actual loss. The threatened loss is basically anxiety producing, whereas actual loss primarily produces depression. Threatened loss includes threats to one's integrity, such as threatened loss of a body part, and threatened loss of a loved object. Actual loss includes death of a loved one, actual loss of a body part or body integrity. Productive worrying helps one to overcome the anxiety of a threatened loss. Grieving is necessary to overcome actual loss and depression.

Worrying motivates the person in crisis to seek a solution. The person who fails to worry may be apathetic or may be denying the threat; therefore, such a person is not motivated to seek help or a solution to the problem. Grieving helps the person through the mourning process, enabling new relationships (Caplan, 1961; Rapoport, 1965).

The nurse may assist the client in productive worrying or grieving through crisis intervention, covered later in this chapter. The nurse may also help the apathetic person or the person using denial by suggesting that there is a problem. She may indicate that worry work needs to be done in order to find solutions to the problem. The nurse should be willing and ready to discuss the crisis event when the client indicates readiness.

Jane suffered a loss of self-esteem when she failed in school. Anxiety and worry over her future as provider of a livelihood for herself and the child motivated Jane to seek a solution to her problems.

Types of Crises

There are two major types of crises; these are maturational (also known as developmental or internal) and situational (also known as accidental or external). Maturational crises occur in the process of moving through the stages of development. Between the stages, there is a crucial period of cognitive and affective upset in which the person must turn one way or another (Erikson, 1959). Many changes or transitions are occurring rather rapidly during these times of a person's life. An example is the phase of adolescence. Numerous developmental tasks must be completed in psychosocial and physical areas to prepare the person for young adulthood. Prolonged hospitalization of an adolescent may produce a crisis, since this interferes with the opportunity to master psychosocial developmental tasks during the dormant period of hospitalization.

A situational or accidental crisis occurs when a stressful external event disrupts one's life; the change is sudden, and the person is unable to cope in the usual manner (Erikson, 1959). Relationships with others are altered. Examples of situational crises include divorce, death of a loved one, loss of a significant object, physical illness or change in body image due to loss of body part or body function.

Jane apparently suffered both types of crises. Developmentally, as a young adult, her plans for establishing an independent life of her own through a job and career were interrupted. The financial problems could be seen as a situational crisis. Both interrupted her life style to the point that she could no longer cope in her usual manner. Her expectations of herself changed.

Sequence of Stages

A person experiencing a crisis goes through a sequence of stages (Hirschowitz, 1973). The sequential stages are similar to the stages of grief as described by Engel (1964) or Kubler-Ross (1969). Initially, the person experiences the stage of impact, usually lasting from a few hours to a few days. Feeling shocked, the individual's first reaction may be to freeze (become immobilized) or to mobilize for fight or flight. Anxiety level is high at this point in the crisis.

Secondly, such a person recoils from the situation and may feel rage, depression or shame or may try to hide or deny feelings, pretending that the situation does not exist or is not as bad as it actually is. This stage usually lasts one to four weeks.

Finally, one reaches the stages of adjustment and reconstruction and experiences hope for the future. Goals are adjusted, and expectations are realistic. The person generally begins functioning adequately within four to six weeks; however, complete reconstruction may take longer. There may be overlapping of stages, as well as a vascillation between stages.

Jane experienced the first stage when the dean told her she had failed in her classwork. She became immobilized, wanting someone to tell her what to do. In the second stage, she felt shame and depression. Previously enjoying success in school, she now saw herself as a failure. In the third stage, Jane began talking with the dean and learned that she could go back to school in the summer. She was still far from reconciling her feelings with reality, but she began to see possibilities for a successful resolution of her crisis, and once again began to hope for the future.

Operational Steps

Crisis may be studied through the development of steps used to formulate an operational definition. An operational definition outlines the steps of a concept as it occurs to the person involved and then summarizes the steps in a definition (Burd, 1963). Through this method, one gains a more specific understanding of what the person is experiencing.

The operational steps that follow end with a positive resolution of the crisis:

1. The person is in a state of equilibrium or homeostasis.
2. A sudden, hazardous event occurs, changing one's self-expectations with respect to others (frequently related to a threatened or actual loss).
3. The person feels an increased level of anxiety or depression.

4. Usual problem-solving methods and coping mechanisms do not produce a solution.
5. Anxiety or depression continue to increase.
6. Helplessness, frustration, confusion follow.
7. One seeks help from significant others or from professionals.
8. Emergency coping devices that are new or unusual are tried.
9. The problem is solved, or the goals are relinquished.
10. Anxiety and/or depression are decreased so that the person is able to function as well as or better than before the crisis occurred.

Consideration of Jane's situation in light of the steps of the operational definition reveals how her crisis developed.

1. Considering the normal amount of stress surrounding her divorce, Jane managed to maintain a state of relative equilibrium, until she was formally faced with the reality of failing her course work.
2. Failing her course work, Jane thought, would cause her parents, classmates and faculty to think less of her. Experiencing decreased self-esteem, she wanted to avoid facing others.
3. Jane felt shame and guilt for failing. She was anxious about her finances and depressed about the school work.
4. After her husband left, there was no one close she could turn to for immediate help. Her parents lived some distance away, and she did not feel comfortable confiding in her classmates.
5. With no one to turn to, Jane seemed to despair, saying repeatedly, "I don't know what I'm going to do."
6. In the dean's office, it was obvious that Jane felt helpless and hopeless.
7. The dean directed Jane to professional help.
8. The therapist became Jane's support and helped her look at possible solutions to her problems. These were solutions that Jane had not been able to find on her own.
9. Jane was able to go back to school, and her financial problems became manageable.
10. Her anxiety and depression decreased, and she began regaining her self-respect.

Crises are resolved positively or negatively in one to six weeks. If

Jane had not received help in step 7, her life could have been quite different. Had her anxiety and despair continued, she might have become desperate to the point of hurting herself. She could also have changed her life goals and accepted an unskilled labor job, rather than continuing her pursuit of a career. While it is crucial for a person in crisis to receive help at the right time, the help does not necessarily have to come from a professional person; but it must come from someone who cares. Gerald Caplan says that a crisis is a turning point toward or away from mental disorder (Caplan, 1964). Help at the right time works to prevent negative resolution of crisis, such as further problems and personality deterioration or disintegration (Rapoport, 1965); therefore, crisis intervention by the nurse or significant other becomes preventive psychiatry. The new pattern of coping that the person works out in dealing with the crisis becomes an integral part of the repertoire of problem-solving responses and increases the chances of dealing more or less realistically with future hazards (Caplan, 1964). Once the crisis is over, the individual returns to a steady state and then is less open to intervention or help.

NURSING INTERVENTION

Assessment and Data Base

The same items listed for assessment in Chapter 6, "The Nursing Process as a Framework for Psychiatric Nursing," should be used for the data base of a person in crisis.

Standard I of the ANA Standards for Psychiatric-Mental Health Nursing Practice states that "data are collected through pertinent clinical observations based on knowledge of the arts and sciences, with particular emphasis upon psychological and biophysical sciences" (Congress for Nursing Practice, 1973). The data base for a person in crisis may have to be gathered over a period of time, in a series of interviews, or from significant others. The person may be functioning at a high level of anxiety, may be confused, disoriented and unable to relate the desired information upon first meeting. If the person is verbal, the nurse needs to be able to assess thought processes, thought content and whether or not one is in contact with the total environment.

If significant others accompany the person to the crisis center or hospital, the nurse notes communication patterns between the person in crisis and the significant others, whether the person is able to speak adequately or if someone else does all the talking. Some impressions about intellectual level and clearness of sensorium may be gained by listening to the language used, noting whether or not words are enunciated clearly. When thinking about this, the nurse must allow for cultural differences. Not only are words pronounced differently in various cultures, but the same words may have different meanings. For example, to most people in the United States, "signify" means to point out; however, in some segments of the population the term means to degrade another by clever use of words. Awareness of the possible differences in word interpretations will help the nurse make an accurate assessment of the person's condition.

Observation of nonverbal behavior provides clues to the person's feelings of self-worth, as seen in dress, posture and general appearance; anxiety level, as noted in gestures and facial expression; organizational abilities, as noted in dress and makeup; and affect or feeling tone, as seen in facial expression. These observations help the nurse therapist decide how much distress the person is in and what intervention may be necessary.

Whether the person's social life has changed in relation to the crisis is noted. If one has withdrawn from all contacts, the chances for outside support are negligible. Support from friends and family increases chances for a positive resolution of the crisis.

A medical assessment should be included, since problems in this area may influence coping abilities and, indeed, may be a part of the crisis situation.

The client, or the accompanying significant person, should be encouraged to discuss the reasons for coming to the crisis center or hospital. A description of problems and symptoms is vital. Such a description provides the nurse therapist with information regarding the amount of disruption the crisis is causing in the person's life and indicates the level of distress being experienced. This information helps in formulating the problem list and the nursing diagnosis.

The precipitating event is particularly significant in a crisis situation, since this is frequently the core of the problem. Sometimes just discussing it helps the person put it in better perspective and, thus, causes a reduction in anxiety level. The person should be encouraged to discuss the event in detail, covering the who, what, when and where the situation, and the resulting actions, thoughts and feelings regarding the situation.

How the person handles stress should be noted. A query on what one does in difficult situations and why that did not work, or why one was not able to do that in the current situation will help in assessing both strong and weak coping abilities. Encouragement to use one's strengths when planning intervention should follow appraisal of how one has handled problems in the past, and how successes and failures will influence attempts to solve the current crisis.

Additionally, support systems should be appraised. Friends and relatives are crucial in solving crisis situations, and the person should be encouraged to elicit their help. Frequently, it is advisable to include significant others in therapy sessions. Caplan says that family or significant others will support the individual in choosing ways of handling the problem, consonant with the cultural traditions and in keeping with the present needs of the group as a functioning system which satisfies its members' intragroup needs (Caplan, 1964). The family should be given direction in helping the person in crisis to deal with a problem, rather than avoid it or restrict activity to tension-relieving mechanisms. Significant others often have a major effect in determining how the person will deal with a crisis and, therefore, will influence the outcome. The people who most strongly affect an individual during crisis are those who meet needs for love and dependence (Caplan, 1964).

The person's self-assessment can give clues to feelings of self-worth. It is important that the therapist determine if the person is homicidal or suicidal before ending the session. A person with ideas about hurting himself or others must be referred to a physician or hospital.

The person's awareness of the problem he is experiencing must be evaluated. A person in crisis often distorts the significance of the situation, giving it more importance than necessary. Such a person knows there is a problem but, often, does not view it in proper perspective.

During the initial visit, the therapist completes as much of the assessment as is feasible considering the person's anxiety level and tolerance. Assessment is continued in each following visit to help clarify problems or as new data indicate the necessity of further assessment.

Problem List and Nursing Diagnosis

From the assessment data, the therapist and person in crisis decide which problem areas are to be worked on and in what order, depending upon the person's ability to decide at the time. Standard II of the ANA Standards for Psychiatric-Mental Health Nursing Practice states that "clients are involved in the assessment, planning, implementation and evaluation of their nursing care program to the fullest extent of their capabilities" (Congress for Nursing Practice, 1973). Problems causing immediate discomfort are usually given first priority; these include anxiety and suicidal or homicidal tendencies. After the problems are identified, the nurse therapist can make nursing diagnoses.

Intervention

It is important that the nurse therapist make plans and begin intervention to solve the crisis during the first session. Again, this is done in conjunction with the client, if the client is able to participate. The client should leave the session with the idea that the crisis can be overcome and with a plan for working toward its solution (Aquilera and Messick, 1974). The problem list, the nursing diagnoses and plans are refined or clarified in each additional session. It is to be hoped the patient learns how to avoid such a crisis in the future or how to cope with unavoidable hazardous events so that they do not become crises.

Discussing phases of development in advance of the time when crisis often occurs can be a valuable learning experience which may prevent problems in the future. This is sometimes referred to as anticipatory guidance (Cyr and Wattenberg, 1965). The ANA Standards for Psychiatric-Mental Health Nursing Practice emphasize health teaching in Standard IV. This states: "Individuals, families, and community groups are assisted to achieve satisfying and productive patterns of living through health teaching" (Congress for Nursing Practice, 1973).

Crisis intervention is considered an abbreviated technique, as compared to psychoanalysis. The objective is to assist the client in solving present problems, to be able to function at an equal or higher level than before the crisis occurred. Therapy usually lasts from one to six sessions. The therapist is often more direct and specific and participates more in the therapy than in traditional psychotherapy, actively helping the client seek a solution to the problem (Aquilera and Messick, 1974). Primary prevention is an important goal in crisis intervention. The helping person tries to counteract harmful circumstances, before they have a chance to produce ill health. An attempt is made to help the person cope with hazardous life stages or events in such a way that maladaptation is prevented (Robischon, 1967).

When considering crisis intervention, the nurse might be interested in specialized areas, such as suicide intervention, rape crisis counseling and divorce counseling. These specialities are relatively recent compared to the traditional role of the nurse in psychiatry. Since results of the nursing effort are usually seen in a shorter period of time, as compared to general psychiatric care, these areas hold particular interest for many nurses.

Progress notes are maintained with each client visit, using the SOAP (subjective, objective, assessment and planning) format. Such a format makes time spent with the client purposeful and goal directed. Both parties know what they are working on, what progress has been made and what needs to be done.

STANDARD IX

Standard IX summarizes the nursing role in crisis intervention. Psychotherapeutic interventions are used to assist clients to achieve their maximum development.

Rationale

People with mental health problems fashion many of their patterns of living and relating to others on a psychopathologic basis. In order to help clients achieve better adaptation and improved health, a nurse assists them in identifying that which is useful and that which is not useful in their modes of living and relating. Alternatives available to them are identified.

Assessment Factors

1. Useful patterns and themes in the client's interactions with others are reinforced.
2. Clients are assisted in identifying, testing out and evaluating

more constructive alternatives to unsatisfactory patterns of living.
3. Principles of communication, problem-solving, interviewing and crisis intervention are employed in carrying through psychotherapeutic intervention.
4. Knowledge of psychopathology and its healthy adaptive counterparts is used in planning and implementing programs of care.
5. Limits are set on behavior that is destructive to self or others, with the ultimate goal of assisting clients to develop their internal controls and more constructive ways of dealing with feelings.
6. Crisis intervention is used to reduce panic of disturbed patients.
7. Long-term psychotherapeutic relationships with clients are undertaken.
8. Colleagues are utilized in evaluating the progress of the psychotherapeutic relationships and in formulating modification of intervention techniques.
9. Nursing participation in the therapeutic relationship is evaluated and modified as necessary.

NURSING INTERVENTION WITH JANE

Data Base

The nurse therapist utilized the foregoing items to form a data base for Jane's crisis intervention. When Jane entered the office, the therapist began dealing with the problem which seemed most pressing. She observed that Jane was ready and willing to talk about what was bothering her. As Jane talked, the therapist noted that her statements seemed logical; therefore, she concluded that her thought processes were clear. She was obviously in contact with her environment and showed no signs of disorganization or confusion. Her intellectual functioning was adequate. Jane was anxious. She fidgeted with her hand tissue and indicated she was in despair, stating that she did not know what she was going to do. Her facial expression was one of sadness; she appeared fatigued. Her dress was clean and orderly.

Regarding Jane's social life, the nurse therapist noted that she had friends in her classes, but that her husband had been her main "sounding board" until the divorce. Since then, she had kept most of her feelings to herself. Some of her classmates had tried to help by asking her to study with them, but finding a babysitter had been a problem, so she was not able to meet with them.

Medically, Jane was fatigued and somewhat thin but appeared to be in relatively good health. The nurse therapist made a note to check into this further.

The dean of the college of nursing had told the nurse therapist why Jane was coming to the center. When Jane arrived, she gave more detail. She had failed in school, had financial problems and was in acute psychological distress. She was unable to cope with the situation and needed help.

Jane discussed the precipitating event with the nurse therapist. The therapist asked her what had happened to get her started and Jane willingly told her.

Jane's primary mode of handling stress had been to talk it out with her husband. Since this was no longer a possibility, she had begun to form closer relationships with classmates but still did not feel comfortable relating her major problems to them or accepting their help.

Self-assessment, at first, indicated that Jane was a failure. She could not be a good mother if she could not support her child and herself. She stated that she had no thoughts of hurting herself or anyone else. The nurse therapist noted that Jane was very much aware of her problem, but that she was not able to cope with it at the time of her first visit.

Problem List and Nursing Diagnoses

During the first interview, the therapist asked Jane to list her problems and put them in the order in which they should be solved. Jane said she just wanted to be able to support herself and her daughter. She said she wanted a good job. Then she said she was tired and needed rest. The nurse therapist asked if she were nervous or anxious. Jane admitted she was and that she would like to get over that, too.

The therapist then listed problems in the following order, and Jane agreed that the order was all right, and the problems were the ones she wanted to solve:

1. Inadequate finances—(not enough alimony to support her and her child in a comfortable way and a loan that must be repaid, beginning in September).
2. Lack of job education and security.
3. Anxiety—(moderate level; perhaps severe level at the time of entering the counseling center).
4. Fatigue.
5. Weak support system—(needs close friends to rely on in times of need).

This was the problem list after the first visit. It would be clarified and elaborated upon during successive visits.

The nurse therapist developed the following nursing diagnoses from the assessment and problems list:

1. Economic insecurity related to a loan and inadequate alimony.
2. Unable to fulfill educational goals related to financial pressures.
3. Moderate level of anxiety related to scholastic failure and financial pressures.
4. Fatigue related to inadequate rest and sleep.
5. Inadequate support system related to divorce, lack of close family or friends.

These would change with successive visits, as problems were solved and more assessment data were obtained.

When planning interventions, the therapist helped Jane look at exactly what she wanted and what the possibilities were and directed her intervention toward those goals. Her plans were as follows:

1. Inadequate finances (problem); economic insecurity related to a loan and inadequate alimony (diagnosis).
   a) Discuss repayment of loan with bank officials. Make an appointment the next day.
   b) If delaying repayment of the loan is not possible, consider getting a loan through the college of nursing and paying the bank loan with money received from working this coming semester.
   c) Look for a job, so that Jane can work full-time until summer school begins. Think about part-time work during school, if absolutely necessary. Discuss this in more detail, second session.

    d) Possibly discuss budgeting during second session.
    e) Discuss with the dean of the college of nursing the possibility of taking the examination to become a licensed practical nurse, second session.
2. Lack of job education and security (problem); unable to fulfill educational goals related to financial pressures (diagnosis).
    a) Discuss with the dean the possibility of entering nursing school in the summer. Make an appointment tomorrow.
    b) If reentering nursing school is not a possibility, then consider changing major to a similar occupation.
3. Anxiety (problem); moderate level of anxiety related to scholastic failure and financial pressures (diagnosis).
    a) Encourage ventilation of thoughts and feelings regarding problems.
    b) Encourage detailed description of precipitating event.
    c) Develop a feasible plan for solving problems so that Jane feels there is hope for relief (incorporated in problems 1 and 2).
    d) Develop support system so that anxiety may be dealt with before reaching crisis stage in the future (included in problem 5).
    e) Review the steps in the development of crisis and the felt anxiety, so that Jane can see the process and learn ways to help prevent such problems in the future.
4. Fatigue (problem); fatigue related to inadequate rest and sleep (diagnosis).
    a) Reduce anxiety to a level conducive to sleep (by ventilating to others, making plans to solve problems and following through with those plans).
    b) Go to bed at regular hours each night.
    c) Avoid eating large meals four hours before retiring.
    d) Do a relaxing activity before going to bed (such as reading).
    e) Eat a balanced diet at regular times.
    f) Plan time for herself to do a pleasurable activity each day.
    g) Check with her to see if she has had a physical examination recently.
5. Weak support system (problem); inadequate support system related to divorce, lack of close family or friends (diagnosis).
    a) Encourage development of close friendships with classmates, persons she works with, neighbors.

b) Let her know that she can come to the counseling center or call, whenever she feels the need.
c) Encourage her to discuss her academic problems and the reason for them with the faculty and dean, if she returns to nursing school.

The nurse therapist discussed her plans for Jane with other members of the clinical staff at the counseling center. The team, consisting of a psychiatrist, a social worker, a clinical psychologist and another nurse therapist, agreed that these plans should help Jane solve her problems.

Progress Notes—Second Visit

1. Inadequate finances
   Subjective—"The loan officer at the bank said that the loan could be repaid beginning next January, but that it would cost considerably more, since the loan would cover a longer time. I would like to find a better method of financial aid."
   Objective—Carried through with plans from last visit. Looks more confident, less anxious, maintains eye contact.
   Assessment—Bank loan is not satisfactory. Need to explore other possibilities. Discussion of budgeting indicates that she has no problem in this area.
   Plan—Make an appointment with the dean, tomorrow, to consider a loan through the college of nursing and the possibility of taking the examination for a license to practice practical nursing. Begin looking for a job, preferably at a local hospital as a nurse's assistant. Make appointments this week. Will consider part-time work, summer semester, after she sees how difficult her school workload will be.
2. Lack of job education and security
   Subjective—"I talked with the dean, and I plan to enter summer school."
   Objective—Smiled while she was telling me this. Seems pleased.
   Assessment—If she can get her other problems solved, so that she can concentrate on her studies, this should no longer be a problem.
   Plan—Let her know that she can come back to the center, if she has problems in this area in the future.

3. Anxiety
   Subjective—"I feel less anxious than I did when I saw you last. Knowing that I can go back to school this summer helps. Also, the financial problems don't seem so insurmountable as before. I am still jittery at times, and I don't sleep as well as I used to. I think once I get the schooling and finances worked out, I'll be OK. I think I understand how I got in this mess. I believe I'll get help sooner next time I see myself getting into trouble."
   Objective—Facial expression is more relaxed. Does not fidget with hands. Still changes positon in chair frequently but appears more comfortable than last visit.
   Assessment—Anxiety level vascillating from mild to moderate. She understands how her crisis developed and that she will be able to avoid such problems in the future or seek help earlier.
   Plan—Continue working on other problems and check with her next session about anxiety level.
4. Fatigue
   Subjective—"I'm not as anxious as I was. I am sleeping better, but not as well as I used to. I am definitely not as tired as I was. I think I was driving myself too hard. I'm eating better, since I've been at home more."
   Objective—Appears less fatigued, is more energetic.
   Assessment—Is improving in this area.
   Plan—Continue same regime as discussed during the first visit and check on progress, next session.
5. Weak support system
   Subjective—"I haven't had much time to see classmates. I did see Sue. I told her what had happened. She seemed sympathetic. I'll try to see her again soon. There is a new neighbor in our building. She's a little older than I. I think I could like her. I'll see if she can go to the pool with me this week. I did talk with the dean about everything that had happened. She was very understanding and willing to help."
   Objective—Ready to try to make friends to avoid problems in the future.
   Assessment—Somewhat reticent about making new or close friends but sees the necessity.
   Plan—Continue to encourage her to make friends that she can confide in. Check on this in later sessions.

With each session, the therapist used the SOAP system. This gave direction for the time she and her client spent together. They knew what had been accomplished and what still needed working on. Also, at the end of each session, the therapist and client reviewed the problems list and changed it as they saw fit.

Although the precipitating event in Jane's case was quite clear, this is not true with all clients. Sometimes the client is not sure what precipitated the current problem. Also, one may be embarrassed or hesitant to reveal personal problems upon first meeting the nurse therapist. So the first sessions may be spent clarifying what the problem really is. Direct questioning about life events for the past two weeks may be necessary in order to help the client piece together the crisis situation. The nurse therapist should note recurring themes in the client's description of recent events (Mitchell, 1977). Clarifying the problem, as soon as possible, aids in beginning the problem-solving process and the actual solution of the problem.

PRINCIPLES

The foregoing includes a broad discussion of crisis. The statements that follow summarize the principles found in this chapter:

1. A crisis causes a sudden alteration in an individual's expectations of himself with respect to others.
2. A crisis has a duration of at least several days and usually four to six weeks.
3. A crisis cannot be handled by the individual with his usual patterns of coping.
4. There are two major types of crisis, maturational and situational.
    a) A maturational crisis occurs in the process of moving through the stages of development. In each stage, there is a crucial period in which the person must turn one way or another. Changes are occurring rapidly.
    b) A situational crisis occurs when a stressful event disrupts one's life. Usual coping abilities are not adequate. Relationships with others are altered.
5. A crisis may result from a threatened or actual loss. A

threatened loss usually causes anxiety; whereas an actual loss causes depression. Worry work is necessary to overcome anxiety, and grief work is necessary in overcoming depression.
6. The steps which occur when a person experiences a crisis are impact, recoil, and adjustment and reconstruction
   a) Impact is a state of shock lasting from a few hours to a few days, and the person experiences either a fight, flight or frozen reaction.
   b) Recoil is a state of turmoil lasting from one to four weeks, and the person experiences rage, anxiety, depression, guilt or shame.
   c) Adjustment and reconstruction is a state of reconciliation and resolution, is sufficiently completed so that the person can function within four to six weeks of the onset of the crisis and gives hope for the future.
7. Development of operational steps helps in understanding what a client is experiencing and may be a valuable learning tool to help the person see how the current crisis situation arose. Areas for prevention may be pointed out to the client, when looking at the steps.
8. Since crises are solved positively or negatively in one to six weeks, it is important that the person receive help, so that chances are increased that the crisis may be solved positively.
9. When the nurse is working with a person in crisis:
   a) Determine the level of anxiety and assist in problem-solving and anxiety management.
   b) Develop a plan for problem-solving with the client during the first visit to decrease client anxiety.
   c) Determine the level of depression and refer the person to a physician or a hospital, if the person is homicidal or suicidal.
   d) Allow for cultural differences when assessing, since the same words can have different meanings and words may be pronounced differently.
   e) Help the person describe the precipitating event in detail, including feelings, so that the problem may be clarified and put in proper perspective.
   f) Determine the person's usual coping methods and assist in finding different ways of handling or preventing crisis.
   g) Encourage involvement of the client's support system to in-

crease the chances for a positive resolution of the crisis.
h) Assist the person in using the crisis as a learning situation.

BIBLIOGRAPHY

Aquilera, Donna C., and Messick, Janice. *Crisis Intervention—Theory and Methodology.* 2d ed. St. Louis: The C.V. Mosby Co., 1974.

Burd, Shirley. "The Development of an Operational Definition Using the Process of Learning as a Guide," in *Some Clinical Approaches to Psychiatric Nursing.* Edited by Shirley F. Burd and Margaret A. Marshall. New York: The Macmillan Co., 1963, pp. 330-332.

Caplan, Gerald. *An Approach to Community Mental Health.* New York: Grune & Stratton, Inc., 1961.

———. *A Conceptual Model for Primary Prevention: Principles of Preventive Psychiatry.* New York: Basic Books, Inc., 1964, pp. 26-55.

Congress for Nursing Practice. *Standards of Psychiatric-Mental Health Nursing.* Kansas City, Mo.: American Nurses' Association, 1973.

Cyr, Florence E., and Wattenberg, Shirley H. "Social Work in a Preventive Program of Maternal and Child Health," in *Crisis Intervention: Selected Readings.* Edited by Howard J. Parad. New York: Family Service Association of America, 1965, pp. 88-99.

Engel, G. L. "Grief and Grieving," *American Journal of Nursing,* LXIV, No. 9 (September, 1964), 93-96.

Erikson, Eric. *Identity: Psychological Issues.* New York: International Universities Press. Vol. 1, No. 1, (January, 1959).

Hirschowitz, Ralph. "Crisis Theory: A Formulation," *Psychiatric Annals,* III, No. 12 (December, 1973), 36-47.

Kubler-Ross, Elizabeth. *On Death and Dying.* New York: The Macmillan Co., 1969.

Mishel, Merle. *Crisis Theory and Crisis Therapy Applied in a Nurse-Patient Situation.* Regional Clinical Conferences. New York: American Nurses' Association, 1965.

Mitchell, Carol. "Identifying the Hazard: The Key to Crisis Intervention," *American Journal of Nursing,* LXXVII, No. 7 (July, 1977), 1194-1196.

Rapoport, Lydia. "The State of Crisis: Some Theoretical Considerations," in *Crisis Intervention: Selected Readings.* Edited by Howard J. Parad. New York: Family Service Association of America, 1965, pp. 22-31.

Robischon, Paulette. "The Challenge of Crisis Theory for Nursing," *Nursing Outlook,* Vol. 15 (July, 1967), 28-32.

CHAPTER 18

Case Presentations For Application Of The Nursing Process

DIRECTIONS FOR CASE PRESENTATIONS

Read each of the following psychiatric nursing cases and make decisions regarding assessment, planning and strategies for implementation of care. Each case presents a limited amount of background information which, seemingly, has had an impact on the client's current state of functioning. Data are provided which indicate clues as to current functioning. While no direct nurse-patient interaction is described, the reader can elicit both subjective as well as objective data from the descriptive information. It is expected that the reader will utilize theories of personality development, growth and development as well as clinical formulations in planning intervention strategies.

CASE #1: JUDY KANE—23-YEAR-OLD FEMALE WITH DIAGNOSIS OF SIMPLE SCHIZOPHRENIA

Both Judy and her 21-year-old sister were adopted as infants by Mr. and Mrs. Kane. Currently, Mr. Kane, an accountant, and Mrs. Kane, a housewife, are in their middle 50s. Mr. Kane describes his childhood as one of many losses and few emotional supports. Orphaned at age 10, he lived in various foster homes and children's homes until he was sixteen and able to begin educational preparation for a career in accounting. Mrs. Kane describes her childhood as a time of many illnesses. Her sickness behavior carried into the adult years, necessitating that Mr. Kane "protect" her from worries and hardships.

Both of Judy's parents are described by the psychiatrist and social workers as depressed persons, conservative and conforming in orientation. Mrs. Kane displays considerable hypochondriacal behavior, thus serving as an "unwell" role model for Judy. Neither parent gives a clear medical or social developmental history for Judy. They describe their older daughter thusly: "She has done better than we ever expected her to do in the first place." Mrs. Kane says that the family has always done what Judy wants, since she was "sick so much." Mr. Kane admits that he has given his daughter as many tasks and household responsibilities as he dares.

In sharp contrast, Judy's younger sister experienced success and considerable peer support in school. She had a large circle of friends in high school and is currently married and expecting her first child.

Judy was characterized as an easily upset and colicky infant. Poorly coordinated, she learned to walk later than is normally expected, at age 2. An asthmatic, Judy was often ill with upper respiratory infections as a child. Due to her shyness, she was frequently teased by peers and called a "mama's baby." Although her grades in the elementary school years were good, academic achievement decreased in the upper grades. In college, despite considerable effort, Judy was barely able to achieve passing grades. Mr. and Mrs. Kane believed that Judy's poor coordination and weak eyesight led to her intense social isolation and low academic achievement.

Upon her first admission to the hospital three years prior, the diagnosis was obsessive-compulsive disorder with a discharge diagnosis of chronic undifferentiated schizophrenia. Psychological assessment by the physician revealed her to exhibit autism, looseness of association, ambivalence, depersonalization and a distinct lack of interpersonal warmth. Judy viewed her first hospitalization as a chance to rest and clarify her thinking. She was also aware that the college she attended had requested she withdraw because of "unusual behavior." Psychological testing revealed a hostile, dependent pattern of interaction with significant others, lacking any form of emotional closeness.

Two years after the first admission, Mr. and Mrs. Kane contacted a psychiatrist because Judy suddenly began worrying about bowling, school, a job and boys. One night soon after the college session resumed, she began emitting animal noises and disrobing in public areas of the dormitory. At this time, a diagnosis of simple schizophrenia was made.

CASE #2: CHERYL JONES—28-YEAR-OLD FEMALE WITH DIAGNOSIS OF DEPRESSION

Twenty-eight-year-old Cheryl Jones, the middle child of a retired military family, has an older sister and younger brother. She reports crying episodes with no known cause and generalized depressed feelings for the past ten years. She states that she is "afraid to go out, because she might begin crying in front of other people." She also admits to thoughts of killing herself and, at times, wishes she had never been born. Cheryl generally eats well but when she is depressed she abstains from eating and, subsequently, loses weight rapidly.

Cheryl complains of a constant headache "covering her entire body". She wears glasses and says that she experiences diplopia without the corrective lens. She began menarche at age 13 and denies ever having sexual intercourse, stating that she does not date.

Cheryl evidences a depressed facies with flattened affect and often utilizes the defense mechanism of denial. She is withdrawn and unwilling to interact with other patients. Most of her interactions with staff and nursing students are limited to short sentence responses. Spontaneous comments are rare for Cheryl.

Mrs. Jones stated that following a normal pregnancy and delivery, no problems evolved until Cheryl was 9 months old, at which time the child began crying frequently for no apparent reason. When Mrs. Jones attempted to comfort Cheryl, the child's response was to "fight her." These crying episodes continued until age 3 when it was learned that Cheryl needed glasses for double vision. After she was fitted with glasses, Cheryl ceased the crying episodes until age 6. Even with her visual problems, Cheryl walked, talked and was toilet-trained at normal developmental stages. Although Cheryl once again began experiencing the crying episodes at age 6, she did well in school. There were two occasions when her crying reached hysterical proportions. Both instances occurred when Cheryl was in sex education classes in school and became upset over the stimulating feelings she was having due to the course content. Psychiatric assistance was sought on a short-term basis at each occurrence of the hysterical crying.

Mrs. Jones thinks that Cheryl is jealous of her brother and sister but gets along well with her parents. Cheryl's older sister is married and lives in an adjacent community, yet visits the family most weekends.

Psychological assessment reveals that much of Cheryl's crying is disproportional to the environmental context in which it occurs. She is oriented to time, place and person, with no evidence of hallucinations or delusions. Cheryl's life style seems to reflect feelings of alienation from others with crying resulting from frustrating situations. There also seems to be a strong family dependency bond, as exhibited by the older daughter's frequent visits and Cheryl's need to control the family with her tears. Mrs. Jones presents herself as a "push-over" in regard to her children, allowing them to push her around and dictate to the family, rather than expressing her angry or contradictory feelings.

Assessment further reveals that Cheryl has a prorated verbal I.Q. of 100. Both her judgment and abstract reasoning abilities are consistent with other scores; no unusual or bizarre responses were obtained in the evaluation by the psychologist. Findings from the Rorschach test exhibited markedly immature percepts, with responses more consistent with those expected from a young child than from a 19-year-old girl.

Cheryl's sex role identity is quite diffuse. On projective tests, she associated femininity with weakness, passivity and being easily manipulated. Cheryl states that her mother was "sick a lot" and takes a passive stance in regard to her father. Hence, to model after her mother would mean to identify with passivity and illness. Cheryl's behavior pattern is to elicit anger from peers or members of the staff and then assume a passive stance. She borders on being fearful of others and is quite afraid of emotional involvement. She is shy, meek and awkward in meeting others. On one hand, she solicits the attention of the staff by speaking as they pass; yet, on the other hand, she seems unable to engage in conversation, once she has the nurse's attention.

CASE #3: JOHN JONES—25-YEAR-OLD MALE WITH A DIAGNOSIS OF SIMPLE CHILDHOOD SCHIZOPHRENIA WITH PARANOID IDEATION AND DEPRESSION

John's presenting problem upon entering the institution was a long history of stealing and breaking into automobiles. He is known to have stolen keys and key rings from stores and various people since he was 8 years old. He has been arrested three times in the past two years; the charges were dropped at each arrest. Following these incidents, John began leaving home late at night, breaking into several cars, hot wiring and driving them around, then returning the car and sneaking into his house.

The social history indicates that Mr. Jones presents himself as a precise, aloof, dogmatic and obsessive person. Mr. Jones describes an inability to show affection toward John. Mrs. Jones is described as an overweight woman who used amphetamines for a number of years for weight control. She tended to blame John for everything that went wrong in the household. John gets along well with his 17-year-old sister, who presents no obvious emotional problems.

Five years prior to the present hospitalization, the Jones' obtained a divorce. John lived with his father after the divorce, and his sister lived with his mother. John has infrequent contact with his mother.

Past history reveals that John was taken to the Child Guidance Center for emotional testing and observation at age 8. It was at this time that he was diagnosed as having childhood schizophrenia. In addition, an ulcer was found which was thought to be of psychogenic origin.

One year prior to hospitalization, John appeared less withdrawn and depressed when a 23-year-old female moved near him. She befriended John, and immediately his stealing and driving of other people's automobiles ceased. John seemed happy, until his friend married and moved away. At this time, his depression and withdrawal were more pronounced than on any previous occasion.

A Rorschach test revealed loose associations of a psychotic variety with depressive features, active hostility expressed in emotional outbursts, rigid concern for detail, free-floating anxiety and an extensive fantasy life. Additionally, his coping defenses were viewed as rapidly deteriorating, with large amounts of guilt and resentment surfacing. John was observed to retreat into daydreaming to escape the harsh facts of reality.

John's response to the female nurse working with him was similar to the watchfulness a small child has for his mother. John kept the nurse in sight at all times and appeared downcast when she spent time with other patients.

CASE #4: BOB BROWN—43-YEAR-OLD MALE WITH DIAGNOSIS OF DEPRESSION

Bob Brown was born in a small southern town to a family that urgently wanted a child. The couple had waited for a child for several years and the mother, overjoyed by the birth of her son, took him to every social event that the town had. She spent a great deal of her time fixing Bob up and showing him off to friends and relatives. Mr. Brown, Bob's father, had a very demanding job and spent most of his time away from the family. Mr. and Mrs. Brown could never seem to find time to do things together and with Bob.

Mrs. Brown wanted Bob to stay perfect at all times, in case someone might come by. Being a child, Bob occasionally played outside and got dirty or spilled something. Mrs. Brown would, on such occasions, scold him severely and tell him that he never did anything right. Bob had insufficient parental acceptance. He was not given praise and was frequently told that he never did anything right. He was constantly frustrated, because he could not live up to his mother's suggestions and expectations.

As Bob began to meet children, he soon found that he did not know how to play with the other children, and he felt ineffective in trying to get to know them. He began to stay home and stated that he preferred to be at home.

When Bob was old enough to work in his father's business, he took a position as a clerk. He found that he could handle this job with a little assistance from other workers. Bob's father decided to turn the business over to him when Bob was 40 years old and Mr. Brown was 68 and ready to retire. Two years later, due to various unforeseen happenings in the economy, the business went bankrupt.

The combined forces of Bob's childhood and this adult trauma mobilized turmoil in him, overwhelming him with intense feelings of melancholy, inadequacy, guilt, inferiority and worthlessness. He reports a loss of interest in all activities, diminished drive, a loss of ambition and difficulty in concentrating. He states that he ruined the whole business and is an awful person. Looking sad and tired, he emphasizes his past as well as present shortcomings. He reports sleep disturbances with fitful dozing and unpleasant dreams. He has lost about nine pounds in the last month.

CASE #5: MARY C.—15-YEAR-OLD FEMALE WITH DIAGNOSIS OF DRUG ABUSE

Mary C., age 15, has been admitted to the acute psychiatric unit of the city hospital. She was brought to the emergency unit by a boy friend after a party where drugs were freely used. She was unconscious on admission but responded to the administration of stimulants. Mary was assigned to the psychiatric unit at the request of her grandmother, who is her legal guardian. Mary is untidy, withdrawn and hostile when approached.

Mary's mother was a rebellious teenager of 16 when she became pregnant. She refused to identify the baby's father, who was married. After Mary's birth, she presented the baby to her own mother saying, "Here's another chance. See if you can do a better job this time." She then left and contacted her mother infrequently thereafter.

Mary's grandmother, a widow, supported the child and herself working as a clerk in a department store. Mary's physical development was within the limits of normal. As a preschooler, she attended day care centers. In school, she related with others but had few friends. She spent long hours alone after school watching television.

Mary made average grades in school until she was in the seventh grade. At that time, she became attractive to older boys at school. She had few girl friends, but an increasing number of boy friends. She was introduced to marijuana and spent several hours each week smoking with older friends.

Her grandmother was unaware of Mary's older friends and her marijuana smoking but often argued with her over her lack of achievement in school, her ungrateful attitude and her likeness to her "no-good mother". Mary reacted to the arguments with indifference and no change in behavior.

Mary was sexually active but received little pleasure from sex, preferring the dreamy sensations induced by marijuana. At a party she attended, she smoked some pot and became bored. When some white pills were passed around, she took two. Feeling nothing, she took a handful of them. Her boy friend found her lying on the floor and thought she had passed out. When he could not arouse her, he took her to the emergency room and left her there.

APPENDICES

APPENDIX A

Diagnostic and Statistical Manual of Terms*

Acting Out—Expressions of unconscious emotional conflicts or feelings of hostility or love in actions, rather than words. The individual is not consciously aware of the meaning of such acts.

Addiction—Dependence on a chemical substance to the extent that physiological dependence is established. The latter manifests itself as withdrawal symptoms (the abstinence syndrome), when the drug is withdrawn.

Adolescence—A chronological period beginning with the physical and emotional processes leading to sexual and psychosocial maturity, and ending at an ill-defined time when the individual achieves independence and social productivity.

Affect—A person's emotional feeling tone and its outward manifestations.

Affective Disorder—Any mental disorder in which a disturbance of affect is predominant (including depressive neurosis, major affective disorders and psychotic depressive reaction).

Aggression—A forceful physical, verbal or symbolic action. May be appropriate and self-protective, including healthful self-assertiveness, or inappropriate to the situation.

Agitated Depression—A psychotic depression accompanied by constant restlessness.

Agitation—Severe restlessness; a major psychomotor expression of emotional tension.

Alienation—The state of estrangement the individual feels in cultural settings he views as foreign or unacceptable.

Ambivalence—Coexistence of two opposing drives, desires, feelings or emotions toward the same person, object or goal. These may be conscious or partly conscious.

---
*Printed by permission of the American Psychiatric Association (Washington, D.C., 1975) from *Psychiatric Glossary*.

Amnesia—Pathological loss of memory; forgetting. A phenomenon in which an area of experience is forgotten and becomes inaccessible to conscious recall.

Anal Character—A personality type that manifests excessive orderliness, miserliness and obstinacy.

Anomie—Apathy, alienation and personal distress resulting from the loss of goals previously valued.

Anorexia Nervosa—A syndrome marked by severe and prolonged inability to eat, with marked weight loss, amenorrhea (or impotence) and other symptoms resulting from emotional conflict and biological changes.

Antabuse (Disulfiram)—Drug used in the treatment of alcoholism. It blocks the normal metabolism of alcohol and produces increased blood concentrations of acetaldehydes which cause very unpleasant reactions, including pounding of the heart, shortness of breath, nausea and vomiting.

Anxiety—Apprehension, tension or uneasiness that stems from the anticipation of danger, the source of which is largely unknown or unrecognized.

Apathy—Disinterest or lack of attention to self and environment.

Association—Relationship between ideas or emotions.

Aura—A premonitory, subjective sensation (e.g., a flash of light) that often warns the person of an impending headache or convulsion.

Autism—Form of thinking marked by extreme self-absorption and egocentricity, in which objective facts are obscured, distorted or excluded in varying degrees.

Autoeroticism—Sensual Self-gratification. Characteristic of, but not limited to, an early stage of emotional development.

Behavior Therapy—Any treatment approach designed to modify the patient's behavior directly, rather than to correct the dynamic causation.

Blocking—Sudden inability to recall that which is familiar.

Blunting—Dulling of emotional response.

Castration—Removal of the sex organs. In psychological terms, the fantasized loss of the penis.

Castration Anxiety—Due to fantasized danger or injuries to the genitals and/or body.

Catatonic State—Characterized by immobility with muscular rigidity or inflexibility and, at times, by excitability.

Catharsis—The therapeutic release of ideas through a "talking out" of conscious material accompanied by the appropriate emotional reaction.

Cathexis—Attachment, conscious or unconscious, of emotional feeling and significance to an idea or object, most commonly a person.

Cerea Flexibilitas—The "waxy flexibility" often present in catatonic

schizophrenia, in which the patient's arm or leg remains passively in the position in which it is placed.
Cerebral Arteriosclerosis—Hardening of the arteries of the brain, sometimes resulting in an organic brain syndrome that may be either primarily neurologic in nature or primarily mental, or a combination of both.
Character Defense—Any character or personality trait which serves an unconscious defensive purpose.
Character Disorder—A personality disorder manifested by a chronic and habitual pattern of reaction that is maladaptive, in that it is relatively inflexible, limits the optimal use of potentialities and often provokes the very counterreactions from the environment that the subject seeks to avoid.
Commitment—A legal process for admitting a mentally ill person to a mental hospital. The legal definition and procedure vary from state to state.
Community Mental Health Center—A health service delivery system first authorized by the Federal Mental Retardation Facilities and Community Mental Health Centers Construction Act of 1963, to provide a coordinated program of continuing mental health care to a specific population.
Compensation—A defense mechanism, operating unconsciously, by which the individual attempts to make up for real or fantasized deficiencies.
Complex—A group of associated ideas that have a common strong emotional tone.
Compulsion—An insistent, repetitive, intrusive and unwanted urge to perform an act that is contrary to the person's ordinary wishes or standards.
Compulsive Personality—A personality characterized by excessive adherence to rigid standards (inflexible, overconscientious).
Confabulation—The filling in of memory gaps with made-up stories.
Conflict—A mental struggle that arises from the simultaneous operation of opposing impulses, drives or external (environmental) or internal demands.
Confusion—Disturbed orientation in respect to time, place or person.
Conscience—The morally self-critical part of the self, encompassing standards of behavior, performance and value judgments.
Conscious—That part of the mind or mental functioning of which the content is subject to awareness or known to the person.
Conversion—A defense mechanism, operating unconsciously, by which intrapsychic conflicts that would otherwise give rise to anxiety are, instead, given symbolic external expression.
Convulsive Disorder—Primarily the centrencephalic seizures, grand mal

and petit mal, and the focal seizures of Jacksonian and psychomotor epilepsy.

Coping Mechanisms—Ways of adjusting to environmental stress without altering one's goals or purposes; includes both conscious and unconscious mechanisms.

Countertransference—The therapist's partly unconscious or conscious emotional reaction to his patient.

Death Instinct (Thanatos)—In Freudian theory, the unconscious drive toward dissolution and death; coexists with and is in opposition to the life instinct (Eros).

Decompensation—Deterioration of existing defenses, leading to an exacerbation of pathological behavior.

Defense Mechanism—Unconscious intrapsychic process serving to provide relief from emotional conflict and anxiety.

Deja Vu—Sensation that what one is seeing one has seen before.

Delirium—Acute reversible mental state characterized by confusion and altered, possibly fluctuating, consciousness due to an alteration of cerebral metabolism with delusions, illusions and/or hallucinations.

Delirium Tremens—Acute and sometimes fatal brain disorder caused by withdrawal or relative withdrawal from alcohol, usually developing in 24-96 hours.

Delusion—A firm, fixed idea not amenable to rational explanation; maintained against logical argument, despite objective contradictory evidence.

Dementia—Irreversible mental state characterized by decreased intellectual function, personality change, impairment of judgment and, often, changes in affect.

Dementia Praecox—Obsolete descriptive term for schizophrenia.

Denial—Defense mechanism, operating unconsciously, used to resolve emotional conflict and allay anxiety by disavowing thoughts, feelings, wishes, needs or external reality factors that are consciously intolerable.

Dependency Needs—Vital needs for mothering, love, affection, security and warmth; may be a manifestation of regression when they reappear openly in adults.

Depersonalization—Feelings of unreality or strangeness concerning either the environment or the self or both.

Depression—When used to describe mood, depression refers to feelings of sadness, despair and unhappiness. As such, depression is universally experienced and is a normal feeling state.

Deprivation, Emotional—A lack of adequate and appropriate interpersonal and/or environmental experience, usually in the early developmental years.

Deterioration—Worsening of a clinical condition, usually expressed as progressive impairment of function.

Detoxification—Treatment by use of medication, diet, rest, fluids and nursing care to restore physiological functioning after it has been seriously disturbed by the overuse of alcohol, barbiturates or other addictive drugs.

Disorientation—Loss of awareness of the position of the self in relation to space, time or other persons.

Displacement—A defense mechanism, operating unconsciously, in which an emotion is transferred from its original object to a more acceptable substitute, used to allay anxiety.

Dissociation—A defense mechanism, operating unconsciously, through which emotional significance and affect are separated and detached from an idea, situation or object.

Double Bind—A type of interaction in which one person demands a response to a message containing mutually contradictory signals, while the other is unable either to comment on the incongruity or to escape from the situation.

Drive—Basic urge, instinct, motivation.

Drug Dependence—Habituation to, abuse of and/or addiction to a chemical substance.

Drug Interaction—The effects of two or more drugs being taken simultaneously, producing an alteration in the usual effects of either drug taken alone.

Echopraxia—The pathological repetition, by imitation, of the movements of another.

ECT (electroconvulsive treatment)—A form of psychiatric treatment in which electric current, insulin, carbon dioxide or Indoklon is administered to the patient and results in a loss of consciousness or a convulsive or comatose reaction to alter favorably the course of the illness.

Ego—In psychoanalytic theory, one of the three major divisions in the model of the psychic apparatus, the others being the id and superego. The ego represents the sum of certain mental mechanisms, such as perception and memory, and specific defense mechanisms.

Ego Ideal—That part of the personality that comprises the aims and goals of the self; usually refers to the conscious or unconscious emulation of significant figures with whom the person has identified.

Electra Complex—An infrequently used term describing the pathological relationship of a woman with men, based on unresolved developmental conflicts partially analogous to the Oedipus complex in the man.

Emotion—A feeling such as fear, anger, grief, joy or love which may not always be conscious.

Empathy—An objective and insightful awareness of the feelings, emotions and behavior of another person, their meaning and significance.
Encopresis—Incontinence of feces.
Enuresis—Incontinence of urine.
Epilepsy—A disorder characterized by periodic motor or sensory seizures or their equivalents and sometimes accompanied by a loss of consciousness or by certain equivalent manifestations; may be idiopathic (no known organic cause) or symptomatic (due to organic lesions).
Euphoria—An exaggerated feeling of physical and emotional well-being not consonant with apparent stimuli or events.
Exhibitionism—A man exposing his genitals to women or girls in socially unacceptable situations.
Existential Psychiatry—A school of psychiatry evolved from orthodox psychoanalytic thought; stresses the way in which man experiences the phenomenological world about him and takes responsibility for his existence.
Extrapsychic—That which takes place between the psyche (mind) and the environment.
Extrapyramidal System—The portion of the central nervous system responsible for coordinating and integrating various aspects of motor behavior or bodily movements.
Family Therapy—Treatment of more than one member of the family simultaneously in the same session. The treatment may be supportive, directive or interpretive.
Fantasy—An imagined sequence of events or mental images (for example, daydreams).
Fear—Emotional and physiological response to recognized sources of danger, to be distinguished from anxiety.
Fetishism—A sexual deviation characterized by attachment of special meaning to an inanimate object (or fetish) which serves, usually unconsciously, as a substitute for the original object or person.
Fixation—The arrest of psychosexual maturation. Depending on degree, it may be either normal or pathological.
Flight of Ideas—Verbal skipping from one idea to another. The ideas appear to be continuous but are fragmentary and determined by chance or temporal associations.
Folie a Deux—A condition in which two closely related persons, usually in the same family, share the same delusion.
Free Association—In psychoanalytic therapy, spontaneous, uncensored verbalization by the patient of whatever comes to mind.
Fugue—Personality dissociation characterized by amnesia and involving actual physical flight from the customary environment or field of conflict.

Functional Disorder—A disorder in which the performance or operation of an organ or organ system is abnormal, but not as a result of known changes in structure.

General Systems Theory—A theoretical framework that views events from the standpoint of the "systems" involved in the event. Systems are groups of organized, interacting components.

Gestalt Psychology—A German school of psychology that emphasizes a total perceptual configuration and the interrelations of its component parts.

Globus Hystericus—An hysterical symptom in which there is a disturbing sensation of a lump in the throat.

Grief—Normal, appropriate emotional response to an external and consciously recognized loss. It is usually self-limited and gradually subsides within a reasonable period of time.

Hallucination—A false sensory perception in the absence of an actual external stimulus; may be induced by emotional and other factors such as drugs, alcohol and stress.

Homeostasis—Self-regulating biological processes which maintain the equilibrium of the organism.

Homosexual Panic—An acute and severe attack of anxiety based upon unconscious conflicts involving homosexuality.

Homosexuality—Sexual orientation towards persons of the same sex; not a psychiatric disorder, as such.

Hyperactivity—Increased or excessive muscular activity seen in diverse neurological and psychiatric disorders.

Hyperventilation—Overbreathing associated with anxiety and marked by reduction of blood carbon dioxide, subjective complaints of lightheadedness, faintness, tingling of the extremities, palpitation and respiratory distress.

Hypnotic—Any agent that induces sleep. While sedatives and narcotics, in sufficient dosage, may produce sleep as an incidental effect, the term "hypnotic" is appropriately reserved for drugs employed primarily to produce sleep.

Hypomania—A psychopathological state and abnormality of mood falling somewhere between normal euphoria and mania. It is characterized by increased happiness, optimism, mild to moderate pressure of speech and activity and a decrease in the need for sleep.

Id—In Freudian theory, that part of the personality structure which harbors the unconscious instinctual desires and striving of the individual.

Ideas of Reference—Incorrect interpretation of casual incidents and external events as having direct reference to one's self.

Identification—A defense mechanism, operating unconsciously, by which an individual patterns himself after another.

Identity Crisis—A loss of the sense of the sameness and historical continuity of one's self, and inability to accept or adopt the role the subject perceives as being expected of him by society; often expressed by isolation, withdrawal, extremism, rebelliousness and negativity.
Illusion—The misinterpretation of a real experience.
Impulse—A psychic striving; usually refers to an instinctual urge.
Incorporation—A primitive defense mechanism, operating unconsciously, in which the psychic representation of a person, or parts of him, are figuratively ingested.
Insight—Self-understanding of one's attitudes and behavior.
Instinct—An inborn drive (self-preservation and sexuality).
Intellectualization—The utilization of reasoning as a defense against confrontation with unconscious conflicts and their stressful emotions.
Intelligence—Capacity to learn and to utilize appropriately what one has learned.
Interpretation—The process by which the therapist communicates to the patient understanding of a particular aspect of his problems or behavior.
Intrapsychic—That which takes place within the psyche or mind.
Introjection—A defense mechanism, operating unconsciously, whereby loved or hated external objects are taken within oneself symbolically. The converse of projection. May serve as a defense against conscious recognition of intolerable hostile impulses.
Isolation—A defense mechanism, operating unconsciously, in which an unacceptable impulse, idea, or act is separated from its original memory source, thereby removing the emotional charge associated with the original memory.
Kleptomania—Compulsion to steal.
Korsakoff's Psychosis—A disorder of central nervous system metabolism due to a lack of vitamin B_1 (thiamine) seen in chronic alcoholism. Characterized by confabulation, and grossly impaired memory function with deficient new learning ability.
La Belle Indifference—Literally, "beautiful indifference"; seen in certain patients with hysterical neurosis, conversion type, who show an inappropriate lack of concern about their disabilities.
Labile—Pertaining to rapidly shifting emotions.
Latent Content—The hidden (unconscious) meaning of thoughts or actions, especially in dreams or fantasies.
Latent Homosexuality—A conditon characterized by unconscious homosexual desires.
Lesbian—A homosexual woman.
Libido—The psychic drive or energy usually associated with the sexual instinct.
Lithium Carbonate—The particular lithium salt usually used in the treat-

ment of acute manic states and in the prevention of future episodes in individuals with recurrent affective disorders, which may be either unipolar (depression or mania only) or bipolar (both mania and depression occasionally occurring).

Loosening (of associations)—A thinking disorder or disturbance in associations, in which thinking becomes over-generalized, diffuse and vague, progressing unevenly toward a goal and generally failing as an adequate vehicle of communication with others.

LSD (lysergic acid diethylamide)—A potent drug that produces psychotic symptoms and behavior.

Magical Thinking—A person's conviction that thinking equates with doing.

Major Affective Disorders—A group of psychoses characterized by severe disorders of mood—either extreme depression or elation or both—that do not seem to be attributable entirely to precipitating life experiences.

Mania—Formerly used as a nonspecific term for any kind of "madness." Currently used as a suffix, with any number of Greek roots, to indicate a morbid preoccupation with some kind of idea or activity and/or a compulsive need to behave in some deviant way.

Manic-Depressive Psychosis—A major affective disorder characterized by severe mood swings and a tendency to remission and recurrence.

Manifest Content—The overt or remembered content of a dream or fantasy, as contrasted with latent content, which it conceals and distorts.

Masochism—Pleasure derived from physical or psychological pain inflicted either by one's self or by others.

Masturbation—Genital manipulation for the purpose of sexual stimulation.

Mental Health—A state of being, relative rather than absolute, in which a person has effected a reasonably satisfactory integration of his instinctual drives.

Mental Retardation—Significantly below average intellectual functioning, which may be present at birth or become evident later in the developmental period, and is always characterized by impaired adaptation in one or all of the areas of learning, social adjustment and maturation.

Mental Status—The level and style of functioning of the psyche, used in its broadest sense to include intellectual functioning, as well as the emotional, attitudinal, psychological and personality aspects of the subject.

Methadone—A synthetic narcotic. It may be used as a substitute for heroin, producing a less socially disabling addiction, or it may be used to aid in the withdrawal from heroin.

Migraine—A syndrome characterized by recurrent, severe and usually one-sided headaches, often associated with nausea, vomiting and visual disturbances.

Milieu Therapy—Socioenvironmental therapy in which the attitudes and behavior of the staff of a treatment service and the activities prescribed for the patient are determined by what the patient's emotional and interpersonal needs are presumed to be.

Monamine Oxidase (MAO) Inhibitors—A group of antidepressant drugs that inhibit certain brain enzymes and raise the level of serotonin.

Mutism—Refusal to speak for conscious or unconscious reasons.

Narcissism—Self-love as opposed to object-love (love of another person).

Narcotic—Any opiate derivative drug, natural or synthetic, that relieves pain or alters mood.

Neologism—A new word or condensed combination of several words coined by a person to express a highly complex idea often related to his conflicts.

Nervous Breakdown—A nonmedical, nonspecific euphemism for a mental disorder.

Neurosis—An emotional maladaptation arising from an unresolved, unconscious conflict. The anxiety is either felt directly or modified by various psychological mechanisms to produce other, subjectively distressing symptoms.

Object Relations—The emotional bonds that exist between an individual and another person, as contrasted with his interest in, and love for, himself.

Obsession—A persistent, unwanted idea or impulse that cannot be eliminated by logic or reasoning.

Occupational Therapy—An adjunctive therapy that utilizes purposeful activities as a means of altering the course of illness.

Oedipus Complex—Attachment of the child to the parent of the opposite sex, accompanied by envious and aggressive feelings toward the parent of the same sex.

Organic Brain Syndrome—Any mental disorder associated with or caused by disturbance in the physiological functioning of brain tissue at any level of organization—structural, hormonal, biochemical, electrical, etc.

Orientation—Awareness of one's self in relation to time, place and person.

Overcompensation—A conscious or unconscious process in which a real or imagined physical or psychological deficit inspires exaggerated correction.

Panic—Acute, overwhelming anxiety; can be life-threatening due to exhaustion.

Paranoid—An adjective applied to individuals who are overly suspicious.

Parasympathetic Nervous System—That part of the autonomic nervous system that controls the life-sustaining organs of the body under normal, danger-free conditions.

Partial Hospitalization—A psychiatric treatment for patients who require hospitalization but not on a full-time basis (day hospital, night hospital, weekend hospital).

Passive-Dependent Personality—A disorder manifested by marked indecisiveness, emotional dependency and lack of self-confidence.

Pedophilia—A sexual deviation involving sexual activity with children as the objects.

Personality—The characteristic way in which a person behaves; the ingrained pattern of behavior that each person evolves, both consciously and unconsciously, as his style of life or way of being, in adapting to his environment.

Personality Disorders—A group of mental disorders characterized by deeply ingrained maladaptive patterns of behavior, generally life-long in duration and, consequently, often recognizable by the time of adolescence or earlier.

Perversion—An imprecise term used loosely to designate sexual variance.

Phobia—An obsessive, persistent, unrealistic intense fear of an object or situation.

Pleasure Principle—The psychoanalytic concept that man instinctually seeks to avoid pain and discomfort and strives for gratification and pleasure.

Prevention—In traditional medical usage, the prevention of a disorder. The modern trend is to broaden the meaning of prevention to encompass also the amelioration, control and limitation of disease. (Often categorized as: primary, secondary and tertiary).

Primary Gain—The relief from emotional conflict and the freedom from anxiety achieved by a defense mechanism.

Primary Process—In psychoanalytic theory, the generally unorganized mental activity characteristic of unconscious mental life. Seen in less disguised form in infancy and in dreams.

Problem-oriented Record—A simple, conceptual framework to expedite and improve the medical record. The record is structured to contain four logically sequenced sections: a) the data base, b) the problem list, c) the plans and d) the follow-up.

Projection—A defense mechanism, operating unconsciously, whereby that which is emotionally unacceptable in the self is unconsciously rejected and attributed (projected) to others.

Psychodrama—A technique of group psychotherapy in which individuals express their own or assigned emotional problems in dramatization.

Psychomotor Excitement—Generalized physical and emotional overactivity in response to internal and/or external stimuli, as in hypomania.

Psychomotor Retardation—A generalized slowing of physical and emotional reactions.

Psychophysiological Disorders—A group of disorders characterized by physical symptoms that are caused by emotional factors and that involve a single organ system, usually under autonomic nervous system control.

Psychosexual Development—Generally, a term encompassing all of the influences from prenatal life onward, including biological, cultural and emotional, that affect the sexuality of the individual throughout the life cycle.

Psychosis—A major mental disorder of organic or emotional origin in which the individual's ability to think, respond emotionally, remember, communicate, interpret reality and behave appropriately is sufficiently impaired, so as to interfere grossly with his capacity to meet the ordinary demands of life.

Psychosurgery—Surgical intervention to sever fibers connecting one part of the brain with another or to remove or to destroy brain tissue with the intent of modifying or altering disturbances of behavior, thought content or mood for which no organic pathological cause can be demonstrated by established tests and techniques.

Psychotherapy—A generic term for the treatment of mental and emotional disorders based primarily upon verbal or nonverbal communication with the patient.

Rationalization—A defense mechanism, operating unconsciously, in which the individual attempts to justify or make consciously tolerable, by plausible means, feelings, behavior and motives that would otherwise be intolerable.

Reaction Formation—A defense mechanism, operating unconsciously, wherein attitudes and behavior are adopted that are the opposites of impulses the individual harbors either consciously or unconsciously.

Reality Principle—In psychoanalytic theory, the concept that the pleasure principle, which represents the claims of instinctual wishes, is normally modified by the inescapable demands and requirements of the external world.

Regression—The partial or symbolic return to more infantile patterns of reacting.

Remotivation—A group treatment technique administered by nursing service personnel in a mental hospital; of particular value to long-term, withdrawn patients by way of stimulating their communication skills and interest in their environment.

Repression—A defense mechanism, operating unconsciously, that banishes unacceptable ideas, affects or impulses from consciousness or that keeps out of consciousness what has never been conscious.

Retardation—Slowing down of mental and physical activity; most frequently seen in severe depressions.
Ritual—Any psychomotor activity sustained by an individual to relieve anxiety.
Sadism—Pleasure derived from inflicting physical or psychological pain or abuse on others.
Schizophrenia—A large group of disorders, usually of psychotic proportion, manifested by characteristic disturbances of thought, mood and behavior.
Secondary Gain—The external gain that is derived from any illness, such as personal attention and service, monetary gains, disability benefits and release from unpleasant responsibility.
Secondary Process—In psychoanalytic theory, mental activity and thinking characteristic of the ego and influenced by the demands of the environment.
Sedative—A broad term applied to any agent that quiets or calms or allays excitement.
Senile Dementia—A chronic organic brain syndrome associated with generalized atrophy of the brain due to aging.
Sensorium—Synonymous with consciousness.
Separation Anxiety—The fear and apprehension noted in infants when removed from their mother (or surrogates) or when approached by strangers.
Sexual Deviation—The direction of sexual interest toward objects other than persons of the opposite sex and/or toward sexual acts not associated with coitus.
Sibling—Term for a full brother or sister.
Sibling Rivalry—The competition between siblings for the love of a parent or for other recognition or gain.
Socialization—The process by which society integrates the individual and the way in which the individual learns to become a functioning member of that society.
Sociopath—An unofficial term for antisocial personality.
Sublimation—A defense mechanism, operating unconsciously, by which instinctual drives, consciously unacceptable, are diverted into personally and socially acceptable channels.
Substitution—A defense mechanism, operating unconsciously, by which an unattainable or unacceptable goal, emotion or object is replaced by one that is more attainable or acceptable.
Succinylcholine—A potent drug used intravenously in anesthesia as a skeletal muscle relaxant.
Superego—In psychoanalytic theory, that part of the personality structure associated with ethics, standards and self-criticism.

Suppression—The conscious effort to control and conceal unacceptable thoughts, impulses, feelings or acts.

Therapeutic Community—A term of British origin, now widely used, for a specially structured mental hospital milieu that encourages patients to function within the range of social norms.

Transference—The unconscious assignment to others of feelings and attitudes that were originally associated with important figures (parents, siblings) in one's early life.

Transsexual—A disturbance of gender identity in which the person feels a lifelong discomfort with his or her own sex and a compelling desire to be of the opposite sex.

Transvestitism (Transvestism)—Sexual pleasure derived from dressing or masquerading in the clothing of the opposite sex.

Trauma—An extremely upsetting emotional experience that may aggravate or contribute to a mental disorder.

Unconscious—That part of the mind or mental functioning of which the content is only rarely subject to awareness.

Undoing—A defense mechanism, operating unconsciously, in which something unacceptable and already done is symbolically acted out in reverse, usually repetitiously, in the hope of relieving anxiety.

Voyeurism—Sexually motivated and often compulsive interest in looking at or watching others and, particularly, looking at genitals.

Withdrawal Symptoms—Physical and mental effects of withdrawing drugs from patients who have become habituated or addicted to them.

Word Salad—A mixture of words or phrases that lack comprehensive meaning or logical coherence, commonly seen in schizophrenic states.

APPENDIX B

Standards of Psychiatric-Mental Health Nursing Practice*

STANDARD I

Data are collected through pertinent clinical observations based on knowledge of the arts and sciences, with particular emphasis upon psychosocial and biophysical sciences.

Rationale

Clinical observation is a prerequisite to realistic assessment of a client's needs and for the formulation of appropriate intervention. Observations can be facilitated through knowledge derived from a broad general education. In addition, scholarship acquired in the study of psychosocial and biophysical sciences fosters acuity of perception and alerts the nurse to psychologic, cultural, social and other relevant clinical data.

Assessment Factors

1. Data collecting activities involve observation, analysis and interpretation of behavior patterns of clients which indicate a need for growth promoting relationships.
2. Data collecting activities involve identification of significant areas in which clinical data are needed
3. Data collecting activities involve utilization of knowledge derived from appropriate sources to gain a comprehensive grasp of the client's experience.
4. Data collecting activities involve inferences drawn from obser-

---
*Printed by permission of American Nurses Association (Kansas City, Mo., 1973).

vations which contribute to a formulation of therapeutic intervention.
5. Data collecting activities involve inferences and treatment observations which are shared and validated with appropriate others.

STANDARD II

Clients are involved in the assessment, planning, implementation and evaluation of their nursing care program to the fullest extent of their capabilities.

Rationale

To a very large degree, the therapeutic process is a learning process. The same principle that applies to learning also applies to therapy; that is, the learner or client must be an active participant in the process. The ability to participate in such a process will vary from person to person and, at times, even within the same person. The word "therapy" is used here in its broadest sense; that is, any behavior or planned activity that promotes growth and well-being. Thus, "nursing care program" and "nursing therapy" are interchangeably used, although it is recognized that many other forms of therapy exist.

Assessment Factors

1. Clients' capabilities to participate at any given time are assessed, always keeping in mind the ultimate goals mutually determined by the client and nurse.
2. Plans for achieving and reexamining the goals are developed with the client, making whatever readjustments are necessary to progress toward them.
3. Problems are identified in collaboration with the client to determine needs and to set goals.
4. Progress of clients toward mutual goal achievement is assessed.

STANDARD III

The problem-solving approach is utilized in developing nursing care plans.

Rationale

A nursing diagnosis is based on pertinent theories of human behavior. It is used to plan therapeutic intervention taking into consideration the characteristics and capacities of the individual and his environment in order to maximize the treatment program for the client.

Assessment Factors

1. The individual's reaction to the environment is observed and assessed.
2. Themes and patterns of the behavior are observed and assessed.
3. Nursing care plans are used as a guide to nursing intervention.
4. Nursing care plans are interpreted to professional and nonprofessional persons giving care.
5. Observations and reports of others are incorporated in the nursing care plans.
6. Nursing care plans are designed, implemented and reviewed systematically by the nursing staff.

STANDARD IV

Individuals, families and community groups are assisted to achieve satisfying and productive patterns of living through health teaching.

Rationale

Health teaching is an essential part of a nurse's role in work with those who have mental health problems. Every interaction can be utilized as a teaching-learning situation. Formal and informal teaching methods can be used in working with individuals, families, the community and other personnel. Emphasis is on understanding mental health problems as well as on developing ways of coping with them.

Assessment Factors

1. The needs of individual, family and community groups for health teaching are identified and appropriate techniques are used in meeting these needs.
2. The principles of learning and teaching are employed.
3. The basic principles of physical and mental health and interpersonal and social skills are taught.
4. Experiential learning opportunities are made available.
5. Opportunities with community groups to further their knowledge and understanding of mental health problems are identified.

STANDARD V

The activities of daily living are utilized in a goal directed way in work with clients.

Rationale

A major portion of one's daily life is spent in some form of activity related to health and well-being. An individual's developmental and intellectual level, emotional state and physical limitations may be reflected in these activities. Therefore, nursing has a unique opportunity to assess and intervene in these processes in order to encourage constructive changes in the client's behavior so that each person may realize his full potential for growth.

Assessment Factors

1. An appraisal is made of the client's capacities to participate in activities of daily living based on needs, strengths and levels of functioning.
2. Clients are encouraged toward independence and self-direction by various skills such as motivating, limit setting, persuading, guiding and comforting.
3. Each person's rights are appreciated and respected.

4. Methods of communicating are devised which assure consistency in approach.

STANDARD VI

Knowledge of somatic therapies and related clinical skills are utilized in working with clients.

Rationale

Various treatment modalities may be needed by clients during the course of illness. Pertinent clinical observations and judgments are made concerning the effect of drugs and other treatments used in the therapeutic program.

Assessment Factors

1. Pertinent reactions to somatic therapies are observed and interpreted in terms of the underlying principles of each therapy.
2. A patient's responses are observed and reported.
3. The effectiveness of somatic therapies is judged and subsequent recommendations for changes in the treatment plan are made.
4. The safety and emotional support of clients receiving therapies is provided.
5. Opportunities are provided for clients and families to discuss, question and explore their feelings and concerns about past, current or projected use of somatic therapies.

STANDARD VII

The environment is structured to establish and maintain a therapeutic milieu.

Rationale

Any environment is composed of both human and nonhuman resources which may work for or against the person's well-being. The nurse works with people in a variety of environmental settings, e.g. hospital, home, etc. The milieu is structured and/or altered so that it serves the client's best interests as an inherent part of the overall therapeutic plan.

Assessment Factors

1. The effects of environmental forces on individuals are observed, analyzed and interpreted.
2. Psychological, physiological, social, economical and cultural concepts are understood and utilized in developing and maintaining a therapeutic milieu.
3. Communications within the environment are congruent with therapeutic goals.
4. All available resources in the environment are utilized when appropriate in therapeutic efforts.
5. Nursing participation and its effectiveness in establishing and maintaining a therapeutic milieu are evaluated.

STANDARD VIII

Nursing participates with interdisciplinary teams in assessing, planning, implementing and evaluating programs and other mental health activities.

Rationale

In addition to the nurse, the number and variety of people working with clients in the mental health field today make it imperative that efforts be coordinated to provide the best total program. Communication, planning, problem-solving and evaluation are required of all those who work with a particular client or program.

Assessment Factors

1. Specific knowledge, skills and activities are identified and articulated so these may be coordinated with the contributions of others working with a client or a program.
2. The value of nursing and team member contributions are recognized and respected.
3. Consultation with other team members is utilized as needed.

4. Nursing participates in the formulating of overall goals, plans and decisions.
5. Skills are developed in small group process for maximum team effectiveness.

STANDARD IX

Psychotherapeutic interventions are used to assist clients to achieve their maximum development.

Rationale

People with mental health problems fashion many of their patterns of living and relating to others on a psychopathologic basis. In order to help clients achieve better adaption and improved health, a nurse assists them to identify that which is useful and that which is not useful in their modes of living and relating. Alternatives available to them are identified.

Assessment Factors

1. Useful patterns and themes in the client's interactions with others are re-enforced.
2. Clients are assisted to identify, test out and evaluate more constructive alternatives to unsatisfactory patterns of living.
3. Principles of communication, problem-solving, interviewing and crisis intervention are employed in carrying through psychotherapeutic intervention.
4. Knowledge of psychopathology and its healthy adaptive counterparts are used in planning and implementing programs of care.
5. Limits are set on behavior that is destructive to self or others with the ultimate goal of assisting clients to develop their own internal controls and more constructive ways of dealing with feelings.
6. Crisis intervention is used to reduce panic of disturbed patients.
7. Long-term psychotherapeutic relationships with clients are undertaken.
8. Colleagues are utilized in evaluating the progress of the psycho-

therapeutic relationships and in formulating modification of intervention techniques.
9. Nursing participation in the therapeutic relationship is evaluated and modified as necessary.

STANDARD X

The practice of individual, group or family psychotherapy requires appropriate preparation and recognition of accountability for the practice.

Rationale

Acceptance of the role of therapist entails primary responsibility for the treatment of clients and entrance into a contractual agreement. This contract includes a commitment to see a client through the problem he presents or, if this becomes impossible, to assist him in finding other appropriate assistance. It also includes an explicit definition of the relationship, the respective roles of each person in the relationship, and what can realistically be expected of each person.

Assessment Factors

1. The potential of the nurse to function as a primary therapist is evaluated.
2. The accountability for practicing psychotherapy is recognized and accepted.
3. Knowledge of growth and development, psychopathology, psychosocial systems and small group and family dynamics is utilized in the therapeutic process.
4. The terms of the contract between the nurse and the client, including the structure of time, place, fees, etc., that may be involved, are made explicitly clear.
5. Supervision or consultation is sought whenever indicated and other learning opportunities are used to further develop knowledge and skills.
6. The effectiveness of the work with an individual, family or group is routinely assessed.

STANDARD XI

Nursing participates with other members of the community in planning and implementing mental health services that include the broad continuum of promotion of mental health, prevention of mental illness, treatment and rehabilitation.

Rationale

In our contemporary society, the high incidence of mental illness and mental retardation requires increased effort to devise more effective treatment and prevention programs. There is a need for nursing to participate in programs that strengthen the existing health potential of all members of society. In this effort cooperation and collaboration by all community agencies becomes imperative. Such concepts as early intervention and continuity of care are essential in planning to meet the mental health needs of the community. The nurse uses organizational, advisory or consultative skills to facilitate the development and implementation of mental health services.

Assessment Factors

1. Knowledge of community and group dynamics is used to understand the structure and function of the community system.
2. Current social issues that influence the nature of mental health problems in the community are recognized.
3. High risk population groups in the community are delineated and gaps in community services are identified.
4. Community members are encouraged to become active in assessing community mental health needs and planning programs to meet these needs.
5. The strength and capacities of individuals, families and the community are assessed in order to promote and increase the health potential of all.
6. Consultative skills are used to facilitate the development and implementation of mental health services.
7. The needs of the community are brought to the attention of appropriate individuals and groups, including legislative bodies and regional and state planning groups.

8. The mental health services of the agency are interpreted to others in the community. There is collaboration with the staff of other agencies to insure continuity of service for patients and families.
9. Community resources are used appropriately.
10. Nursing participates with other professional and non-professional members of the community in the planning, implementation and evaluation of mental health services.

STANDARD XII

Learning experiences are provided for other nursing care personnel through leadership, supervision and teaching.

Rationale

As leader of the nursing team, the nurse is responsible for the team's activities, and must be able to teach, supervise and evaluate the performance of nursing care personnel. The focus is on the continuing development of each member of the team.

Assessment Factors

1. Leadership roles and responsibilities are accepted.
2. Team members are encouraged to identify strengths and abilities. A climate is provided for the continuing self-development of each member.
3. A role model in giving direct nursing care is provided for the team.
4. The supervisory role is used as a tool for improving nursing care.
5. The client's needs, as well as the abilities of each member of the nursing team, are evaluated and assignments are based on these evaluations.

STANDARD XIII

Responsibility is assumed for continuing educational and professional development and contributions are made to the professional growth of others.

Rationale

The scientific, cultural and social changes characterizing our contemporary society require the nurse to be committed to the ongoing pursuit of knowledge which will enhance professional growth.

Assessment Factors

1. There is evidence of study of one's nursing practice to increase both understanding and skill.
2. There is evidence of participation in in-service meetings and educational programs either as an attendee or as a teacher.
3. There is evidence of attendance at conventions, institutes, workshops, symposia and other professionally oriented meetings and/or other ways to increase formal education.
4. There is evidence of systematic efforts to increase understanding of psychodynamics, psychopathology and avenues of psychotherapeutic intervention.
5. There is evidence of cognizance of developments in relevant fields and utilization of this knowledge.
6. There is evidence of assisting others to identify areas of educational needs.
7. There is evidence of sharing appropriate clinical observations and interpretations with professionals and other groups.

STANDARD XIV

Contributions to nursing and the mental health field are made through innovations in theory and practice and participation in research.

Rationale

Each professional has responsibility for the continuing development and refinement of knowledge in the mental health field through research and experimentation with new and creative approaches to practice.

Assessment Factors

1. Studies are developed, implemented and evaluated.
2. Responsible standards of research are used in investigative endeavors.
3. Nursing practice is approached with an inquiring and open mind.
4. The pertinent and responsible research of others is supported.
5. Expert consultation and/or supervision is sought as required. Judgment is used in assessing abilities as well as limitations to engage in research.
6. The ability to discriminate those findings which are pertinent to the advancement of nursing practice is demonstrated.
7. Innovations in theory, practice and research findings are made available through presentations and/or publications.

APPENDIX C
Sample Process Recording

Data	Thoughts	Feelings	Needs	Principles and Revisions
N: "What is gong on with you, Joe?"	He looks kind of lonesome lying there by himself. I wonder if he feels like talking?	1. curiosity 2. empathy 3. challenge	1. to know 2. to get closer to him 3. to feel competent 4. to test skills	1. Giving a broad opening, offers an invitation to talk. 2. By observing that someone may want to talk and pointing this out, you let the person know you care enough to listen. Revision: "Is there something you would like to talk about, Joe?"
P: "Oh, I don't know. It seems like you're pretty interested in me."	1. I have things to say, but I'm not going to unless I know you like me. 2. Does she really like me? 3. Can I trust her?	1. timid 2. decreased self-esteem 3. sensitive 5. scared	1. to increase self-esteem 2. to talk 3. feel relaxed 4. acceptance	1. Before a person can open up, he must be able to trust. 2. A threat to a person's self-esteem decreases his desire to communicate. 3. Anxiety decreases one's ability to communicate (high levels).
N: "Sure, I'm interested. I'd like to get to know you better, and it kind of seems like you're unsure about talking to me. Is there something you would like to say?" (Long period of silence where Joe was restless and avoided eye contact.)	I want him to know that I can accept him. I hope this is the right thing to say.	1. curiosity 2. anxiety 3. confusion 4. interest 5. decreased competency	1. to say the right thing 2. to convey acceptance 3. to decrease anxiety	1. Focusing on someone's feelings may help him see what is going on with him. 2. Accepting another as worthwhile may increase his sense of security.

(Continued)

Sample Process Recording (Continued)

Data	Thoughts	Feelings	Needs	Principles and Revisions
P: "What kind of music do you like?"	I feel responsible for the conversation, but I am not sure I want to talk.	1. anxiety 2. responsibility 3. threatened	1. acceptance 2. to change subject to less threatening topic	1. Changing the subject is a device to decrease anxiety. 2. A threat to self is a source of increased anxiety. 3. Silence may increase anxiety.
N: "Oh, I like most kinds."	He sure is uncomfortable with silence. Why am I going along with his change of topic?	1. confusion 2. frustration 3. uneasy	1. decrease anxiety 2. figure out what is going on	1. Talking on a superficial level often gives one time to gather thoughts. 2. Superficial topics allow both parties to decrease anxiety. Revision: "Joe, you seem uneasy with this conversation."
(Conversation about music continues for several minutes. I couldn't find the words *at this time* to get the topic back on the previous track, because of increased anxiety.)				
P: "Do you have a boyfriend?"	It really seems like she likes me. I wonder if I am special to her. People don't usually pay attention to me.	1. curious 2. interest 3. increased self-esteem	1. cared about 2. loved 3. noticed	Testing a person is a form of gathering data.
N: "No, but I have lots of boys who are friends."	Help!	1. anxiety 2. confusion 3. helpless 4. incompetent	1. competency 2. not to hurt his feelings	1. Anxiety decreases effectiveness. 2. Getting too personal can be threatening to a person's sense of self. Revision: "What makes you ask?"

Appendix C / 585

P: "Can I be your boyfriend?"	I want her to like me. This will tell me if she thinks I am special. I need somebody.	1. hopeful 2. nervous 3. shy	1. love 2. acceptance 3. to be like other kids	1. Being accepted by one's peers increases self-esteem. 2. Relationships with the opposite sex are particularly important to the adolescent.
N: "Joe, I would like you to be a friend, but maybe not what you are referring to as a boyfriend."	What do I say? Where is the instructor when I need her? I've got to be honest but gentle.	1. anxiety 2. empathy 3. cautious	1. competency 2. caution 3. decreased anxiety	1. Honesty is essential in establishing a trusting relationship. 2. Belittling a person's feelings is threatening to a sense of self. Revision: "Joe, I would feel more comfortable being a friend rather than a girlfriend."
P: "Well, that's the way I feel, too."	I wonder if I said the right thing?	1. defensive 2. hurt 3. rejected	1. acceptance 2. appropriateness 3. to be cared about	1. Decreased ego strength causes one to compromise his wishes. 2. To gain acceptance an individual must behave in socially accepted ways.
N: "I enjoy getting to know people, and I would like to get to know you."	How can I let him know that I still think a lot of him? I hope he will understand.	1. anxiety 2. frustration 3. incompetent	1. understanding 2. competence	1. Increased anxiety decreases communication. 2. Therapeutic communication often may not consist of answers to questions, but of reflections of the patient's own remarks. Revision: "You feel what way, Joe?"

(Continued)

Sample Process Recording (Continued)

Data	Thoughts	Feelings	Needs	Principles and Revisions
P: "Do you still think I am trying to hide something from you?"	I hope she is not mad at me. Does she think there is something strange about me?	1. worry 2. timidity 3. apprehension 4. confusion	1. acceptance 2. to test intentions	1. People with decreased self-esteem often wonder what others think about them. 2. Past experiences with mistrust lead to future difficulties in trusting.
N: "Hiding something?"	I wonder if he is projecting? What is he getting at?	1. curiosity	1. knowledge 2. increased rapport	1. Reflective comments may foster therapeutic communication. 2. Reflective comments shift the emphasis back onto the patient.
P: "It seems like you think I am hiding something."	What is she thinking? I wonder if she is like a lot of people who say they want to help but don't.	1. anxiety 2. apprehension 3. threatened	1. to be cared about 2. trust 3. non-threatening relationship	1. Before people open up, they must know they are accepted.
N: "No, Joe, I would like to get to know you, but we can take it slowly."	Maybe I am moving too fast, because he seems threatened.	1. disappointed 2. angry at self 3. hopeful	1. to feel competent 2. to decrease anxiety	1. Letting someone know you can take a relationship slowly can decrease their feelings of threat and anxiety.

Appendix C / 587

P: "Oh, that sounds good."		2. An intact sense of self is essential to optimum functioning. Revision: "I still don't understand what you mean by hiding something. Could you explain this?"
Well, I got out of that one. Boy, I want to take it slow.	1. relief 2. decreased anxiety	1. to decrease threat 2. to end conversation 3. to be accepted
		1. A statement of agreement often ends a conversation.

INDEX

Index

Abstract reasoning, 419, 425
  decreased in organic brain syndrome, 419
  difficulty in, 420, 425
Abusive behavior, 381
  physical, 381
  verbal, 381
Acalculia, 399
Acceptance, 93-94, 133-139, 211
  of death, 93-94
  of differences in others, 134
  of suicidal persons, 211
Acetazolamide, 449
  in epilepsy, 449
  toxic effects, 449
Ackerman, Nathan, 486
Acting out, 292-294
  in antisocial personality disorder, 292-294
Action for Mental Health, 514
Activity group therapy, 494-499
Acute dystonic reaction, 467
Addiction, 335
Adolescent, 72-78
  age span, 72
  body image, 73-74
  developmental tasks, 72
  identity, 72
  independence from parents, 77-78
  self-concept, 73
  sexual identity, 73
  vocational choice, 77
Adult, 78-94
  middle age, 81-89
  older age, 89-94
  young, 78-81
Advice giving, 120
  as a barrier to effective communication, 120
  "sermonettes," 120-121
Affect, 284, 357
  inappropriate, 357
  isolation of, 284

Affective disorder, 360
Aggression, 149-152, 197, 293-294
  in antisocial personality disorder, 293-294
  anxiety and, 149
  in depression, 197
  differentiated from violence, 151
  frustration leading to, 149
  handling of, 151
  limits for, 150
  release of, 149
Agranulocytosis, 471
Akathisia, 467
Akinesia, 467
Al-anon, 333
Al-a-teen, 333
Alcohol (see Alcoholism)
Alcoholics Anonymous, 328, 333
Alcoholism, 328-335
  case study of, 342-352
  chronic, 348
  classification, 330-331
  clinical course, 330-331
  definition, 328
  delirium tremens in, 332
  dependency in, 329
  etiology, 329
  malnutrition, 331
  nursing intervention, 333-335
  personality traits, 329
  test level for intoxication, 328
  treatment, 332-333
Allen, Clifford, 300
Allport, G.W., 16
Ambivalence, 118
Amitriptyline, 469
Amnesia, 258
Amobarbital, 475
Amytal (see Amobarbital)
Anal phase, 30
  ages, 30
  personality traits, 30
  toilet training, 30

Anders, Robert, 293
Anectine, 476
Anger, 196-197, 204-205
   in depressed persons, 196-197, 204-205
   as retroflexed rage, 197
Anosognosia, 396
Antabuse, 332
Anti-anxiety drugs, 474-475
Anticathexis, 22
Anticonvulsant drugs, 446-450
Antidepressant drugs, 469-473
Antisocial personality disorder, 287-294
   case study, 316-324
   characteristics, 290
   common factors in, 287-290
   etiology, 288-289
   manipulative behavior, 291-292
   nursing management, 290-294
   parent-child relationship, 288-290
Anxiety, 2, 12, 23, 128, 139-142, 248-255, 260, 266, 349, 543, 544
   in alcoholism, 349
   characteristics of, 140-141
   classification of, 250
   in crisis, 543-544
   definition, 2
   differentiated from fear, 249
   and mechanisms of defense, 23
   mild, 187-188, 250
   moderate, 188, 250
   in neuroses, 248-255, 257, 266-272
   normal, 249
   nursing intervention, 251-254, 266, 271
   operational definition, 141-142
   panic, 188
   in phobic neurosis, 260
   physiological signs of, 251
   severe, 188, 250
   signs and symptoms of, 141-142, 251
   stages of, 141-142
   student reaction, 2, 5, 128
   types of behavior evoked by, 251
Anxious patient (see Anxiety)
Aphasia, 383, 399
Appel, Kenneth, 514
Appetite, 199, 217
   alterations in depression, 199, 217
Apraxia, 388, 393
Aristotle, 195
Assessment, 147-148, 167-191
   activity, 173
   of attitude, 173

   general appearance, 173
   interview tool, 171-177
   medical, 174
   in nursing process, 166, 192
   of psychophysiological dysfunction, 238-245
   of self, 176-177
   social, 174
   of support systems, 175-176
Associative shifting, 38-39
Asthenic personality, 281
Atropine, 476
Autonomy, 32, 56
Aventyl (see Nortriptyline)
Awareness, 7, 9, 128, 177
   of self, 7, 9, 128

Beers, Clifford, 512
Behavior, 173, 483-484, 536
   nonverbal, 173, 536
   therapy, 483-484
Behaviorist theory, 38-44, 297
   associative shifting, 38
   classical conditioning, 40
   connectionism, 38
   counterconditioning, 41
   extinction, 41
   implications for nursing, 45
   operant, 39
   operant conditioning, 39
   probability of response, 39
   Skinner's theory of operant conditioning, 39-41
   in treatment of fetishism, 297
   Wolpe's behavior theory, 41-45
Bell, J., 486
Benadryl (see Diphenhydramine)
Benjamin, Harry, 309
Benzedrine (see Racemic amphetamine)
Benzodiazepines, 474
Berne, Eric, 493
Bertalanffy, Ludwig von, 220, 224-225
Bleuler, Eugene, 364
Blindness, 258-259
   in hysterical neurosis, 258-259
Blocked Personal Growth Theory, 255
Blocking, 172
Blues, 193, 199
   in depression, 193
   symptoms of, 193
Body image, 73-74
Bormann, Ernest, 109
Bowen, Murray, 486

Brink, Pamela, 339
Bristol Social Adjustment Guides, 294
Burgess, Ann, 311, 313-314
Butaperazine, 463
Butler, R.N., 94
Butyrophenone, 463-464

Caplan, Gerald, 516, 535
Castration fear, 69
Cataplexy, 456
Catatonia, 366
Cathexis, 21-22
Celontin (see Methsuximide)
Cephalocaudal muscular development, 61
Ceserpidine, 463
Chloral hydrate, 332, 475
  in alcoholism, 332
Chlordiazepoxide, 332, 451, 474
  in alcoholism, 332
Chlorpromazine, 332, 463-468
  in alcoholism, 332
  contraindications, 465
  drug action, 464-465
  extrapyramidal signs of, 467
  side-effects, 465, 469
  subjective discomfort, 465
Clarification, 114
Clark, Terri, 314
Client-centered therapy, 45-46, 488-489
Climacterium, 86
Cognitive development, 64, 68, 72
  of preschool child, 68
  of school-age child, 72
  of toddler, 64
Cognitive theory, 36-38, 56-57
  developmental stages in, 36-37
  implications for psychiatric nursing practice, 37-38
Communication, 98-125, 171-172, 213
  blocks to, 117-122
  effectiveness of, 122-124
  language, 103-104
  listening, 108-109
  modes of, 109
  nonverbal, 98
  observation, 105-107
  patterns, 171-172
  process of, 98-103
  silence, 107
  of suicidal persons, 213
  techniques, 112-117
  therapeutic, 98-125
  tools of, 103
  verbal, 100
Community Mental Health Centers Act, 514-515
Community mental health nurse, 516-524
Compazine (see Prochlorperazine)
Compensation, 27
Compulsion, 264
Concrete attitude, 411, 421
Condensation, 24
Confidentiality, 129-130
Confrontation, 113
Confusion, 188-189
Congruency, 111
Conn, Canary, 311
Connectionism, 38
Conscience, 20
Constipation, 206, 217, 339
  in depression, 206, 217
  in drug dependence, 339
  nursing plan, 217
Conversion, 24, 225-226, 248, 257-259
  anesthesia type, 257-258
  "la belle indifference," 258
  in neuroses, 257-260
  origin, 24
  paralysis, 258
  reaction, 225-226
  symptoms, 257-259
Convulsions, 450-452, 466
  from phenothiazines, 466
  nursing care, 450-452
Cooper, Kenneth, 243
Coprophagia, 300
Coprophilia, 300
Corsini, Raymond J., 23
Crisis, 530-548
  definition, 530
  developmental, 532, 546
  and loss, 531
  maturational, 532, 546
  nursing intervention, 535, 536
  operational steps, 533, 534
  precipitating event, 536
  stages, sequence of, 532-533
  support systems in, 537
  types of, 532
Crisis intervention, 528-548
  case study of, 528-530
Cultural differences, 104-105
  in communication, 104-105
Cumming, E. and Henry, W.E., 94

Cyclothymic mood swings, 277
Cyclothymic personality, 277-278

Deja vu, 262
Deliriform, 406
Delirium, 405-407, 425-431
 accompanying infections, 426
 clinical manifestations, 430-431
 management, 431-435
 pathophysiology, 426-430
 symptoms, 405-406
Delirium tremens, 332
Delusions, 172, 357
 of grandeur, 357
 of persecution, 357
 of reference, 357
Dementia, 406-408, 414, 419-421
Dementia praecox, 364
Dementiform, 406-407
Denial, 13, 23, 28, 361
 defined, 28
 in mania, 361
Dependence, 329
 in alcoholism, 329
Depersonalization, 262-263
 contrasted with deja vu, 262
 manifestations of, 262
 in neuroses, 262-263
 nursing care, 263
 transient, 262
Depression, 193-219, 349, 361, 551-552, 554
 in alcoholism, 349
 case study, 551-552, 554
 and decreased self-esteem, 195
 drug-induced, 197
 dynamics of, 195-197
 neurotic, 215-219, 261
 nursing management, 199-207, 215, 219
 psychotic, 361
 symptoms of, 198-200
Dereflection, 491
Desensitization, 260, 297
 for fetishism, 297
 in phobic neurosis, 260
 systematic, 260
Desipramine, 470
Despair, 34, 200
 in depressed persons, 200
 in psychosocial theory, 34
Detoxification, 332
Detre, Thomas, 387, 406, 431, 444, 446

Developmental sequence, 61
Developmental tasks, 57-59, 63
Dexedrine (see Dextroamphetamine)
Dextroamphetamine, 449, 470
 in epilepsy, 449
 toxic effects, 449
Diagnostic and Statistical Manual, 194, 247, 273-274, 295-296, 302
Diamox (see Acetazolamide)
Diazepam, 450, 473
Dilantin (see Diphenylhydantoin)
Diphenhydramine, 473
Diphenylhydantoin, 332, 447
 in alcoholism, 332
 in epilepsy, 447
 toxic effects, 447
Discipline, 66, 69-70
 overpermissive, 70
 permissive, 69
 of preschool child, 69-70
 of toddler, 66
Disengagement, 94
Disorientation, 387, 389, 411-414, 420, 425
 in organic brain syndrome, 387, 411, 420
 to person, place, time, 390, 420, 425
Displacement, 13, 23, 28, 260
 defined, 28
Dissociation, 29, 248
Dissociative, 258-259
 amnesia, 258
 fugue state, 258
 in hysterical neurosis, 259
 multiple personality, 259
 somnambulism, 259
Dix, Dorothea, 511-512
Door-openers, 180
Doriden (see Gluthethimide)
Double-bind, 369, 486
Doubling, 500
Doubt, 32
Doxepin, 469
Drug dependence, 335-342, 556
 case study, 556
 clinical course, 337-339
 etiology, 336
 hepatitis, 339
 nursing intervention, 339-342
 nutrition, 339, 341
Dubos, Rene, 519
Durkheim, Emile, 207-208
Dyskinesia, tardive, 468

Dysmnesia, 390, 408, 425
Dyssocial behavior, 295

Eaton, Merrill, 228, 302
Echolalia, 172
Ectonyl (see Pargyline)
Edwards Personal Preference Scale, 227
Ego, 18-21, 34, 62
  alien, 18
  ideal, 20
  integrity, 34, 89-90
Ego Defense Mechanisms, 23-29
Ehmann, Virginia, 132
Elavil (see Amitriptyline)
Electroconvulsive therapy, 475-476
  contraindications, 476
  procedure, 475-476
  side-effects, 476
Emotional specificity, 229
Empathy, 119, 131-133
  communication of, 133
  in contrast to sympathy, 132
  definition, 131
  in the nursing process, 131
Emptiness, 200
Energy, 21
  in id, 21
  psychic, 20-22
Engel, G.L., 532
Environment, 154, 157, 173, 213
  contact with, 173, 213
  in nurse-patient relationship, 154
  therapeutic, 157
Environmental mastery, 56
Epilepsy, 435-454
  acquired, 438-439
  clinical manifestations, 439-440
  drug treatment, 540-543
  etiology, 437-439
  focal, 443-445
  grand mal, 440
  idiopathic, 438-439
  incidence, 436-437
  management, 446-450
  nursing care, 450-454
  petit mal, 438, 441-443
  psychological considerations, 445-446
  role of stress, 439
Epileptiform, 406, 435-454
Equanil (see Meprobamate)
Erikson, Eric, 31, 82, 89, 94, 146, 359
Erogenous zones, 29, 62, 65-66
  of infant, 62

  of preschool child, 66
  of toddler, 65-66
Eros, 207-208
Ethchlorvynol, 474
Ethosuximide, 448
Ethylphenylhydantoin, 447
  in epilepsy, 447
  toxic effects, 447
Evaluation, 122-124, 166, 185-186
  of communication effectiveness, 122-124
  in nursing process, 166, 185-186
  in psychophysiological disorders, 240
Ewing, John, 331
Exhibitionism, 299
Existentialistic theory, 50-52
  implications for nursing practice, 51-52
Explosive personality, 281
Extrapyramidal signs, 467
  from phenothiazines, 467

Failure, 200
Family, 63-65, 67-72, 78
  of adolescent, 73-78
  of preschool child, 67-69
  of school-age child, 70-71
  of toddler, 63-65
  of young adult, 79-80
Family therapy, 486-487
Fantasy, 67
  of preschool child, 67
Fear, 9-10, 249, 371-372
  differentiated from anxiety, 249
  of losing control, 10
  of psychiatric patients, 9
  of rejection, 10
  in schizophrenia, 371-372
  of unknown, 9
Feelings, of student nurse, 8
Fetishism, 296-298
  behavior therapy for, 297
  definition, 296
  desensitization, 297
  etiology, 297
  nursing care, 298
Flight of ideas, 172, 360
  in mania, 360
Fluphenazine, 462
Focal epilepsy, 443-445
  aura, 444
  jacksonian seizure, 445
  psychomotor, 443-444

temporal lobe, 443
Focusing on specifics, 115
Formal operational stage (see Cognitive theory)
Frankl, Victor, 490
Freedman, Alfred, M., 194
Freud, Sigmund, 17, 20, 22-23, 29, 58, 207-208, 255-256, 481-482, 512-513
Frontal lobe syndrome, 398

Gemonil (see Metharbital)
Generativity, 34, 82
  of middle-aged adult, 62
  in psychosocial theory, 34
Gestalt, 224, 489-490
  concepts related to stress, 224
  theory, 489-490
  therapy, 489-490
Glaser, Gilbert, 438
Glasser, William, 148, 492
Glutethimide, 475
Goffman, Irving, 514
Grand mal epilepsy, 440-441
  clonic phase, 441
  epileptic cry, 440
  postictal stage, 441
  prodromal phase, 440
  seizures, 440-441
Grief, 193-194
Grieving, 189, 531
  acute, 189
  anticipatory, 189
  in crisis situation, 531
  delayed, 190
Group therapy, 484-485
Guilt, 33, 196-197, 202
  feelings of, in depression, 196-198, 202
  in neurotic depression, 216
  in psychosocial theory, 33

Habituation, 335
Haldol (see Haloperidol)
Hallucinations, 173, 357, 455
Haloperidol, 463
Hariton, Barbara, 301
Health, 223-225
  contributing factors, 224
  and illness, 223-225
Hebephrenia, 365
Hepatitis, 339
Hexafluorodiethyl ether, 477
Hierarchy of human needs, 164
Holmstrom, Lynda, 313

Homosexuality, 302-308
Hooker, Evelyn, 304
Hormonyl (see Ceserpidine)
Horney, Karen, 255-256
Human ecology, 516-520
Humanistic theory, 44-50
Humor, 153-154
Hypnosis, 483
Hypochondriacal, 263-264
  neurosis, 263-264
  secondary gain, 263
  symptoms, 263
Hysteria, 257-260
  amnesia, 258
  anesthesia, 257
  dissociative type, 258
  fugue state, 258
  multiple personality, 259
  in neurosis, 257-260
  paralysis, 258
  somnambulism, 258
Hysterical personality, 282-283
  characteristic behavior, 282
  nursing intervention, 282-283

Id, 18-22
Ideal self, 73
Ideas of reference, 173
Identification, 11, 23-25
  defined, 25
  origin, 24
  with psychiatric patients, 11
  types of, 25-26
Identity, 33, 72
Imagery, 243
Inadequate personality, 274-275
Incorporation, 26
Indecisiveness, 205, 216
Indoklon therapy, 476
Industry, 33
Infant, 58-63
  age span, 58
  basic needs, 58
  capability of, 58
  cephalocaudal muscular development, 61
  developmental tasks of, 58-60
  oral needs of, 62
  parenting, 61-63
  physical development, 61-62
  pleasure principle in, 62
Inferiority, 33
Initiative, 33

Insomnia, 217-218, 270-271, 349-350
  in alcoholism, 349-350
  in depression, 217-218
  in neuroses, 270-271
  nursing intervention, 217-218, 270-271
Instinct, 20
  defined, 20
  features of, 20
Insulin shock therapy, 476
Integration, 56
Interview, 127
Intimacy, 34
Introjection, 23-24, 26
Involutional melancholia (see Involutional psychotic reaction)
Involutional Psychotic Reaction, 363-366
Involvement, 12-14, 130-131
  definition, 130
  objectivity in, 130
  stages of, 131
Isocarboxazid, 470
Isolation, 28, 34
Isolation of affect, 284

Jacksonian seizure, 445
Jahoda, Marie, 55
Janov, Arthur, 491
Jarecki, Henry, 387, 406, 431, 444, 446
Johari Window Concept, 110
Jones, Maxwell, 501
Juvenile period, 70
  age span, 70
  peer relationships, 70

Kalish, Beatrice, 132-133
Kallman, Franz, 304
Kaplan, Harold, I., 194
Kinsey, Alfred, 303
Kiritz, Stewart, 226
Kolodny, Rodney, 304
Kubler-Ross, E., 94, 532

La belle indifference, 258
La Bicetre Hospital, 511
Lachman, Sheldon, 226, 231-236
Latency, 70
Lazare, Aaron, 311, 314
Lesak, Muriel, 386
Lesbian, 303
Lesions, in organic brain syndrome, 396-403
  cerebral cortex, 397-398
  frontal lobe, 398-399
  occipital lobe, 399-400
  parietal lobe, 399
  subcortical, 396
  temporal lobe, 401-403
Levels of consciousness, 22, 393
  conscious, 22
  preconscious, 22
  unconscious, 22
Librium (see Chlordiazepoxide)
Life assessment, 83-84
Limbic system, 402-403
Listening, 108-109, 211
Liston, Mary, 519
Lithium carbonate, 473-474
  for mania, 473-474
  side-effects, 473-474
  toxicity, 473-474
Lobotomy, 477-478
  frontal, 477
  transorbital, 478
Logotherapy, 490-491
Loneliness, 371
Luminal (see Phenobarbital)

Maladaptive Learning Theory, 256
Malingering, 225-226
Mania, 360-361
  flight of ideas in, 360
  hypomania, 361
  physical behavior in, 360
Manic-depressive psychosis, 361
Manipulation, 190, 291-294, 380
  in antisocial personality disorder, 291-294
  in psychoses, 380
Marplan (see Isocarboxazid)
Maslow, Abraham, 45, 47-51, 82, 90-91, 164, 255
Masochism, 299-301
Masters, W.H. and Johnson, V.E., 76, 88
Masturbation, 76
Matthews, W.B., 436
May, Rollo, 50-51, 139
Mayers, M.G., 180
McLean Hospital, 512
McMahon, A.W., 227
Mebaral (see Mephobarbital)
Mechanisms of defense (see Ego defense mechanisms)
Mellaril (see Thioridazine)
Memory, 385-386, 404

immediate, 386
impaired, 404
in organic brain syndrome, 385
recent past, 386
remote, 386
Menopause, 86-88
Mental health, 519
Mephobarbital, 448
Meprobamate, 474
Mereness, Dorothy, 23-24
Mesantoin (see Methylphenylethylhydantoin)
Methamphetamine, 470
Metharbital, 448
Methedrine (see Methylphenidate)
Methsuximide, 449
Methylphenidate, 470
Methylphenylethylhydantoin, 447
Meyer, Adolf, 512
Middle-aged adult, 81-99
  family, 83-84
  generativity, 82
  life assessment, 83
  physiological changes, 85-89
  self-evaluation, 83-84
  stagnation, 82
  work, 85
Millay, Edna St. Vincent, 195
Miller, Henry, 436
Minnesota Multiphasic Personality Inventory, 227
Mirroring, 500
Model of positive personality development, 54-55
Monoamine oxidase inhibitors, 470-472
Moos, R.H., 226
Moreno, J.L., 497
Multiple personality, 259
Mutism, 172

Narcolepsy, 454-456
Nardil (see Phenelzine)
Nausea, 206
Navane (see Thiothixene)
Nembutal (see Pentobarbital)
Neologism, 172
Neonate, 61
Neugarten, B.L., 89
Neurasthenic neurosis, 262
Neurosis, 194, 215-219, 247-273
  anxiety, 257
  classification, 257-266
  depressive, 194, 215-217, 261

differentiated from psychoses, 248
hypochondriacal, 263-264
hysterical, 257-260
manifestations of, 247
obsessive-compulsive, 264-266
phobic, 260-261
theories of etiology, 255-256
Noctec (see Chloral hydrate)
Non-progressive brain syndrome, 404-405
Norpramin (see Desipramine)
Nortriptyline, 470
Nurse-patient relationship, 127-162, 519
  components, 520
  as essence of nursing practice, 156
  evaluating effectiveness of, 160
  orientation phase, 154-155
  termination, 159-160
  working phase, 155-159
Nursing diagnosis, 179-182
Nursing goals, 181-182
Nursing orders, 182
Nursing process, 164-186
  assessment, 166-192
  definition, 165
  evaluation, 166, 185-186
  implementation, 166-184
  planning, 166
  and problem solving approach, 165
  in psychophysiologic disorders, 237-245
  purpose of, 166

Obsession, 172, 248, 264-266
  definition, 172, 264
  in obsessive-compulsive neurosis, 264-266
Obsessive-compulsive neurosis, 264-266
  guidelines for communication, 265
  nursing intervention, 265
Obsessive-compulsive personality, 283-286
  characteristics, 283-284
  isolation of affect, 284
  nursing intervention, 284-285
Oculogyric crisis, 467
Odum, Eugene, 517
Oedipal conflict (see Oedipal situation)
Oedipal situation, 66, 68-69
Older adult, 89-94
  acceptance of death, 93-94
  changes in life style, 90
  developmental tasks, 90

psychological changes, 91-93
phychological changes, 91-93
Operant conditioning, 39
Oral stage (see Infant)
Oral zone, 29
  functions of mouth, 29-30
  oral personality types, 30
Organ language, 228
Organic brain syndrome, 384-457
  changes in personality, 394-395
  deliriform syndromes, 425
  delirium, 405-407
  diagnosis, 385
  epilepsy, 435-454
  location of lesion, 396-403
  memory, 385-387
  nursing actions, 416-425
  orientation, 387-388
  perception, 385
  spatial ability, 388
  tissue destruction, 395-396
  verbal ability, 388
Organic psychoses, 384
Osborne, Oliver, 515
Overcompensation, 23
Oxazepam, 475

Paradoxical intention, 491
Paraldehyde, 332
Paralysis, 258
Paranoia, 259, 366, 371-377
Paranoid, 279-280
  nursing intervention, 278-279
  personality, 278-279
Parenting, 62
Pargyline, 469
Parnate (see Tranylcypromine)
Passive-aggressive personality, 279-280
Pavlov, I.P., 38, 482
Peganone (see Ethylphenylhydantoin)
Penis envy, 69
Pentobarbital, 475
Perception, 56, 105-106, 190-191, 385
  alteration in, 190-191
  in communication, 105-106
  in organic brain syndrome, 385
  of reality, 56
Percy, Charles, 90
Perls, Frederick, 489
Perphenazine, 463
Personality, 16-31
Personality disorders, 273-294
  antisocial personality disorders, 287-294

asthenic, 281
cyclothymic, 277-278
differentiation from neurosis, 274
differentiation from transient situational disorders, 274
dyssocial behavior, 295
explosive, 281
hysterical, 282-283
inadequate, 274-275
obsessive-compulsive, 283-286
paranoid, 278-279
passive-aggressive, 279-281
schizoid, 275-277
Personality type, 229
Petit mal epilepsy, 438, 441-443
  akinetic seizures, 442
  myoclonic seizures, 442
  precipitating factors, 442
Phallic phase, 30, 66
Phenelzine, 470
Phenmetrazine, 470
Phenobarbital, 448, 475
Phenothiazines, 463
Phillips, Bonnie, 159
Phobia, 248
Phobic neurosis, 260-261
  nursing management, 260-261
  role of anxiety, 260
  and systematic desensitization, 260
  use of displacement, 260
  use of projection, 260
Photosensitivity, 471
Physiotherapy, 478
Piaget, Jean, 32-38, 92
Pincus, J.H., 387
Pinel, Philippe, 511
Placidyl (see Ethchlorvynol)
Play, 64, 67, 71
  preschool child, 67
  school-age child, 71
  toddler, 64
Pleasure principle, 19, 62
Pre-adolescent, 70
Preludin (see Phenmetrazine)
Preoperational stage (see Cognitive theory)
Preschool child, 66-70
  age span, 66
  cognitive development, 68
  developmental tasks, 67-70
  emotional development, 68
  erogenous zone, 66
  fantasy, 67

Oedipal situation, 66, 68-69
penis envy, 69
physical development, 67
play, 67
safety, 67
sibling rivalry, 68
Primal therapy, 302, 491-492
Primary gain, 225
Primary prevention, 516, 520, 539
Primary process, 18-19
Primidone, 448
Principles, 509
  of behavior, 8, 15
  for care of clients with alcoholism, 352
  for care of clients with personality disorders and sexual deviations, 324-325
  for care of neuroses, 272
  of crisis intervention, 546-547
  for effective communication, 124-125
  for intervention in depression, 218
  for intervention in psychophysiological disorders, 245
  for nurse-patient relationship, 161, 187
Problem-oriented record, 166-184
Process recording, 8, 12, 583-587
  sample, 583-587
Prochlorperazine, 463
Progressive brain disease, 403-404
Progressive relaxation techniques (see Imagery)
Projection, 13, 23-24, 26, 260
  defined, 26
  origin, 24
  pathological use in paranoid reactions, 26
  in phobic neurosis, 260
Prolixin (see Fluphenazine)
Promazine, 463
Proxemics, 98
Pseudoparkinsonism, 468
Psychic energy, 20-23, 248
  defined, 20
  in neuroses, 248
Psychoanalysis, 481-482
Psychoanalytic psychotherapy, 482-483
Psychoanalytic theory, 17-31, 35, 195-196, 255-256, 355-356, 481-482
  compared to psychosocial theory, 31-32, 35, 56-57
  Freudian theory, 17-31
  implications for nursing practice, 35
  in neuroses, 255-256

  in psychoses, 355-356
  related to depression, 195-196
Psychodrama, 497-500
Psychomotor stimulants, 472-473
Psychopharmacology, 462
Psychopath (see Personality disorders)
Psychophysiological disorders, 220-246
  cardiovascular, 233
  case study, 240-245
  causes of, 226
  contributing factors, 224
  definition, 225
  emotional specificity, 229
  endocrine, 235
  gastrointestinal, 233
  genitourinary, 234
  musculoskeletal, 234-235
  nursing management, 237-245
  organ language, 228
  personality type, 229
  physical symptoms of, 232-245
  psychoanalytic theory of, 228-229
  role of learning in, 231-232
  role of stress in, 229-232
  systems theory, 220-223
  treatment of, 237-240
  undischarged emotion, 229
Psychoses, 194, 354-383
  affective disorders, 360
  defined, 354
  depressive reaction, 194
  developmental sequence, 355
  functional, 356
  involutional psychotic reaction, 363-364
  manic-depressive, 361
  organic, 356
  paranoia, 362-363
  psychotic depression, 361-362
  schizophrenia, 364-369
Psychosexual theory (see Psychoanalytic theory)
Psychosocial theory, 31-35
  compared to psychoanalytic theory, 31-32, 56-57
  stages, 32-35
Psychosomatic, 224-225
  (also see Psychophysiological disorders)
Psychosurgery, 477-478

Racemic amphetamine, 470
Rachman, S., 297

Rape, 311-315
    acute phase, 313, 314
    definition, 311
    nursing intervention, 313
    patterns of, 310-311
    reorganization phase, 314-315
    trauma syndrome, 313
    victims, 313
Rationalization, 23-24, 27
Rauwolfia alkaloids, 463-465
Reaction formation, 23-24, 27
Real self, 73, 79
Reality principle, 19
Reality therapy, 148, 492-493
Reassurance, 118
Refusal to eat, 206
Regression, 24-25
Rejection, 119, 202
    in depression, 202
    of patient's point of view, 119
Relationship, 128-162
    nurse-patient, social vs. professional, 128-129
    therapeutic, 128-162
Repoise (see Butaperazine)
Repression, 23-24
Reserpine, 463
Responsibility, 146-147
Restating, 114
Retroflexed rage, 197
Rheumatoid arthritis, 234-235
Ritalin (see Methylphenidate)
Rogers, Carl, 44, 79, 84, 108, 132, 488, 518
Rogers, Martha, 222-223
Role, 3, 33, 79, 128, 499-500
    confusion, 33
    expectations in young adulthood, 79
    playing, 499
    reversal, 499
    therapeutic nursing role, 128
    threat, 3
Roth, Martin, 427, 438
Ruesch, J., 98
Rush, Benjamin, 511

Sadism (see Sadomasochism)
Sadness, 193, 198, 200, 216
Sadock, Benjamin, 194
Sadomasochism, 299-302
    etiology, 300-301
    nursing intervention, 301
    treatment modalities, 301

Safety, 64, 67
    of infant, 64
    school-age child, 71-72
    toddler, 67
Satir, Virginia, 486
Schizo-affective, 366
Schizoid personality, 275-277
    description, 275-276
    nursing intervention, 276-277
Schizophrenia, 364-383, 549-553
    case study, 549-553
    catatonic, 366
    childhood experiences in, 368
    defenses used, 367
    etiology, 367-369
    hebephrenic, 365
    onset, 366
    paranoid, 366, 371-377
    schizo-affective, 366
    simple, 365
School-age child, 70-72
    age span, 70
    cognitive development, 72
    developmental tasks, 70
    emotional development, 72
    gang, 71
    juvenile period, 70
    latency stage, 70
    physical development, 70
    play, 71
    pre-adolescent stage, 70
    safety needs, 71-72
Secobarbital, 475
Seconal, 475
Secondary gain, 225, 259, 263
    in hypochondriacal neurosis, 263
    in hysterical neurosis, 259
    in malingering, 225
Secondary prevention, 516, 520
Secondary process, 18-19
Sedative-hypnotic drugs, 475
Self-actualized, 46-47, 55, 89, 164
Self-awareness, 7, 9, 128
Self-concept, 17, 63, 73, 190
    of adolescent, 73
    and alteration in body image, 190
    development during toddler stage, 63
Self-destruction, 207
Self-esteem, 49-51, 82, 195-197, 200, 208, 350
    in alcoholics, 350
    decreased in depression, 195-197, 200
    in Humanistic theory, 49-51

peak experience, 49
in suicidal persons, 208
Self-evaluation, 83-84
Selye, Hans, 224-225
Sensorimotor stage (see Cognitive theory)
Sensorium, 172, 213
Serax (see Oxazepam)
Serpasil (see Reserpine)
Sexual deviation, 273, 295-327
  coprophagia, 300
  coprophilia, 300
  definition, 296
  exhibitionism, 299
  fetishism, 296-299
  homosexuality, 302-308
  masochism, 299-301
  pedophilia, 298-299
  sadomasochism, 299-302
  transsexuality, 303
  voyeurism, 299
Sexual identity, 74-76
Shame, 152-153
  general nursing actions, 153
  in psychosocial theory, 32
  range of reactions, 152
Sibling rivalry, 68
Silence, 107-108
  inability to tolerate, 119-120
  types of, 107-108
Sinequan (see Doxepin)
Skinner, B.F., 38
Slater, Eliot, 427, 440
Sleep, 191, 199, 206-207
  disturbances in depression, 199, 206-207
  insomnia in depression, 217, 218
  rest activity, 191
Soliloquy, 500
Soma, 461
Somatic therapy, 461-479
Somatization, 228
Somnambulism, 259, 456
Sparine (see Promazine)
Stagnation, 34, 82
Standards of Psychiatric-Mental Health Nursing Practice
  Standard I: 167-168, 535, 569
  Standard II: 168-169, 538, 570
  Standard III: 178, 570
  Standard IV: 184-185, 538, 572-573
  Standard V: 148, 572
  Standard VI: 461, 573

Standard VII: 147-148, 573-574
Standard VIII: 183-184, 573-574
Standard IX: 539-540, 575-576
Standard X: 480-481, 576
Standard XI: 520-522, 577-578
Standard XII: 524-525, 578-579
Standard XIII: 522-524, 578-579
Standard XIV: 525, 579-580
Status epilepticus, 452-453
Stelazine (see Trifluoperazine)
Stimulus-response, 40
Stress, 196, 228
  and depression, 196
  in psychophysiological disorders, 228-232
Stressors, 229-232, 239
  negative, 229
  positive, 229
  in psychophysiological disorders, 229, 239
  response to, 230
Sublimation, 24, 28
Substitution, 28
Suicide, 207-212
  clues to impending attempt, 209-210
  nursing management for prevention, 208-212
Sullivan, H.S., 132
Summarizing, 116-117
Superego, 19-22, 63
Suppression, 24
Symbolization, 24, 29
Sympathy, 132
Systems theory, 220-223, 516-520
  and community mental health, 516-520
  definition of, 221
  and human ecology, 516-520
  linear model, 221-222
  open, 222
  in psychophysiological disorders, 220, 223
  subsystems, 223
  suprasystems, 223

Tansley, A.C., 517
Termination, 159-160
  common reactions to, 160
  evaluation process, 159-160
  of nurse-patient relationship, 159-160
  reasons for, 159
Tertiary prevention, 516, 520
Thanatos, 207-208

Therapeutic community, 500-503
Thioridazine, 463
Thiothixene, 463
Thorazine (see Chlorpromazine)
Thorndike, E.L., 38, 483
Thought process, 171-172, 191, 206
  degree of associations, 172
  and disordered thinking, 172
  impaired, 191
  slowed in depression, 206, 217
  in suicidal persons, 213
  and verbal ability, 171
Thoughts, 8, 172, 214
  content of, 172, 214
  of student nurses, 8
Threat, 140-141
  anxiety due to, 140-141
  to biological integrity, 140
  in schizophrenia, 140
  to self-system, 140
Tissue destruction, 395-396
Toddler, 63-66
  age span, 63
  anal period, 63
  attention span, 64
  cognitive & emotional development, 64
  developmental task of, 63
  discipline of, 66
  physical development, 63
  play, 64
  safety, 64
  self-concept, 63
  separation from parents, 65
  superego development, 63
  toilet training, 63, 65-66
Topographical theory, 22
Touch, 104
Transactional analysis, 493-494
Transient situational personality disorder, 274
Transsexuality, 303, 308-311
  etiology, 309
  hormonal therapy, 310
  nursing care, 310-311
  surgical therapy, 310
Tranylcypromine, 470
Tricyclic antidepressants, 470-471
Tridione (see Trimethadione)

Triflupromazine, 463
Trilafon (see Perphenazine)
Trimethadione, 449
Trust, 32, 142-146
  component of nurse-patient relationship, 142
  lack of, 32
  nursing actions to promote, 143
  in psychosocial theory, 32
Tucker, G.J., 387
Tuke, William, 511

Ujhely, Gertrud, 139
Undischarged emotion, 229
Undoing, 23, 29

Valium (see Diazepam)
Value clarification, 503-507
Verbalizing the
  implied, 116
Violence, 293-294, 381
Voicing doubt, 116
Voyeurism, 299

Watson, J.B., 38-39
Weed, Lawrence, 184
Wernicke's encephalopathy, 428
Wertham, F., 301
Withdrawal, 199, 203
  in depression, 199, 203
  nursing intervention, 203
  symptoms of, 203
Wolpe, Joseph, 483
Word salad, 172
Worry, 531
Worthlessness, 201, 216
Wynne, L.C., 486

Yerkes-Dodson law, 370
York Retreat, 511
Young adult, 78-81
  age span, 78
  developmental tasks, 78-81
  family development, 78-80
  need for intimacy, 78-79
  work, 80-81

Zarontin (see Ethosuximide)